T0260537

Clinical Psychiatry in Imperial Germany

A volume in the Series
CORNELL STUDIES IN THE HISTORY OF PSYCHIATRY
  A series edited by
  Sander L. Gilman
  George J. Makari

Clinical Psychiatry
in Imperial Germany

A History of Psychiatric Practice

Eric J. Engstrom

CORNELL UNIVERSITY PRESS | *Ithaca & London*

First published 2003 by Cornell University Press

Printed in the United States of America

Library of Congress Cataloging-in-Publication Data

Engstrom, Eric J.
  Clinical psychiatry in imperial Germany : a history of psychiatric practice / Eric J. Engstrom. — 1st ed.
    p. ; cm. — (Cornell studies in the history of psychiatry)
  Includes bibliographical references and index.
  ISBN 0-8014-4195-1 (alk. paper)
  1. Psychiatry—Germany—History—19th century. 2. Mental illness—Germany—History—19th century.
  [DNLM: 1. Psychiatry—history—Germany. 2. History of Medicine, 19th Cent.—Germany 3. Mental Disorders—history—Germany. WM 11 GG4 E5c 2003] I. Title. II. Series.
  RC450.G4 E54 2003
  616.89'00943'09034—dc22

                                                          2003019788

Cloth printing   10 9 8 7 6 5 4 3 2 1

For my family and friends

■

and everyone interested in the history of psychiatry

Contents

Acknowledgments

Over the years my research has been supported by numerous individuals. Many of them will have long since forgotten my queries and visits, but in ways likely unbeknownst to them, they have all helped to move me further along toward the completion of this book. I list them here in acknowledgment of their assistance and as an expression of my gratitude for their generosity: Rolf Baer, Susan Barnett, Axel Bauer, Cornelia Becker, Jost Benedum, Udo Benzenhöfer, German Berrios, Johanna Bleker, Wenche Blomberg, Marie-Luise Bott, Allan M. Brandt, Gerhard Buchkremer, Peter Burger, Wolfgang Burgmair, John Burnham, Craig Calhoun, Hildegard Christian, Thorsten Dette, Wolfgang Eckart, Gerhard Fichtner, Wolfgang Gerke, Christoph Gradmann, Luigi Grosso, Michael Hagner, Volker Hess, Paul Hoff, Axel Huentelmann, Konrad Jarausch, Teresa Jesionowski, Adelheid Kasbohm, Gundolf Keil, Cheryce Kramer, Lloyd Kramer, Gert-Eberhard Kühne, Mario Lanzcik, Martin Leonhardt, George Makari, Gregory Mann, Michael McVaugh, Christian Mundt, Melissa Oravec, Herman Rapaport, Donald Reid, Diane Richardson, Thomas S. and Linn M. Royster, Michael Schmidt-Degenhard, Catherine Rice, Volker Roelcke, Kai Sammet, Frank Sander, Wolfgang Schäffner, Gustav Schimmelpennig, Heinz-Peter Schmiedebach, Annette Sundermann, Juan Tetzeli, Achim Thom, Nancy Tomes, Paul Unschuld, Rüdiger vom Bruch, Keith Wailoo, Matthias Weber, Rolf Winau, Susanne Zimmerman.

Several foundations and institutions have supported my research at various stages. I have been enormously fortunate to have been associated with each of them: the Fulbright-Hays Doctoral Dissertation Research Abroad Program, the Carolina Society of Fellows, the DeWitt Wallace Readers Digest Fund, the Deutsche Forschungsgemeinschaft, the Stiftung der Deutschen Forschungsanstalt für Psychiatrie, the Max-Planck-Institut für Psychiatrie in Munich, the departments of history at the University of North Carolina at Chapel Hill and at the Humboldt University in Berlin, the Institute for the History of Medicine at the Free University in Berlin, the Department of Psychiatry of Weill Medical College of Cornell University in New York, and Cornell University Press.

The employees of numerous libraries and archives have helped me to locate references and collect materials. I have benefited from their professionalism in countless ways and owe a great debt of gratitude, especially for the librarians and archivists at the Zweigbibliothek für Wissenschaftsgeschichte of the Humboldt University, the Staatsbibliothek Preussischer Kulturbesitz (Haus 1), the Zentral Universitätsbibliothek der Humboldt Universität, the General Landesarchiv Karlsruhe, the Geheimes Staatsarchiv Preussischer Kulturbesitz, the Bayerische Staatsbibliothek, and the Bayerisches Hauptstaatsarchiv

I extend special thanks to the students of my seminars on Madness in Imperial Germany at the Humboldt University in Berlin and the participants of *the* Reading Seminar at the Institute for the History of Medicine at the Free University.

Eric J. Engstrom

Berlin

Abbreviations

AfPN	*Archiv für Psychiatrie und Nervenkrankheiten*
AJW	Archiv des Juliusspitals Würzburg
AZP	*Allgemeine Zeitschrift für Psychiatrie und psychisch-gerichtliche Medizin*
BHStA	Bayerisches Hauptstaatsarchiv
BKW	*Berliner Klinische Wochenschrift*
BWG	*Berichte zur Wissenschaftsgeschichte*
CA	*Charité Annalen*
CblAVT	*Correspondenz-Blätter des Allgemeinen ärztlichen Vereins von Thüringen*
CblDGPgP	*Correspondenz-Blatt der deutschen Gesellschaft für Psychiatrie und gerichtliche Psychologie*
DGPgP	Deutsche Gesellschaft für Psychiatrie und gerichtliche Psychologie
DMW	*Deutsche Medicinische Wochenschrift*
GDNÄ	Gesellschaft Deutscher Naturforscher und Ärzte
GLA	Badisches Generallandesarchiv
GSR	*German Studies Review*
GStA PK	Geheimes Staatsarchiv Preussischer Kulturbesitz
GuG	*Geschichte und Gesellschaft*
GWU	*Geschichte in Wissenschaft und Unterricht*
HP	*History of Psychiatry*
HZ	*Historische Zeitschrift*
If	*Der Irrenfreund*
JMH	*Journal of Modern History*
JSH	*Journal of Social History*
MCblWAL	*Medicinisches Correspondenz-Blatt des Württembergischen ärztlichen Landesvereins*
MdJKU	[Badisches] Ministerium der Justiz, des Kultus und Unterrichts
MFin	Finanzministerium
MGG	*Medizin, Geschichte und Gesellschaft*
MgUMA	[Preussisches] Ministerium der geistlichen, Unterrichts- und Medizinal-Angelegenheiten
MInn	Innenministerium
MMW	*Münchener Medicinische Wochenschrift*

MPI	Historisches Archiv des Max-Planck-Instituts für Psychiatrie
MschrKS	*Monatsschrift für Kriminalpsychologie und Strafrechtsreform*
MschrPN	*Monatsschrift für Psychiatrie und Neurologie*
PKUH	Psychiatrische Universitätsklinik Heidelberg
PNW	*Psychiatrisch-Neurologische Wochenschrift*
SBB2	Staatsbibliothek Preussischer Kulturbesitz (Haus 2)
SMIKSA	[Bayerisches] Staatsministerium des Innern für Kirchen- und Schul-Angelegenheiten
StadtAM	Stadtarchiv München
StadtF	Stadtarchiv Freiburg
StF	Staatsarchiv Freiburg
StM	Staatsarchiv München
UAB	Universitätsarchiv Bonn
UAE	Universitätsarchiv Erlangen
UAF	Universitätsarchiv Freiburg
UAG	Universitätsarchiv Giessen
UAH	Universitätsarchiv Heidelberg
UAHa	Universitätsarchiv Halle
UAHUB	Universitätsarchiv der Humboldt Universität
UAJ	Universitätsarchiv Jena
UAM	Universitätsarchiv München
UAT	Universitätsarchiv Tübingen
UAW	Universitätsarchiv Würzburg
UBE	Universitätsbibliothek Erlangen
UBM	Universitätsbibliothek München
UBT	Universitätsbibliothek Tübingen
VdI	Verein deutscher Irrenärzte
ZBHkS	*Zeitschrift für die Beurteilung und Heilung der krankhaften Seelenzustände*
ZblNP	*Zentralblatt für Nervenheilkunde, Psychiatrie und gerichtliche Psychopathologie*; after 1890: *Zentralblatt für Nervenheilkunde und Psychiatrie*
ZgNP	*Zeitschrift für die gesamte Neurologie und Psychiatrie*

Clinical Psychiatry in Imperial Germany

CHAPTER 1

Introduction

I n the spring of 1868, one of Prussia's most prominent and influential psychiatrists, Heinrich Laehr, took up his pen and wrote a spirited and polemical defense of his young profession. In the manuscript which he produced, Laehr sketched his vision of a clinical hospital as follows:

> The clinical hospital must be geographically isolated, enclosed by its own generous and pleasant terrain, to offer manifold opportunities to preoccupy the patient according to the specific state of his health or illness, to allow for a complete separation of different groups of illnesses, so that no patients are disturbed by the commotion of others; the doctor must comprise the pinnacle of the institution, the head of the household, dedicate himself wholly to it, reside in it, set an example for the entire personnel of loyal execution of duties, so that at all times the patient is more or less conscious that only *one* authority governs the healthy and the sick and that the trustworthy authority of the doctor protects him.[1]

Laehr's vision of a clinical hospital captured much of the ethos of midnineteenth century German mental asylums. These were institutions of discipline and care, expressions of both bourgeois moralism and solicitude. Their directors were patriarchs, reigning as an ambiguous blend of physician, judge, father, and teacher over an institutional model-family; their internal organization was rigidly hierarchical and segmented into distinct social and administrative spaces; and their exacting house rules effected a certain bedlamic order designed to synchronize the rhythm and cadence of daily life. They also had at their disposal a wide spectrum of therapeutic means which extended from moral persuasion, isolation, and punishment to physical labor, dietetics, and mental distraction. Indeed, the institution itself represented one primary color in this therapeutic spectrum, its organization and orderly functioning being designed to restore coherence and equanimity to otherwise chaotic lives. Its ultimate purpose was the mental reconstruction of these lives, an arduous operation that could be executed only outside contemporary society, distant from its distractions and corrupting influences. To this end there was method to the peripheral location of asylums, in rural seclusion far from the madding civic crowd, on the geographic and moral fringe of respectable, urbane society. It was there that the mad lived and died, that young physicians were acculturated to their patients' madness, and that alienism was nurtured as a blend of medical and moral science. Well into the 1870s, such asylums—usually bursting at the seams with their charges—comprised the focal points of professional authority in German psychiatry.

Despite all this, by the end of the nineteenth century, entirely different institutions had come to represent the epitome of professional power and knowledge in German psychiatry. Less than forty years after Laehr had outlined his vision, Emil Kraepelin had described the clinical hospital in wholly different terms. The organic and familial character of the mid-century asylums had given way to an educational and research institute:

> The unique character of patient treatment in a clinic is naturally determined by the goals of teaching and scientific research. The facilities, the administration, and the treatment should be exemplary in order to infuse its doctors with the spirit of scientific discovery and generous empathy. It is furthermore the task of the clinic, as far as our current knowledge allows, to introduce young students systematically to a very difficult field of study, to provide them with the key to the scientific understanding of mental diseases and to teach them to recognize those diseases early and treat them competently. Therefore, the core of all instruction must be clinical psychiatry, which can never be learned from books and lectures, but rather only by individual examination and observation of as many patient cases as possible.[2]

Unlike large rural asylums, university psychiatric clinics were significantly smaller institutions. They were usually situated in an urban environment and, optimally, as close to other academic clinics and to the central train station as possible. Their directors were members of university medical faculties who understood themselves to be not just physicians or administrators, but natural scientists as well. As part of the corporate structure of the university, these institutions placed a premium on teaching and scientific research. University clinics were conceived and constructed as elite institutions where state-of-the-art medical technologies were developed and applied toward a solution of the persistent and troublesome social "problem" of insanity (*Irrenproblem*). They were model institutions that were built by the state with the intent of solving a socio-medical problem and in the hope of projecting an image of psychiatry as a scientific, research-oriented, and medical discipline.[3]

Laehr's asylum and Kraepelin's university clinic embodied two different psychiatries with often antithetical priorities, objectives, and tasks.[4] Many asylum psychiatrists, or alienists as they were called, viewed with deep skepticism the emergence of elite academic institutions and tried to thwart their construction. They doubted that physicians could engage in serious medical research if they did not live and work at close quarters with their patients as integral members of an institutional family. They were skeptical of the claim that clinical demonstrations in large lecture halls and in front of dozens of male students posed no danger to patients' mental health. And they were concerned that urban hospitals, far from facilitating the treatment and care of mental patients, aggravated their plight and thus led to increased levels of insanity. For their part, academic psychiatrists countered that it was precisely the asylum's rural locale that had become an albatross around the profession's neck. They argued that overcrowded asylums could not adequately deliver either the medical or the intellectual environment that research and teaching needed if it was to flourish. As a consequence, both the patient and psychiatric science had suffered, the social "problem" of insanity had worsened, and the profession's image had deteriorated to a regrettable nadir.

Out of these disputes between alienists and academics—disputes which to this day have marked the psychiatric profession in Germany—there evolved a new kind of mental hospital: the university psychiatric clinic. This study investigates the conflict-ridden and entangled emergence of these hospitals and the profound transformation of psychiatric work that accompanied them. The histories of these clinics are complex and heterogeneous. The expansion of asylum psychiatry in the first half of the nineteenth century did not necessarily advance the discipline's standing within academic medicine. Indeed, psychiatry's institutionalization in asylums outside of the university did as much to undermine as to facilitate its rise to academic parity alongside other medical disciplines. For decades, professional training and research lay firmly in the hands of the alienists, while academicians rarely had access to more than a handful of patients, let alone much practical experience in treating them. As late as the mid-1870s, academic clinics—conceived as institutions of learning and scientific research—did not exist. In the words of one observer, academic psychiatry itself had virtually "no tradition."[5] Students of medicine in 1860 could count themselves lucky if, upon graduating, they had seen even a single mental patient. For students in search of specialized training in psychiatry, there was little alternative to entering the gainful employment of a state or private institution and learning their craft in hands-on, day-to-day practice from the asylum's director.

Although surprisingly diverse in their historical origins, the development of psychiatric clinics usually reflected this dichotomous situation between rural asylums and academic hospitals. The institutional roots of most psychiatric clinics extend back either to early educational training programs in the rural asylums or to psychiatric wards in academic hospitals for internal medicine.[6] In general, clinics developed in the space between these two institutions and their legitimacy needed to be asserted as well as defended on both fronts. The degree to which clinics managed to establish their autonomy vis-à-vis other hospitals was reflected in their architectural and administrative organization. While varying widely over time and place, prior to World War One they can be classified roughly into categories of largely independent institutions (Halle, Kiel, Breslau, Heidelberg, Leipzig, Freiburg, Greifswald, Munich, Würzburg, Tübingen), of separate wards within urban hospital complexes (Berlin, Straßburg, Königsberg), and of wings in provincial asylums (Göttingen, Bonn, Marburg, Erlangen).

Regardless of the heterogeneous forms that they assumed, and in spite of their belated appearance relative to other academic clinics, from the late 1870s there followed a steady stream of ministerial proclamations and ceremonial inaugurations that by the outbreak of World War One had brought clinics and full academic chairs in psychiatry to nearly every Imperial German university town. Early clinics were constructed in the states of Baden (Heidelberg, 1878), Thuringia (Jena, 1879), and Saxony (Leipzig, 1882); by 1891 Prussia had followed suit with a new clinic in Halle; and with the opening of the clinics in Munich (1904) and Berlin (1901–5) this wave of construction finally crested, so that by 1914 some eighteen university clinics had been built or at least substantially renovated. Boasting such impressive, modern hospitals and the full professorships and growing student populations that accompanied them, psychiatry had by the early twentieth century established itself as an independent academic discipline and effectively had captured core professional tasks that had long been the sole preserve of the alienists.

These clinics became loci about which the nascent discipline increasingly congealed and expanded and on which the prestige and influence of late nineteenth and twentieth-century psychiatry came to rest. Their construction was of pivotal significance in the development of German psychiatry and represented a fundamental redistribution of power and labor within the profession. They facilitated a very different way of perceiving and interpreting madness. They were the location of new modes of sensibility, as well as new methodological approaches that differed significantly from those of alienists. Consequently, they provide an especially useful and accessible framework of historical analysis—analysis of often intangible transformations in the organization of psychiatric practice. It is with the intent of investigating these transformations that this book seeks to locate the origins and to track the emergence of university clinics, to describe their organization and structure, and assess their significance in the development of the psychiatric profession in Imperial Germany.

Economies of Power and Knowledge

University psychiatric clinics were disciplinary institutions in the most general sense of their being facilities in which a complex system of procedures, techniques, and instruments governed and conditioned the conduct of their populations.[7] The obvious targets of these disciplinary systems were the patients themselves. Clinics imposed strictures upon patients that were different from those that had led to their social marginalization and institutionalization in the first place. As the mad passed the threshold of the clinic and turned into "patients," their status as objects of social stigmatization (although certainly not eliminated) was displaced and overlain with a new status, that of being the objects of direct medical intervention and scientific inquiry. That status brought with it an array of disciplinary procedures including a well ordered hospital regime and intensive examination. These procedures were designed to restore patients to normalcy and thereby to "solve" the social "problem" of madness.

When conceiving of university psychiatric clinics in these disciplinary terms, it is, however, important to emphasize that power relationships enveloped the entirety of the institution and not just the doctor-patient relationship. It has often been argued that psychiatric hospitals and the doctors who worked in them acted to discipline the mental patient.[8] But what has less generally been considered is that psychiatric institutions exerted disciplining influence on staff, students, and doctors as well. Medical rounds, house ordinances, daily work routines, ward reports, policies of admission and discharge, examination procedures, laboratory methods, etc. all represented diverse components of this institutional regime. Of course different actors were enmeshed in the clinic's disciplinary web in different ways and to different degrees. But everyone was caught up in that web: it touched not only patients, but those engaged in scientific research, teaching, and therapy as well. As Michel Foucault has emphasized, disciplinary power as asserted through the institutional procedures of normalization was not simply repressive; it was also generative of standardized practices and professional selves.[9] The disciplinary regimes of university psychiatric clinics involved a reflexive, cyclical relationship in which knowledge was derived from disciplinary practices and in turn shaped those practices.[10]

If one understands disciplinary regimes in this extended sense, they provide a flexible framework of analysis for a diverse array of clinical relationships, including those between researchers and their scientific objects, between doctors and patients, between teachers and students, and between professionals and society at large. Each of these relationships can be interpreted in disciplinary terms: mircroscopists employ a series of disciplining techniques in order to elicit useful images from their specimens; doctors study and classify psychiatric symptoms within the ordering structures of the hospital and with well defined procedures of examination and documentation; teachers employ didactic tools (lectures, practica, tests) to instill standards of proper conduct and behavior in their students; and to the extent that professional standards are adopted by non-specialists outside the clinic, they also mold the conduct of a wider social polity. In each of these instances disciplinary methods are brought to bear on unruly objects (be they specimens, patients, students, or societies) in an attempt to bring them to order—in short, to render them normal by the standards of the profession.

Such disciplinary techniques tend to have a pejorative ring to them. But in so far as they also represent the pre-conditions for new knowledge, for effective therapy, for informed judgments, and for structured lifestyles, they can also be read in more affirmative terms. Thus, the ambiguity of the term discipline can be profitably exploited to encapsulate value judgments of professional work. In the context of this study, discipline can connote *both* pejorative and affirmative valuations of professional work. As such, the term can be taken to be either value neutral or, preferably, as an invitation to read differing value judgments onto professional work—in other words, to play with alternative interpretations across a variety of spatial and temporal domains. The term represents an attempt to inscribe the moral ambiguity or, better put, the moral contingency of much professional practice more deeply into the history of the psychiatric profession.

It was within the disciplinary regime of their institutions that academic psychiatrists conducted their research and formulated their theories of psychiatric illness. The clinic placed at their disposal a concentrated multitude of patients. It allowed them to examine and observe those patients systematically and with minimal interruption. At the same time, its regime made possible the careful and extensive documentation of each patient's condition. Thus, in many respects, clinics became model institutions that embodied the very conditions of possibility for "true" psychiatric research. They enabled doctors to elicit and capture meaningful signs. Operating on patients' bodies and behaviors, the disciplinary practices of the clinic generated a reservoir of signs deemed essential to the construction of supposedly natural, reified categories of disease.

Academic psychiatrists juxtaposed their clinical work with what they considered to be the haphazard and subjective research of alienists. In the eyes of many academics after 1850, the great detriment of asylum psychiatry had been its physical isolation from the university. That separation had perforce excluded it from the scientific practices and invigorating intellectual exchange of academic life. As a consequence, asylum psychiatry had always been, in the words of one critic, characterized by a kind of "esoteric" knowledge: alienists were capable neither of disseminating "coherent, empirically based knowledge" nor of establishing a "school" of psychiatric thought and practice; what knowledge was generated in the asylums remained so discrete and "isolated" that every student of psychiatry was condemned to repeat anew the mistakes of his predecessors.[11] Indeed, young medical professionals traversing the threshold of the asylum at once perceived themselves in a "mystical environment," oblivious to the principles of academic medical science.[12]

Aside from these difficulties in knowledge production, the efficient means of disseminating that knowledge was also the subject of considerable professional debate. Of course, efforts were on-going to marshal psychiatric knowledge into a coherent and systematic corpus of diagnostic procedures, disease categories, and therapeutic strategies. In 1833 the first substantial bibliography of German language literature in the emerging field of psychiatry was published by Johann Friedreich.[13] The appearance around mid-century of professional journals and associations were additional milestones in this respect. They provided important new forums for scientific discourse and served as channels through which locally generated knowledge could escape the confines of the asylum, be tested by other alienists, and potentially universalized within a larger body of professional expertise.

But as many psychiatrists were quick to point out, these channels of intellectual exchange had not so much consolidated psychiatric knowledge as they had contributed to an explosion of conflicting theories and interpretations. Indeed, German psychiatry developed as a discipline in the late nineteenth century as much in spite of its members' lack of common scientific ground, as it did thanks to any existing consensus. In the words of one self-critical voice in the profession in the late 1880s, psychiatrists couldn't "teach a 'science' in which even the core issues of method, content, and doctrine were in any way generally accepted. The instructor of psychiatry must not only teach, he must above all make his discipline teachable."[14] University psychiatric clinics were designed with the more or less explicit intent of alleviating such deficiencies of knowledge production and distribution. Increasingly, as the century drew to a close, these institutions came to dominate psychiatric education and "theory building."[15] They became the locales in which psychiatric knowledge was generated and tested, disseminated to students, and applied toward the solution of socio-medical problems. University clinics represented new scientific and didactic environments, designed to make the execution of these tasks more efficient and hence to improve the overall efficacy of psychiatric labor.

It is in this sense that clinics can be understood as elaborate economies of power and knowledge. They comprised extensive repertoires of arguments, strategies, administrative structures, financial instruments, and material tools, all of which were designed to maintain well oiled and silently functioning hospital operations, to facilitate effective research, to ensure efficient didactic exchange, and to maximize the social utility of psychiatric means. Constructing such economies of power and knowledge was no simple undertaking and depended on innumerable variables. This is a study of those economies and how academic psychiatrists went about building them.

Histories of Psychiatry

Historians have written the history of nineteenth-century German psychiatry in a number of different ways. Social historians have emphasized the role psychiatry has played in the rise of modern society, especially as an extended arm of the state's apparatus for the repression of socially marginal groups, but also as the expression of bourgeois efforts to define their own rational self-disposition.[16] Others have investigated specific theories or themes within the development of psychiatric thought, structuring their narratives around individual biographies, nosological categories, or theoretical paradigms.[17] Still others have positioned themselves to view a wider angle of developments by analyzing larger cultural phenomenon or the entire spectrum of debates within a specific professional subgroup.[18] And of course there have been a plethora of studies that draw on the records of specific institutions.[19]

These histories can be interpreted within the wider context of the history of German professions. Traditionally, studies on the German professions have been embedded in broader historiographic debates concerning the strength and influence of the middle classes, of liberalism, and more generally of Modernism in nineteenth and twentieth-century Germany. In particular, these studies have considered the historical development and structure of professional organizations; they have looked for signs of democratic and anti-democratic sympathies and ultimately have sought the historical roots and models that help explain professional conduct under National Socialism.[20] Such studies have been primarily interested in the history of professional politics and have not investigated the day-to-day practice of professionals, their intent being instead to assess the social structure and political weight of these groups in German society and politics.

These are important and useful perspectives in the history of psychiatry, and this book is heavily indebted to them, though it is not designed to mimic their methodologies or reproduce their results. It moves away from analyses that focus on the state or the bourgeoisie in order to look more deeply into the institutional bowels of professional practice and assess the relationship between professional power and knowledge. It takes as it primary object the profession itself, i.e. a group of psychiatric practitioners, and employs the institutional framework of the university psychiatric clinic to explore and assess the work of these professionals. It focuses on professional work as disciplinary practice and in doing so throws up a different set of historical questions. What did psychiatrists actually claim to do in their clinics on a day-to-day basis, and what is the relationship between that work and their status as professionals? In what manner did the disciplinary reality of the clinic and its local environment shape professional knowledge and discourse? How were research projects affected by institutional conditions or, in turn, how did scientists try to mold their institutions and their populations to suit their scientific needs? What were the strategies by which professional knowledge was transmitted to students and how were those students subsequently transformed into psychiatric professionals—and, as such, into psychiatric sentinels of madness who could be distributed throughout society at large? And most generally, how were the overlapping and often conflicting contexts of institutional culture, professional interests, and scientific prerogatives negotiated?

Although apparently more distant from other approaches to the history of psychiatry and the professions, these questions are not irrelevant to older historiographic traditions. Certainly, a study of psychiatric clinics can in no way fully assess or adequately explain broader issues concerning the liberal strength and democratic potential in Wilhelmine society and politics. Indeed, it would be a mistake to think it could do so. Nevertheless, although the psychiatric profession's democratic or liberal potential is not the principle concern here, a study of psychiatric clinics can shed light on the fact that this potential was at least in part a product of the organization of its institutions, as well as the knowledge emanating from them. For an inquiry into the clinic's economy of power and knowledge carries with it the implicit assumption that professional politics, far from being exhausted at the level of state or professional organizations, extends much further to encompass both professional practice and expertise. This assumption opens up a deep and extraordinarily rich dimension of historical awareness.

Much is misunderstood about the historical development of the psychiatric profession if its disciplinary practices are either ignored or simply cast in terms of the political apparatus of the state.[21] Many studies have tended to subordinate professional knowledge and practice to state power. They interpret psychiatry as little more than an appendage to the state and psychiatric expertise as the intellectual and scientific legitimation of the state's authority to exercise control over marginal social groups. Others have simply ignored professional power altogether or, if they do consider it, have reduced it to little more than a noble and "natural" derivative of scientific knowledge, investing scant effort in the question of what mechanisms produce that knowledge or what effects its deployment may have had. Such interpretations deflect attention from crucial components of professional development. In this history I am therefore less interested in interpreting the psychiatric profession as an effect or extension of state power, than as the expression of a kind of disciplinary power embedded in local practices and institutions that are designed to maximize normalcy.[22] Moreover, I see clinics not simply as tools of state repression or beneficent monuments to medical science—although they could certainly be both—but rather as executive instruments in the governance of professional selves and as expressions of the functional distribution of labor within the profession. They are the locales in which professional selves are "assembled"[23] and professional work organized.

Professional Tasks and Jurisdictions

In beginning to analyze professional economies of power and knowledge, I am particularly interested in what Andrew Abbott has called the "cultural machinery of jurisdiction."[24] For Abbott, the central phenomenon of professional life is not so much the social or organizational structure of a profession, as it is the linkage, or, in his terminology, the "jurisdiction" between a given kind of work and the particular group of individuals who perform that work. In emphasizing this linkage, he argues that the control or jurisdiction over certain kinds of work comprises the "central organizing reality of professional life." The object or aim of such professional work is, in turn, the resolution or management of problems. The jurisdictional claims which a group makes to performing a given task represent the "cultural machinery of jurisdiction" or the "cultural logic" of professional practice. Among the claims comprising this machinery is a diagnostic claim to classify a problem, an inferential claim to reason about it, and a therapeutic claim to take action on it. All of these claims are intertwined with a system of knowledge, and together they legitimate the profession's social standing, support research, and facilitate academic instruction. Such claims and the knowledge associated with them do not in themselves suffice to ensure the jurisdiction of a particular group over a given task. Abbott goes on to stress the importance of social recognition and competition in a system of professions.[25] In other words, professional success in establishing and maintaining control over these jurisdictions hinges in part upon the ability to compete with other professional groups in a system of professions and especially on the ability of claims to persuade different audiences.

Academic psychiatrists in Germany faced competition from a number of different quarters, and they pitched their claims to several different audiences. Their competitors included among others alienists, private practitioners, representatives of internal medicine, lawyers, and religious orders. The audiences to which they put their claims included ministerial officials, provincial or city governments, patients and relatives, as well as other psychiatrists and professional groups. To varying degrees across different social and legal terrain, German academic psychiatrists advanced their claims and ultimately succeeded in gaining control over important components of professional work. Thus what I am interested in investigating are the claims made to perform certain tasks, i.e. the cultural logic of academic psychiatry. I am asking, what sorts of claims counted and were successful in arguments surrounding the academic clinic? How were those arguments deployed? In what historical context were they advanced? And how did academic psychiatrists justify the diversion of substantial public resources toward the construction, maintenance, and expansion of their institutions?

In the case of psychiatry, the profession's cultural machinery was designed to solve the so-called problem of insanity, a problem that, then as now, burdened in some respect nearly everyone involved with it. The nature and magnitude of the "problem" varied considerably, depending on the standpoint from which one assessed it, and it is important for historians to keep these different perspectives in mind. For the afflicted individual, insanity could mean acute suffering, the collapse of social networks, and the loss of personal autonomy. To be insane was to be socially marginal and disadvantaged: to be confronted with endemic prejudices and often insurmountable obstacles in nearly all spheres of daily life. For the families and relatives, insanity could mean financial ruin, social ostracism, or exhausting nursing care. For the personnel in mental hospitals, the "problem" could be defined in terms of a schism between actual patient conduct on the wards and the expectations of superordinate physicians. For doctors and scientists, insanity meant a medical and scientific "problem." To the *Bildungsbürger* in nineteenth-century Germany, for whom *Geist* constituted the focal point of their personal sensibilities and social identity, the madman's flaunting negation of that concept became an object of particular consternation. For communities and state bureaucrats, the "problem" was framed in terms of financing and administration of care.

Although madness was a problem, I do not wish to suggest that it was *only* a problem. Obviously, it could also enrich the lives of those who confronted it. Depending on one's perspective, insanity could be seized as an opportunity for expanded self-understanding or alternative lifestyles, for tempering familial or other interpersonal relationships, or for securing one's economic livelihood. It could be used as a rhetorical instrument designed to dislodge and undermine political opponents. Or, to adapt an idea of Donna Haraway's, it could be applied toward the construction of the rational self from the irrational other, the *Geist* from the *Ungeist*, the *Bildungsbürger* from the *Irrsinnigen*, in a kind of bedlamic orientalism.[26] Stressing these different perspectives reminds us that insanity is inextricably part of a collection of broader histories of the family, mentalities, poverty, economics, and politics. Assessing insanity from these and other perspectives is a worthwhile undertaking and goes a long way toward helping to untangle contradictory evidence and understanding what insanity in Germany in the half century prior to World War One symbolized and meant.

However, this book is not a history of insanity. It is not a history from the patient's perspective, nor is it an examination of public attitudes and values in relation to madmen and madwomen. Instead, it is the history of the emergence of a group of practitioners and institutions. I will therefore be restricting my attention largely to problems and opportunities as defined by professional psychiatrists and state bureaucrats, as well as to the institutional and administrative context in which they operated. It is within this framework that I will be excavating the historical traces of clinical work and the claims academic psychiatrists advanced in order to secure their privileged jurisdiction over that work.

If this study is organized around a group of professional tasks performed by psychiatrists in university clinics, then just what were those tasks?[27] What kinds of work did they ascribe to themselves in addressing and attempting to solve the problem of madness? Clearly, two of the most important tasks were scientific research and clinical instruction. As members of the German academic community and representatives of a new psychiatry developing against the backdrop of Humboldtian ideals, the bulk of their labor involved laboratory and clinical investigation as well as medical training. From the 1860s, academic psychiatrists increasingly considered themselves research scientists, beckoned to unveil the hidden truths of nature and to accumulate objective medical facts. This sense of calling, coupled with an inclination to collect and systematize psychiatric knowledge, underpinned their efforts to transport and reproduce that same scientific ethos in their students. Assuming the role of professional gatekeepers, academic psychiatrists worked to transform their pupils into scientists and instill stricter standards of professional practice.

A third task, and one closely associated with the enhancement of psychiatry's professional image, was socio-hygienic prophylaxis. As it became increasingly obvious that scientific research in psychiatry had failed to deliver on promises of the significant therapeutic advancement, and as the profession came under intense public pressure in the early 1890s, academic psychiatrists tended to redefine their work in prophylactic terms. Seeking to prevent what they could not cure, many considered it to be their responsibility, not simply as physicians, but also as citizens of a German nation-state, to help "solve" social questions and augment the health and vitality of the German *Volk*.[28] As experts in their field, they brought their theoretical and diagnostic skills to bear on pressing social questions of their day, ranging from overburdened school children and nervousness to alcoholism and national "degeneration."

Obviously, these were not the only tasks academic psychiatrists performed.[29] Nor was their claim to perform them uncontested, and they by no means gained exclusive jurisdiction over them, in all cases. However, as I will be arguing below, in the final decades of the nineteenth century academic psychiatry captured the first two tasks (research and education) to a substantial degree and, as their influence grew, came to play a significant role in the third (socio-hygienic prophylaxis). It is this process of capture and expansion of specific tasks, this inter- and intra-professional differentiation of expert labor, and the concomitant jurisdictional claims made by academic psychiatrists, that I am investigating in an institutional context and that I see as decisive factors in the professional development of the discipline.

In this short list of tasks, two closely related issues are worth noting. Conspicuous by its absence is the work of direct patient care (*Pflege*). From their inception, university psychiatric clinics were so-called curative, not custodial institutions (i.e. *Heil-* rather than *Pflegeanstalten*). They were designed to treat so-called curable patients and not to engage in long-term care. The task of physically caring for patients, a task which so often gave meaning and a sense of belonging to the patients for whom psychiatry (by its own admission) often had no cure, was rarely if ever given institutional priority in these clinics.[30] Instead, this task was relegated to the asylums or remained the responsibility of other institutions, the family, the church, and more generally the private sphere.

Nor were psychiatric clinics founts of therapeutic innovation.[31] With the exception of non-restraint, the adoption of which harbored other significant professional advantages, academic clinics contributed relatively little in the way of new therapeutic procedures and techniques. In other words, therapeutic efficacy hardly suffices to explain the emergence of clinical psychiatry. The ability to supply diagnoses, to posit plausible explanations of madness, and in general to alleviate the social and administrative problems associated with insanity (shortage of trained experts, institutional overcrowding, public scandal, etc.) were all equally, if not more important factors enabling academics to secure their professional standing. In fact, incantations of therapeutic efficacy were often used as red herrings to mask other far more contentious professional disputes. Thus, it is one of the observations of this study that in practice university clinics did not necessarily have to be very effective therapeutic institutions. Or perhaps better stated, the therapeutic task of the clinic was defined in diagnostic and prophylactic terms, or in terms of what I will call "academic therapy."[32] Be that as it may, one need not sit in judgment over the merits of academic therapy to recognize that, to the extent it came to influence German psychiatry in general, it jeopardized and undercut (for better or for worse) the therapeutic culture, which asylums had developed over decades of contact with the mad.

Terminology

The term *Klinik* is notoriously ambiguous and difficult to define. At times it designated simply a hospital building, at times a method of teaching at the bedside, and at times a combination of both. Although in common English usage today the term 'clinic' retains some of the above connotations, it is more likely to be understood in the sense of a group practice designed to diagnose and treat outpatients. In German the term has retained much of its traditional meaning, although it is also used generically to describe an institution specializing in the treatment of particular diseases.[33] Nevertheless, the ambiguity of the term has often served to make it an ideal signifier of the interests and aims of academic psychiatrists. Historically, with the institutionalization of medicine in Germany, a gradual shift in emphasis from a technique of teaching involving bedside demonstration to a geographic locale can be observed, although technically that locale was designated as a *Klinikum*. Throughout the second half of the century a distinction was made between various types of *Klinik*: a *stationäre Klinik*, i.e. a ward or hospital in which students were taught; a *städtische* or *Poliklinik*, which saw students visiting the homes of the patients and then consulting with their instructors, who would themselves rarely see the patients; and finally an *ambulatorische Klinik*, which, as a didactic gathering of patients, relatives, teachers, and students in which patients would be examined and treated, was designed to expand the number of patients available for teaching purposes.[34] Throughout this study, the term "psychiatric clinic" will be employed to mean a facility (1) which is part of the corporate structure of a university, (2) in which professional elites are educated and research into the forms and causes of insanity is conducted, and (3) which possesses some form of institutional control over a corpus of psychiatric patients.[35] Clinical psychiatry is the kind of work performed in such clinics, work which, by this definition, emerged in Germany in the latter half of the nineteenth century. The adjective "clinical" will, however, also be used here in the generic sense of "bedside."

Organization

In chapter 2 this book begins with an overview of the German psychiatric profession in the middle of the nineteenth century. It surveys asylum culture and some of the debates within the community of practitioners. Most importantly, it describes a number of the key problems plaguing alienists, among them institutional overcrowding and the profession's public image. In an attempt to provide a clearer sense of the profession's topography, chapter 2 also outlines several of the most important professional organizations, journals, and training facilities.

Chapter 3 then turns to the seminal debate between Wilhelm Griesinger and German alienists in the late 1860s. An understanding of the issues and dynamics of that debate lays out the groundwork for the remaining chapters of the book. For the dispute was, in essence, a watershed event in the long-running and acrimonious contest over the division of expert psychiatric labor. The chapter locates within the dispute each of the distinct professional tasks at issue, including laboratory and clinical research, professional training, and socio-hygienic prophylaxis. It describes how Griesinger's reform program sought to reorganize professional jurisdictions over these tasks and considers its strategic implications in the context of psychiatric discourse and practice.

Having located the various strands of debate relating to professional work in the late 1860s, subsequent chapters will explore each of these tasks in greater detail, proceeding to sketch their respective transformations over time. In organizing the narrative of these later chapters, I have tried to align the professional tasks at issue with certain temporal and spatial contexts. That is to say, I treat the professional tasks in more or less specific historical periods and institutional spaces. This gives the study an implicit chronological progression through time and a spatial progression through the clinic's architecture. I hasten to point out that this alignment is primarily a narrative device. The discourses and practices at issue cannot be rigidly bounded in either time or space.

Concerning the *historical* periodization of the narrative, chapter 4 treats the 1870s and 1880s when, in the wake of both Griesinger's work and the medicalization of psychiatry, laboratory research exerted powerful influence on psychiatric practice. Chapter 5 deals with the late 1880s and 1890s when, in part as a reaction to the predominance of laboratory science, clinical research became increasingly influential. Chapter 6 then turns to clinical education as it became the subject of ever more intensive debate in the run up to new medical licensing laws in 1901. And finally, chapter 7 investigates the years preceding

World War One when, after a crisis of the profession's image in the 1890s, out-patient or polyclinics became the institutional embodiment of widespread psychiatric concern about socio-hygienic prophylaxis.

With respect to the *spatial* progression of the narrative, each professional task can be associated with a specific institutional space in the psychiatric clinic. These spaces will be investigated in a series of case studies that are furthermore designed to expand the geographic focus of the presentation. Thus, chapter 4 considers the work performed in *laboratories* and delves into the situation at the Charité hospital in Berlin. It was there that one of Germany's most influential neuropathologists, Carl Westphal, held the first full Prussian chair in psychiatry. Chapter 5 investigates that most important space for the practice of bedside science, the *surveillance ward*. It analyses in depth the case of Heidelberg, where Germany's preeminent clinical psychiatrist conducted his research. Chapter 6 studies the *lecture hall* as the locale in which psychiatric knowledge was distributed to students. It places special emphasis on the case of Jena, where one of Germany's staunchest advocates of better academic training, Otto Binswanger, lectured to his students. Chapter 7 then assesses outpatient *polyclinics*—especially that of August Cramer in Göttingen—as the space where the clinic's disciplinary technologies were applied to borderline psychiatric cases and from which they could radiate outward into broader society. The ordering of these different clinical spaces gives this study a centrifugal trajectory, which moves from deep inside the clinic, where psychiatrists alone were allowed to tread (laboratories), to the restricted access of hospital wards (*Wachabteilung*), to the semi-public, academic lecture hall, and finally to that most accessible and open of psychiatric spaces, the polyclinic. This trajectory provides insight into the origins and paths traversed by psychiatric knowledge on its way out of the clinic. It also sheds light on what portions or aspects of professional psychiatrists' larger social and political authority (or lack thereof) might be traceable back to the core institutional organization of the university psychiatric clinics in which they worked.

CHAPTER 2

The Topography of Mid-Nineteenth-Century Psychiatry

Introduction: Psychiatry in the New Era

Under the reign of Friedrich Wilhelm IV, the 1850s had been years of political reaction in Germany. Following the revolutionary upheavals of 1848–49, royal policies had been characterized by police persecution, bureaucratic regimentation, press censorship, and more generally the rigorous law and order policies of the king's chief minister Otto v. Manteuffel. But the reign of Friedrich Wilhelm IV, a man whose "fear of democracy had taken on the quality of madness," effectively ended in 1858 after he suffered a stroke and subsequent insanity.[1] His departure coincided with the dawn of a "New Era" under the regency of his successor, crown prince William, who ascended the Prussian throne as Wilhelm I in 1861. The crown prince's prompt dismissal of Manteuffel and the purge of his reactionary ministry vividly marked a political transition toward a more moderate right-of-center government in Germany's largest kingdom. This political transition spurred public debate and the revival of middle class aspirations of national unification and liberal political reform.

The New Era stood, however, not simply for political change, but also for a period of fundamental socio-economic and demographic transition. The legal, financial, and commercial groundwork which had been laid for the development of a capitalist economy in the 1820s and 1830s had, after faltering in the late 1840s, finally begun to support self-sustaining economic growth. Liberal economic reforms, the customs union of 1834, and, above all, railroad investment in the 1840s had all proven to be powerful engines for the accumulation of capital and the expansion of industrial capacity.[2] Intimately fused with the industrial "take off" were the processes of urban concentration, which picked up markedly in the 1850s, despite record levels of emigration. It was fed by the relaxation or abolition of restrictions on personal movement and a concomitant rise in domestic migration, by demographic and economic pressures in the countryside, by the labor demands of industrialization, as well as by the expansion of transportation and communication networks. Of course, such changes also had far-ranging consequences for the social fabric of German society, as the traditional village and familial bonds were severed and new networks of support and of social organization emerged in urban centers. At the end of the 1850s, all of these and many other factors had transformed Germany, in the words of one historian, into a "society on the move."[3]

Not surprisingly, such socio-political changes decidedly shaped the nature of the problem of madness in Germany and did not go unnoticed among German psychiatrists. Many felt encouraged by the political changes and by improved economic and technological prospects. Railroads expanded the psychiatric hinterland of their institutions and sped up communication with colleagues and patients' relatives; the growing middle class was a financially lucrative clientele for psychiatric services; and the production processes of the factory (machines, steam power) swiftly transformed the character and cadence of daily life in many asylums.[4] Themselves largely members of an educated middle class,[5] psychiatrists shared much of the optimism and the aspirations spawned by these innovations. Consequently, they moved quickly to capitalize on such opportunities, as well as to meet the challenges of the New Era.

As a result, the 1860s became watershed years for psychiatry's professional development. That decade witnessed an intensive effort at professional self-organization and unification: psychiatrists formed one major national and several local professional associations; they established new journals for psychiatric specialists; they moved to standardize legal practice on issues ranging from interdiction to private asylum concessions; they called for full academic chairs in psychiatry; and they worked arduously to reach consensus on diagnostic and statistical categories of mental illness. All of these efforts testify to the intense desires to overcome vexing professional problems. By the middle of the decade the profession was in vibrant flux. It was laboring to escape the "absolutism of doctrinal beliefs and coercion" and now "stood on the verge of a new state of affairs."[6] We will now survey this state of affairs—this professional topography of German psychiatry in the mid-nineteenth-century.

The Asylum

The first half of the nineteenth century has quite correctly come to be identified as the beginning of the institutionalization of the mad.[7] Many of the early psychiatric institutions had been made possible by the *Reichsdeputationshauptschluß* (1803), which had sought to compensate German princes whose territories west of the Rhine had been occupied by Napoleon's armies. This agreement resulted in the dissolution of nearly all ecclesiastic principalities and the secularization of church property, including numerous cloisters and castles. Several such structures were then later used to house early psychiatric institutions in Sonnenstein (1811), Marsberg (1814), Siegburg (1825), Hildesheim (1827), Leubus (1830), and Winnenthal (1834). In the kingdom of Bavaria, asylums were constructed in the former cloisters at Irrsee (1849), Karthaus-Prüll (1851), and a castle in Werneck (1855). From the

1830s this use of existing buildings was complemented by the construction of a series of new institutions in Sachsenberg (1830), Illenau (1842), Nietleben (1844), Erlangen (1846), Munich (1859), to name but a few. As part of a broad reform movement in the first half of the century, all of these institutions were designed as *Heilanstalten,* with curative as opposed to custodial ambitions. As such, they were evidence of the state's commitment to address the problem of madness, using medical and therapeutic means. Yet as the reform movement behind them began to wain, state officials also started to complement them with large custodial institutions. After the 1830s, separate institutions for curable and incurable patients increasingly gave way to institutions that joined both medical and custodial responsibilities, to so-called *Heil- und Pflegeanstalten.*[8]

By one authoritative account, at mid-century there were all together some 77 public institutions for the insane in German lands, discounting Austria-Hungary.[9] About two-thirds (50) of these were physically independent structures, the remainder comprised wards within larger hospitals. Although private institutions were relatively abundant in number (20), they treated less than three percent of the institutionalized population. Over the course of the remainder of the century private asylums grew rapidly both in number (to 120 institutions) and in the volume of patients they treated (to nearly a quarter of all institutionalized patients). However, many of the patients residing in private institutions were charges of the state, since the state was often forced to resort to private care to relieve the pressures on overcrowded public asylums.

It would be a mistake to extrapolate from the institutional expansion in the 1830s and 1840s to the existence of a rational, coherent, centralized system of psychiatric care. On the contrary, Germany's particularist past had contributed to a bewildering panoply of institutions and regulative measures, which often competed with and sometimes contradicted one another. Whereas, for example, in certain German states, such as Baden, Württemberg, Saxony, and the duchies of Oldenburg, Sachsen-Weimar-Eisenach, and Mecklenburg the institutions were run by royal or ducal authorities, in others, such as Prussia, Hessen, and Bavaria they were a provincial or county (*Kreis*) responsibility.[10] Furthermore, administrative jurisdictions within the states themselves, in particular the overlapping authority of the interior ministries (responsible for psychiatric care and internal security) and the education ministries (responsible for universities), contributed to the fragmented and highly contested institutional development of academic psychiatry.[11] The emergence of different types of psychiatric institutions was thus not solely an issue of competing theories or therapeutic techniques, but rather in good part also embedded in the very structures of state bureaucracy and the conflicting interests and priorities of different ministries. Far from representing a monolithic system, the general topography of German psychiatric institutions, in which university clinics came to comprise only one small, though significant aspect, was remarkably heterogeneous. This heterogeneity, coupled with the state's general apathy and a lack of political will, help to explain why national legislation on insanity never materialized in Imperial Germany.

Perhaps the most significant defining characteristic of these early institutions was their location in isolated rural environments.[12] In constructing asylums in the countryside, officials availed themselves not only of medical advice, but also of financial expedience, of the opportunities arising from confiscated church properties, as well as of the social advantages of dispatching "unsightly" relatives to distant invisible asylums. Significantly, these decisions framed decisively what institutionalization came to mean in the nineteenth century: the removal of community members from their familial and village environments and their placement in isolated, distant receptacles. While the interests and mechanisms that governed the process of institutionalization will be considered in greater detail later, at this point it is important to emphasize that decisions to evacuate individuals were made within a complex web of moral responsibilities, financial calculations, and security concerns by families and local officials.

For their part, however, alienists played down the pragmatic financial considerations and ambiguous emotional costs of removing individuals from their families and communities. Instead, they stressed the therapeutic benefits accruing from rural institutions. Convinced of the therapeutic beneficence of the asylum, alienists vigorously condemned the conditions, mistreatment, and neglect suffered by the mad living beyond the institutional pale. Consequently, alienists were quick to advocate the removal of individuals from their families and local communities. The director of the asylum in Siegburg, Maximilian Jacobi, suggested that patients rarely recovered from their illness at home and that their "isolation and wholesale removal from their accustomed environment was almost always the first essential condition to their convalescence."[13] Indeed, according to the logic of early nineteenth-century alienist practice, isolation had a crucial therapeutic role to play. Alienist optimism that madness could be cured was coupled with the conviction that such a cure could be achieved only in the seclusion and quietude of nature, away from the corrupting influences of the patient's own family, friends, and more generally from urban civilization. Asylums located amidst the hustle and bustle of city life were ill-suited to accomplish their therapeutic mission. Only the asylum's physical isolation and the consequent dislocation of patients outside their familiar domestic and civic environment could provide the starting-point from which an effective, rational therapy could then be administered. One had first to lead the mad back to "nature and its simplicity" in order to achieve the ultimate goal of acculturating the mad to a "new, rationally ordered reality."[14] Rural isolation was therefore intended not to effect wholesale disassociation from life outside the asylum, but rather to create the conditions for its idealized and therapeutic duplication. The asylum was designed to reconstruct, in the sanitary isolation of its natural environs, the "fundamental principles of every-day-life."[15]

To this end and in keeping with idealistic preponderance of the age, asylums were conceived and constructed around idealized organic, patriarchal, and economically autarkic model families.[16] Architecturally this meant that, at least in principle, far from assuming the character of hospital wards (as they later would), asylums were to provide the spartan comforts of home. Carl Flemming, for example, took special care in designing the asylum Sachsenberg in Mecklenburg-Schwerin to ensure that the patients' rooms in no way differed from common living quarters.[17] In terms of their inner organization, the duplication of the family meant strict adherence to a daily routine, domestic regulations, and codified roles. The house rules in Winnenthal in Württemberg impressed upon the members of the institutional family how therapeutically essential it was that "strict regulation and order dominate all the domestic work and inner activity" of the asylum.[18] Rigid partitioning of gender-specific labor was likewise deemed important in maintaining the asylum's economic self-sufficiency: without both the female labor at the hearth and male labor in the fields, the economic viability of the entire familial enterprise would be jeopardized.[19] Thus, the asylum was designed not as the antithesis of the family, but rather as its idealized, rational, and orderly reconstitution.

Consistent with this ideal of the family, the relationship between the directors and patients was one modeled after that of a patriarch to his children.[20] The asylum director embodied the virtues of paternal affection and he consciously cast himself in the role of a father tending his flock of puerile charges. The image projected of the relationship between the fatherly asylum director ("*Bartpsychiater*"[21]) and his patients was often one of putative domestic harmony. It was important for the patient to know that "the director resides and lives with him as a fatherly head of the household, protects him, cares for him, and can always stand at his side as a helper and consoler, just as he shares in his small delights and pleasures."[22] As such, the patriarchal character of the asylum represented a lifestyle which saw patients and doctors living together in a common household. The proper maintenance of that household was seen as both the expression and the guarantee of humanitarian principles.

But of course the patriarchal character of the asylum brought with it not just the loving, but also the punitive father. Far from being condemned, autocratic means were openly accepted and deemed necessary in a polity of individuals lacking inner autonomy. The asylum's patriarchal order was an inseparable part of the disciplinary regime of the institution, functioning to instill in patients a "healthy" sense of "cleanliness, measure, order, justice, obedience, morality, and religiosity."[23] The patient's resistance had to be "broken," and he had to be made to feel that he "required instruction and had forfeited the right of self-defense."[24] This imperative helps to explain why the house rules of the asylum in Jena tried to banish the bourgeois scourge of idleness by stipulating flatly, "He who does not work, shall not eat."[25] In the patriarchal orga-nization of the asylum, paternal care alongside strict discipline and punishment were two sides of the same coin, two instruments of a psychological treatment [*psychische Behandlung*] applied toward the domestication of madness.[26]

It is difficult to overstate the degree to which alienists found it advanta-geous to project and sanctify this paternalist regime in terms of a higher or-ganic and idealistic unity under the spiritual leadership of the asylum director. They all spoke of a "spiritual principle," of the "soul of the asylum," and of the necessity that a "single intellect" permeate the entire institution.[27] The di-rector was, as Heinrich Damerow insisted, the paternal embodiment of that "indivisible unity" so essential to the harmonious functioning of the institu-tion. "As the intellect and organism of humans are joined by the soul . . . so too are the intellect and organization of the asylum joined together in a vital unity by the alienist. . . . The more consummately are intellect and organism developed in the asylum, the higher and purer *can* the physician stand before God, the world, and himself with a clear conscience, astride the accomplish-ments derived from the unity of both."[28] This reputed spiritual and organic unity was to envelop the entire institution and permeate its administrative or-ganization to the greater good of its inhabitants.

So great was the influence attributed to the environment of the asylum that the institution itself acquired decisive therapeutic value. Aside from all of the intricate and detailed therapeutic devices that alienists had at their disposal, few if any were deemed more effective than institutionalization itself. Alienists were convinced that a strict disciplinary regime ushered into patients' lives a radical, and therapeutically beneficial rupture. Drawing on an analogy of mad-ness as a dreamlike state, Carl Flemming spoke for many of his colleagues when he maintained that admission to an asylum had

> an awakening effect; at times so much so that for days all mental activity ap-pears to return to its normal state until finally these aroused impressions be-come regular occurrences. The impressions made by the unfamiliar faces, com-portment, speech, and activity of other patients is of considerable effect. . . . [Patients] observe and report on each other. Everyone sees his own reflection in the others; a reflection from which he of course turns away in disgust because he does not want to recognize the distorted image which he sees as his own. In some cases this impression alone is so powerful as to provoke the return to a sober state.[29]

In other words, the simple admission to a psychiatric institution could, in it-self, effect the cure of some psychiatric patients. Alongside the *vis medicatrix naturae* and the professional art of healing (*Heilkunst*), the well-ordered insti-tution also acted as a therapeutic force.

If the asylum was to succeed in its therapeutic mission, it was imperative that its organizational unity be embodied and represented in the omnipotent, undivided authority and moral integrity of the director. This principle (*Direktorialprinzip*) was a legacy of the often insecure position of physicians vis-à-vis powerful hospital boards and civic officials on the one hand, and of statist reforms aimed at counteracting local influence and centralizing political power on the other.[30] At the same time, aspiring psychiatrists also raised this principle to an essential precondition of any therapeutic success or scientific progress. An institution lacking an authoritarian director would neither master the art of healing nor advance the cause of science. Heinrich Laehr held the director's "power of psychic influence to be an important therapeutic tool" and believed he had to make patients sense the "moral and intellectual superiority of the doctor," as well as their "utter dependence" on him.[31] Heinrich Neumann saw the "absolute power" of the director as the very precondition of "psychiatric knowledge."[32] And for August Solbrig the director needed to be a man "armed with as much power as knowledge."[33] Furthermore, the director and the organic unity which he embodied served to counterbalance conflicting scientific theories and expose fallacious tenets, as well as to check the methods of psychiatric practice.[34] In keeping with the ideal of a harmonious, familial unity, it was necessary that the authority of the asylum director remain absolute and unchallenged: his presence had to be visible throughout the institution, at all times and in all places. Any division of that authority, whether it took the form of a separation of medical and administrative responsibilities, of the delegation of authority to assistant doctors, or of the subordination of one director to another, endangered the effectiveness of the institution. For alienists in mid-nineteenth-century Germany the director was the moral keystone of the asylum, and only when the reigns of authority were concentrated in his hands could familial dysfunction be averted.

This ideology of the patriarchal family was fused with a complementary practice of rigid spatial distribution and segregation. While many critics argued that such segregation would only exacerbate patients' illnesses, alienists considered it essential to their therapeutic mission and institutional order. Asylums were usually constructed either for curable or incurable patients and, on occasion, for different sexes (as in Hessen and Saxony) and religious confessions (as in Westphalia). Within the asylums themselves further subdivisions segregated patients in terms of various criteria, always including gender and most commonly also class, cleanliness and/or disruptive behavior, as well as curability and the nature of illness.[35] The larger the asylum the more efficiently could patients be divided into relatively smaller, more individualized units. In distributing patients over the architectural space of the asylum, alienists placed them in the controlled environments thought most suitable to their condition. In other words, patients' symptoms were fitted to asylum architecture in a practice which alienists described as "individualizing" treatment.[36] By way of this spatial accommodation of patients, alienists attempted to confront and account for each individual case, to manage every eventuality, and thereby potentially to normalize every abnormality. For alienists working in large asylums, the practices of architectural segregation and individualization were important and powerful instruments in the domestication of madness.

Alienists saw their professional standing threatened by any challenge to the institutional organization of these state asylums. In the words of Heinrich Damerow, they represented the "acquired, solid property, the fixed capital of contemporary psychiatry."[37] It is therefore hardly surprising that a program attempting to reform these institutions and to augment them with university clinics could not help but be a very controversial matter. As we shall see below, the reform project advanced by Wilhelm Griesinger in 1867 violated the ideology of the patriarchal family, the moral imperative of the *Direktorialprinzip*, and the institutional practice of spatial segregation. Griesinger called into question the basic assumptions of asylum life and in doing so postulated an alternative modus operandi for professional psychiatrists.

Medicalization and Specialization

More and more as the nineteenth century progressed, dealing with the mad became the responsibility of physicians. In this very general sense one can speak of the *medicalization* of madness as a defining characteristic of nineteenth-century psychiatry.[38] What in Germany at the end of the eighteenth century had commonly fallen within the purview of priests, jailors, philosophers, and officers of correction, lay by 1900 largely within the jurisdiction of the medical profession. In other words, whereas at the end of the eighteenth century physicians' claims to speak with authority on the issue of madness enjoyed little more recognition than those of other educated citizens (especially clerics), by the close of the nineteenth century their jurisdiction was far more generally accepted.

The historical development of the medical model in psychiatry—closely associated with the names of Reil, Nasse, Jacobi, Zeller, Flemming, and Griesinger—is well known and need not be revisited in detail here.[39] On the basis of many contemporary sources, it is clear that by the 1860s a very large swath of what observers termed insanity had become the subject of medical attention. Alienists themselves certainly saw it this way, as they eagerly and copiously pronounced their medical convictions.[40] In identifying themselves as physicians, they also fell increasingly into line with the trend away from Galenic conceptions of pathology as the imbalance in the bodily fluids and toward more somatically based precepts of localization. From the 1830s, in concert with developments in general medicine, a rising crescendo of alienists could be heard proclaiming mental disease to be a specific somatic disorder.[41] In the words of one alienist, in "our day and age no one still doubts that madness is a disease. It is a disease of the brain which is no more a disgrace to those afflicted by it than a disease of the chest or abdomen."[42] For the majority of practicing psychiatrists in the 1860s, madness was not simply an illness, it had become a disease with its seat in the human brain.

Such sentiments were common throughout the latter half of the century. However, that they were expressed at all, so frequently, and with such fervent conviction only underlines the deeply contentious nature of the struggle to establish professional standards and to secure psychiatry's status within medicine. Psychiatric practitioners lent their medical convictions constant verbal reaffirmation and in the process did not shy away from castigating their lay competitors. For August Solbrig, only if grounded in medical science would the profession be saved from the "one-sided cult of an aesthetic and pedagogical dilettantism and established on the basis of rational indications."[43] The acceptance of psychiatry as part of the medical profession was made that much easier as long as there existed common enemies to attack. Public demonstration of their medical convictions and calls to "squash the hoary head of charlatanism wherever it shows itself" were effective means of securing the approbation of other physicians and keeping the medical pedigree of the psychiatric profession "forever pure."[44]

But just because psychiatrists wished to be seen as physicians doesn't mean that they were necessarily greeted with open arms by the medical establishment. Indeed, medical faculties were at times reluctant to support academic chairs in psychiatry or the construction of new psychiatric clinics when such projects conflicted with other intra-faculty priorities or threatened to disrupt the balance of power within entrenched professoriats.[45] Internists viewed with great suspicion the professional consolidation of alienist psychiatry and often cast doubt on its legitimacy.[46] Psychiatrists also had to struggle with the difficulties of adopting and applying medical models in their daily work. Psychiatric theories, nosologies, and therapeutic techniques all needed to be brought into harmony with the general medical practices and tenets of the day. Hence, although institutionalized outside of the universities long before most other medical specialties, psychiatry was elevated to academic parity with other major fields (internal medicine, gynecology, and surgery) only after 1901, following its formal inclusion in state licensing examinations.[47] By contrast, the meteoric rise to academic respectability enjoyed by public hygiene was never a serious possibility for psychiatry, because it could not deliver the kind of tangible prophylactic and socio-political results that helped motivate strong state support of the Munich and Berlin based institutes of Max von Pettenkofer and Robert Koch.[48]

Although over the course of the nineteenth century psychiatry eventually did emerge as a medical specialty, its specialization differed in fundamental ways from that of other medical disciplines. The simple model of expanding medical knowledge, which is so often traded as an explanation of the rise of medical specialties and ultimately their academic institutionalization, is one that rather poorly describes the development of psychiatry. Nor does the institutional path taken by most medical specialties in Germany—as they evolved either out of clinics for internal medicine or the private practices of university professors—accurately portray the case of psychiatry. On the contrary, psychiatry as a medical specialty evolved in large part out of the institutional culture of the asylums and the disciplinary strictures applied to their populations. That is, psychiatry came to medicine rather than evolving out of it. Karl Bonhoeffer, later professor of psychiatry at the Charité in Berlin, put the distinction clearly: "the development of psychiatry as a clinical field took a path different from other specialized disciplines. Unlike ophthalmology, otiatrics, and orthopedics, it did not gradually specialize and split off from surgery or, like pediatrics, from internal medicine. Its path was just the opposite, it had to be brought laboriously from outside into the framework of the medical disciplines."[49] Psychiatry's control over an institutionalized population meant that its medicalization coincided with and helped ensure its emergence as a subdiscipline within medicine—both medicalization and specialization became part and parcel of the same historical process.

Among those claiming to speak for the interests of the nascent profession, the question of specialization was an ambiguous and paradoxical affair that tended to pit alienists and academic psychiatrists against each other. Because both were in some sense situated at the periphery of medicine—alienists due to their geographic locale and would-be academic clinicians due to their lack of patients—they both sought professional legitimacy less through redefinition in opposition to general medicine, than through identification (some would argue over-identification) with it.[50] In seeking entry and legitimacy within the broader medical profession, neither had an unbounded interest in arguing the case of psychiatry as a medical specialty. However, and for the same reasons, in advancing their respective claims to speak for the entire profession, alienists and academic internists were prone to accuse one another of the sins of specialization. As a result, paradoxically, the issue of specialization tended to divide the nascent discipline as much, if not more, than it united it.

Alienists themselves were very conscious of the drawbacks of their discipline's early institutionalization in rural asylums. From the 1840s, complaints about the isolated situation of asylums had become common coinage.[51] In 1847, for example, Heinrich Neumann found that the "chains of specialism" had become too weighty and that the time had come for psychiatry to "cast off the excrement," which years of specialization had produced, and return to the fold of general medicine—return to psychiatry's "maternal organism."[52] In the psychiatric section of the *Naturforscherversammlung* in Karlsruhe in 1858, C. F. Flemming, editor of the *Allgemeine Zeitschrift für Psychiatrie*, saw progress depending on the "generalization of psychiatry" and the active participation of practicing physicians.[53] A few years later, in 1864, he lamented that psychiatrists in rural asylums had long been "isolated with their science."[54] Nevertheless, Flemming and others emphasized their links to general medicine and rejected accusations that theirs was in any way a specialized science. In their eyes, the specter of a "biased specialism" had been evaded by psychiatry's adoption of medical principles in the first half of the century.[55] Calling for the restructuring of the *Allgemeine Zeitschrift* toward the practical needs of general physicians, one alienist from Frankfurt insisted that it was "petty regionalism [*Kleinstaaterei*] when we say: We psychiatrists! We wish to remain citizens of our great, common, scientific motherland and speak only of We Physicians! Science as a whole, we ourselves, and especially psychiatry will profit most from this proximity [to general practitioners]."[56] While recognizing their isolation, many alienists also argued that there were sound therapeutic reasons for that isolation and that it implied no break with medicine itself. The tasks of the alienist as the paternal head of the asylum family could not be reduced to those of the academic internist or the natural scientist. To alienists, increasingly trained as general physicians and convinced of the therapeutic efficacy of their institutional regimes, it was not they, but rather representatives of a new, scientific medicine who were guilty of myopic and reductive specialization in that they attended only to the physiological dimensions of a far wider praxis-oriented medical science.

However, academic psychiatrists conceived their struggle for recognition within the medical community to be also a struggle *against* alienist culture—a culture which to them lay beyond the pale of medicine proper. For Wilhelm Griesinger, the recognition that mental patients suffered from neurological or brain diseases had made it paramount that psychiatry escape the "biased specialism . . . and guild-like exclusion" which afflicted rural asylums. If psychiatry was to become a legitimate branch of the medical sciences, then it would have to throw off the "specialized circumscription and closure" characteristic of the profession in the first half of the nineteenth century and wholeheartedly embrace the precepts of general medicine.[57]

In spite of these differences, both academicians and alienists could agree on one important point: psychiatry had to take its rightful place in medical faculties as an integral, yet autonomous part of general medicine. Alienists and academic clinicians alike could concur with Wilhelm Griesinger's successor Carl Westphal when he argued that students and doctors who lacked training in psychiatry were deficient in terms of *general*, not *specialized* medical knowledge.[58] Psychiatry had its own unique methods of observation and investigation that were also essential components in the training of every physician. These arguments, as paradoxical as they at times appeared, all reflected psychiatry's borderline medical status as its practitioners sought to reposition it in relation to general medicine.

Psychiatric Nosology

By the 1860s few were more aware than the practitioners themselves of the glaring deficiencies in psychiatric knowledge, especially the absence of a broadly accepted nosological system. As early as 1850, Karl August Solbrig had complained of there being very "little exact and authoritative literature" in the field.[59] Attributing the chaotic situation of psychiatry to the geographic seclusion of its observers and convinced that nowhere in medicine were the differences of opinion greater, he lamented that in his profession "there were as many different opinions as there were psychiatric practitioners."[60] And C. F. W. Roller, who hoped that an airing of differences at professional meetings could alleviate some of the problems and who even looked with envy to the clear programmatic statements of psychiatrists in other countries, believed that much would be won if only "a consensus could be reached in the more important questions."[61] Yet try as they might, on very many issues no such consensus was to be had.

Pointing out such deficiencies was, of course, easier than eliminating them. One of the theoretical approaches that sought at least to accommodate this nosological heterogeneity was advanced by Heinrich Neumann, then owner of a private clinic and later director of a clinical ward in the Breslau city hospital. Neumann rejected altogether the idea that there existed distinct forms of mental disorder and argued instead that what observers deemed to be such forms were simply different stages of one and the same disease process.[62] He thereby called into question the whole idea of a system of discrete diseases and postulated in its place a "unitary psychosis [*Einheitspsychose*]" under which the entire panoply of clinical symptoms was subsumed, though not systematically organized. In what his critics described as a "non-system," the *Einheitspsychose* had the enormous advantage of being flexible enough to accommodate the most diverse of individual nosological systems. In addition, it lent weight to alienist calls for the earliest possible institutionalization of *all* patients, because it linked curability not to a specific disease type, but rather to rapid intervention in a process which, if left untreated, would end in chronicity. Furthermore, it was ideally suited to the slower pace of asylum life, where there was no a priori need to establish a diagnosis and where the "art" of careful and meticulous observation was still held in higher esteem than the "science" of rapid diagnosis that would later come to characterize university clinics. Finally, it fit in well with professional training in the asylums, which stressed clinical observation while frowning upon systematic lecture courses.[63] It was not in the least for these reasons that Neumann's *Einheitspsychose* enjoyed considerable favor among contemporary practitioners.

However, for an increasing number of psychiatrists in the 1860s, the *Einheitspsychose* theory had been purchased at an inordinately high cost. Eager to point out these costs was one of Neumann's harshest critics, Karl Ludwig Kahlbaum, then second physician at the provincial asylum in Allenberg and later director of a private asylum in Görlitz. Kahlbaum too was frustrated by the vexing differences separating the "cyclopian works" of psychiatrists who, in their "addiction to novelty," had all too often disregarded the insights of their colleagues and predecessors.[64] He believed that no scientific discipline was as backward as psychiatry and that like every "real organism" it too had to develop through historical stages.[65] And so in one of the more heroic efforts at bringing the profession's nosological diversity to heel, Kahlbaum took it upon himself in 1863 to carry out the long neglected rational ordering that he saw as a precondition for the fruitful application of exact scientific methods. For psychiatry to profit from the empirical methods of the natural sciences as anatomy and physiology had, it had first to get its conceptual and terminological house in order. This Kahlbaum attempted to do in an elaborate and rigorous system of numerous classes, families, genera, species, and types of disease. While that system needn't be elaborated here, Kahlbaum's classification represented a wholesale attempt to recast the very vocabulary of the discipline. Indeed, it employed so many neologisms as to make it virtually unrecognizable to practicing psychiatrists. Not the least due to his arcane and unfamiliar terminology, Kahlbaum's nosology was never adopted by his contemporaries, and to his death he remained deeply resentful of their disregard.[66] Finally, what had been conceived as a metahistorical critique of past nosologies and an effort to reestablish clinical psychiatry on a unified basis became instead simply one more in the long history of nosological systems.

Nevertheless, Kahlbaum insisted that his nosology was not of mere theoretical interest, but also of great practical significance. He saw the value of his categories lying in their ability to facilitate a diagnosis and in turn to guide therapeutic action. To abstain from a systematic categorization of diseases as Neumann had, or indeed to reject the abstraction implicit in diagnosis altogether in favor of specific, case by case knowledge, was both futile and scientifically worthless—indeed, it spelled the "end to all diagnosis in the field of psychopathology."[67] Without assigning diagnostic labels, therapeutic action and scientific progress would be severely handicapped. Furthermore, nosologies had great practical benefits for teaching. Kahlbaum attributed the failure of university training to the "awkwardness [*Unbehilflichkeit*] of our science" and a lack of "diagnostic brevity and sharpness."[68] Although he considered the unteachable art of alienist practice important (i.e. the "tact" of the psychiatrist that came only with years of experience), psychiatry had to marshal diagnostic terms and nosological categories that could effectively transport information to students. Precision and clarity demanded explicit words and names. Thus, although his own nosology failed to find general approval, Kahlbaum recognized as others increasingly did as well, that if psychiatry was to flourish, the isolated subjectivity of early theorists would have to give way to a standardized and teachable canon.

Nosological heterogeneity was also problematic in psychiatry's dealings with the legal profession. During the 1850s, Prussian jurists had become increasingly exasperated with the incompetence of physicians called upon to give expert testimony before the bar. Their complaints had even resulted in a ministerial query concerning the quality of psychiatric instruction at German universities.[69] In response to that query, however, medical faculties had expressed their opposition to any expansion of the psychiatric curriculum. Most maintained that students were already so overburdened by the existing curriculum that additional courses in psychiatry would be ill-advised. Kahlbaum, however, sympathized with the frustration of jurists in their encounters with ill-informed and conflicting psychiatric opinion.[70] If psychiatry was to be able to put its case successfully to lawyers, then that case had to be based on a solid, though as yet non-existent scientific consensus within the profession.

The same sentiments were expressed in 1863 by Peter Willers Jessen and his son, both of whom practiced in Kiel. The Jessens, who had been commissioned to compile a comprehensive collection of laws and ordinances governing psychiatric affairs in the different German states, laid out guidelines for psychiatrists acting as expert witnesses in court.[71] Those guidelines made clear just how intractable the dilemma was when psychiatric science was subjected to juridical scrutiny. The Jessens found themselves trying to reconcile divergent alienist nosologies with the need to remain credible experts in the eyes of the court. Consequently, their guidelines ambiguously provided for the use of "any given nosological system" while simultaneously stipulating that the expert witness be in the position to "characterize" specific "known" forms of disease.[72] Nor was a loophole that the Jessens included in their commentary on the guidelines likely to fortify confidence in the rigor of psychiatric science. "Individual cases which do not fall within the abstract disease categories of a nosological system can nevertheless be mental diseases. A negative result can be a result of the deficiencies of the system, but a positive result cannot be. Every nosological system is thus useful when it delivers a positive result, useless when it delivers a negative one. The less frequently the latter case arises in the application of the system, the better that system is."[73] While such statements certainly demonstrated psychiatrists' eagerness to share their expertise in the courtroom, they hardly served to recommend the profession to exacting jurists. If psychiatrists could not reliably diagnose specific mental disorders, then their expertise risked being truncated to a simple determination, yes or no, of mental disorder—a determination that had in part already been made in calling on the expert in the first place and that contributed little in the way of helping to distinguish expert from laic opinion.

Due in part to such difficulties, by mid-century the optimism that had accompanied the reforms and institutionalization in the early decades of the century had begun to wane noticeably. Increasingly, a sense of dissatisfaction and even crisis gripped alienist practitioners. For Carl Flemming, one of the profession's foremost advocates, there were "so many deficits in psychiatry" that just tallying them would take years and mitigating them longer still.[74] Damerow, speaking in 1862, painted a bleak picture of psychiatry's future, believing that "the present therapeutic and custodial institutions had reached the end of their tether."[75] And even such an upbeat observer as Heinrich Laehr conceded in 1865 that psychiatry faced an "emergency."[76]

Overcrowding

The most serious and persistent problem troubling alienists in the 1860s was the overcrowded state of their own institutions.[77] Overcrowding and its many harmful side-effects had become an endemic professional problem. Heinrich Damerow diagnosed that "crisis" at the very heart of alienist psychiatry in 1862, describing the progressive rise in the institutionalized population of incurable patients as "the most oppressive concern, the most sweeping emergency" of his day.[78] Asylums had "silted up" with chronic patients and thereby had been transformed from therapeutic to custodial institutions. In a review of the state of psychiatric affairs in Prussia in 1865, Heinrich Laehr was deeply concerned about the spread of insanity and hence the need to build ever more asylums.[79] Indeed, there were persistent complaints that no sooner had a new asylum been constructed, within a matter of months it was already filled to capacity and beyond. Throughout the latter half of the nineteenth century overcrowded asylums were the rule and not the exception in Germany.

The alienist experience of institutional overcrowding was reinforced by reams of statistical evidence. As any purview of psychiatric journals in the 1850s and 1860s quickly reveals, officials eagerly applied the new science of statistics and accumulated a truly astonishing amount of data on nearly every conceivable attribute of asylum life. As early as the 1840s Heinrich Damerow had been one of the persistent advocates of the value of quantitative information, sparing no opportunity to stress the need to collect statistical data. Complaining about the wholesale lack of reliable information on the insane, he appealed to the Prussian provinces to conduct statistical surveys so that a comprehensive picture of the origins and etiological factors of mental diseases could be determined.[80] In fact, one of the principal objectives which Damerow and his fellow editors set for their new journal, the *Allgemeine Zeitschrift für Psychiatrie,* was to reach a consensus among alienists on statistical categories.[81] Damerow's efforts were complemented by Roller and Laehr, both of whom began compiling information on German asylums in the 1840s.[82]

Beyond the diligent efforts of individual alienists, many German states and provinces had conducted more extensive surveys and censuses which documented the rising numbers of institutionalized insane. Over the course of the nineteenth century these findings were made available to a wider community through census reports and medical publications.[83] Often the initiative for these surveys had come not from the state, but rather from the professional psychiatrists themselves. Indeed, one of Prussia's foremost medical statisticians, Albert Guttstadt, believed that the impulse for early state surveys had come from the asylums.[84] However, the lack of nosological and diagnostic consensus within the profession haunted these initiatives, especially if they moved beyond the simple compilation of institutional admissions and dismissals and attempted to classify patients according to their ailments. If professionals themselves could not agree on specific disease categories or on the meaning of different symptoms, then on what basis could statistical categories be formed? These vexing problems sparked intense debate among alienists in the late 1860s and early 1870s.[85] At the same time, it also became obvious that what state ministries were interested in finding out through statistical surveys did not necessarily correspond to what alienists thought important for their practical work or their professional image, to say nothing of what researchers considered to be relevant and meaningful data.[86]

In spite of these difficulties, statistical evidence of rising institutional populations helped to define a core professional problem and to demarcate boundaries of consensus within the profession. Even if psychiatrists couldn't agree on an exact modus of statistical surveys, they all agreed that psychiatric institutions were overcrowded. And irrespective of the motives driving statistical compilations, numerical data provided psychiatrists with important, empirically derived, and "objective" foundations for their claims. Psychiatrists could now buttress their arguments with tangible numbers and construct quasi-natural ratios of the number of cases of insanity per mille in the general population. These were critical pieces of data in assessing institutional needs and in scaling the dimensions of reform programs. Beyond this, however, in their aggregate and as a result of their wider dissemination, statistics on rising *institutional* populations fueled perceptions of madness as a growing *social* problem. Overcrowding was not necessarily interpreted as a failure of professional practice, but as the institutional manifestation of a far larger social problem in need of additional expert attention.

Having identified and statistically catalogued the problem of overcrowding, contemporary analysts advanced a variety of theories to explain it. For most that rise was a simple byproduct of the general rise in population. For some observers, however, the statistical increase represented an increased frequency of mental illness in Germany and was interpreted as a consequence of modern urban society or, especially after the turn of the century, a more ominous sign of moral decline and national degeneration.[87] For others, more perspicacious in their assessment of statistical findings, it was in large measure a product simply of the heightened attention that medical authorities paid to the issue. Still others interpreted the rise iatrogenically, as a consequence of medical science's own progress: the improved hygienic conditions and more effective diagnostic instruments had reduced mortality rates among institutionalized patients, thereby contributing to the increase. No less professionally self-serving, but far more common, was the conviction that delayed admission to an asylum had transformed many potentially curable patients into incurable, long-term, chronic cases.

Historians assessing the rise in the numbers of institutionalized psychiatric cases have considered many of the same explanations, but have also added others. Some have argued the importance of shifts in the family structure in the wake of the combined pressures of pauperism, domestic migration, and urbanization that may have contributed to a decline in the threshold of tolerance vis-à-vis mentally disturbed relatives.[88] Others have placed greater emphasis on state regulation and repression of the socially marginal.[89] Psychiatry itself has been viewed as contributing to overcrowding, either through the generation of ever more categories of disease, thereby expanding its reach to milder forms of disorder and hence pushing up patient numbers, or through the simple conviction that institutionalization was the sole best means of dealing with the problem of insanity.[90] Improved means of transportation, especially the expansion of railways, certainly also made asylums more accessible. No doubt each of these explanations contributes important perspectives on the phenomena of rising patient populations. Whatever its actual causes, there is no doubt that psychiatrists perceived an increase in psychiatric afflictions and considered their institutions to be severely overcrowded.

Over the years, alienists advanced a number of proposals to manage the problem of overcrowding. In the zero-sum calculations of institutions with fixed numbers of beds and personnel, immediate solutions required either that admissions be stemmed or discharges increased. On the admissions side, directors applied statutory criteria with greater rigor or simply closed their institutions entirely;[91] in terms of discharges, more and more use was made of provisional discharges or transfers to other, often local and/or private institutions. For example, in the Rheine province of Prussia in 1868, provincial officials threatened to have incurable patients returned to their home towns if local officials did not assume responsibility for them within three weeks.[92] Proposed solutions to the longer term problem of overcrowding included closing wards for pensioners in public asylums; farming out of patients to private or local institutions; constructing additional or more specialized facilities; building colonies for the insane, as in Gheel or Clermont; educating local officials and families; improving after-treatment and heightening of public awareness through organizations for relatives and former patients.[93] Thus, in the debates of the 1860s, there existed a wide spectrum of potential solutions to the problem of overcrowding.

It is not especially surprising, however, that in spite of these alternatives alienists remained convinced that their institutions were the most suitable means for the care and treatment of the insane. Because of the importance placed in the asylum as a therapeutic institution, it was second nature for alienists to view them as the logical focus of any attempt at alleviate overcrowding.[94] In this context, what might be termed the *dogma of rapid and early admission* represented one of the most resilient and commonly heard refrains in nineteenth-century psychiatric discourse.[95] That dogma was founded on the conviction that the sooner people could be diagnosed, removed from the detrimental environment of the family or community, and delivered up to the therapeutic offices of the alienist, the better stood their chances of being cured and of making a full recovery. Harnessed to this dogma was also its corollary: the longer a mentally disturbed person remained unidentified and untreated, the more diminished did the effectiveness of the alienist's therapeutic instruments become and the greater was the danger that the afflicted individual would decline into a chronic state. Alienists thus warned incessantly of the ominous therapeutic consequences of delayed admission. In early recognition and rapid admission to a psychiatric institution lay, for virtually every mid-century alienist and academician, the key to solving the vexing problem of overcrowding.[96]

Psychiatry in the Public Mind's Eye

The problem of overcrowding was intertwined with the additional problem of the profession's ever fragile public image. Popular ignorance and reticence (to say nothing of prejudice and hostility) toward psychiatric institutions became, then as now, one of the most intractable problems facing the profession. Hence, alienists tried to dispel what they perceived as the general populace's distorted and sometimes malicious image of madness, its causes, and of the doctors who treated it. In the 1850s and 1860s they campaigned assiduously to root out public misconceptions and prejudice and to enlighten a supposedly ignorant populace. Alienists were convinced that the key to understanding and solving the problem of overcrowding lay in improving public trust. They believed that general suspicion of asylums prevented patients from being institutionalized in time for them to be cured. As a consequence, patients declined into chronic, incurable states and became part of an ever expanding "ballast" that "silted up" their institutions. Engendering public trust—that most valuable and lucrative of professional commodities—could alleviate these difficulties.[97]

For psychiatrists, however, public trust was hard to come by. Most alienists envisioned their profession as being besieged by "hyper-smart philanthropists" and "human saviors" bent on liberating unlawfully institutionalized patients.[98] At the same time, the growing number of mental institutions hiked the potential for rumor and scandal. Psychiatry's image problem was further compounded by the isolation of those institutions. While asylums may have been removed from direct sight, their rural isolation could not shield them from the mind's eye of the public. On the contrary, the very distance of the asylum also served to sustain rumor and provoke florid imaginings. This was all the more so in private asylums for the well-to-do bourgeoisie and aristocracy, where a premium was placed on discretion and circumspection in relations with the outside world. For example, in 1853 the city prefect in Kiel complained that the exclusive asylum Hornheim represented a "state within the state" and that "a mystical shroud of darkness enveloped those detained there."[99] Such secrecy could rapidly fan the fires of public scandal.

Just such a scandal reverberated across German lands in the early 1860s, when Hornheim's director and one of the profession's most prominent authorities, Peter Willers Jessen, became the object of intense public criticism. Jessen was accused of having unlawfully detained patients against their will and was driven to pen an extensive vindication of his asylum. In his defense, Jessen lamented the depth of public misconceptions and the "abusive slander" which had "soiled the honor" of himself and his profession.[100] He was convinced that the public, including local officials and academics, had been hoodwinked by the accusations of a madman. While the details of the case needn't concern us here, it illustrated how the profession's image and public trust hinged decisively on admission policy and on public concerns that patients were being detained against their will.

Similar concerns had prompted state ministries to enhance regulations governing privately owned mental hospitals. For example, in 1859 the Prussian government augmented its periodic inspections of public institutions by extending them to include private asylums as well.[101] The government advised its inspectors to pay special attention to whether admission procedures conformed with existing legal statutes. It justified its action on the grounds that if admissions to all asylums were processed through local judicial or police channels, then many public scandals could be avoided.[102] Such supervision was a logical extension of the state's own custodial responsibilities given that overcrowding had forced provinces to place ever more public charges in private institutions.

The state found support for its actions among alienists working in public institutions. These psychiatrists were more positively disposed toward the state's regulative function and likewise suspicious of independent entrepreneurs and "quacks" plying their trade on the open market. Thus, less liberally minded commentators were more inclined to place the fate of private asylums wholly in the hands of the state. Damerow, for instance, recommended that provincial governments not hesitate to control private hospitals by "limiting or revoking the operating licenses of profit-hungry and wayward facilities."[103] Stricter government guidelines would help put an end to public scandals and purge the profession of its rotten apples.

The owners of private asylums, however, protested against such tightened supervision.[104] Confident of their own professional integrity, they claimed that state inspections unnecessarily fed public suspicions of impropriety in the asylums. Of course, that owners had a considerable financial interest in the good name of their institutions and that they feared state regulation might jeopardize their commercial enterprises was an obvious, though usually unspoken fact. Instead, owners advanced the dogma of early admission in support of their case. They maintained that public controls of admission had a detrimental therapeutic effect because they scared off patients and prevented early institutionalization. Formal admissions procedures placed unwarranted hurdles in the paths of reticent (especially bourgeois) relatives who were loath to appear publicly in front of local officials in order to initiate the institutionalization of a relative.

Debates of this nature reveal how the profession's image was associated with a web of interrelated and often conflicting interests. For one, such debates were infused with issues which dominated wider liberal political and economic discourse in the early 1860s. They exposed the specific paradoxes of that discourse, which expounded, on the one hand, the need for safeguards to individual liberty while, on the other hand, striving to unshackle free enterprise from the chains of governmental regulation. Furthermore, they illustrated the ambiguities of the relationship between professional experts and the state. Depending on which role the state assumed, either as a self-proclaimed guarantor of individual liberties or as a regulative mechanism in a capitalist economy, it might either safeguard or undermine the profession's reputation. The debates also highlighted the fault lines within the profession itself, which divided alienists working in public as opposed to private asylums. In sum, they demonstrated the very complex and tightly interwoven issues shaping the profession's developments and its relationship with the state and other political and socioeconomic issues of the day. The Jessen scandal and these early debates were, however, preludes to still more intensive discussions later in the decade that went to the heart of the question of whether asylums were carceral institutions or simply ordinary medical hospitals—discussions to which I will return in chapter 3.

Professional Journals

Scientific journals represented important instruments in the evolution of psychiatry as a profession.[105] Through the publication of articles and reviews, of professional proceedings, of awards, commendations and appointments, as well as of government regulations and petitions, journals served to bolster the emergence of an imagined professional community. In a discipline whose members were so widely scattered across different institutions, and for whom no formal academic training yet existed, journals were especially important in creating that community and facilitating the negotiation of professional consensus. Furthermore, in reaching a wider audience of specialists, journals served as vehicles for the outward dissemination of locally generated and potentially innovative psychiatric knowledge. Yet, while they provided broad exposure and potential influence for that knowledge, they also opened it to broader comparison and to the critical scrutiny of colleagues, thereby simultaneously imposing and reproducing norms of professional conduct. Each of various specialized journals extended the bounds of debate and facilitated a dramatic expansion in the propagation of specialized knowledge and standards of practice. As the century progressed, the number of journals on the market specializing in neuropathology and psychiatry grew steadily from a mere handful around 1860 to about a dozen German and some forty to fifty international publications by the turn of the century.[106] Taken together, they comprised an expansive and complex topography of professional discourse.

Germany's most influential professional psychiatric journal, the *Allgemeine Zeitschrift für Psychiatrie und psychisch-gerichtliche Medicin* (*AZP*), was founded in 1844 by Heinrich Damerow, Carl Flemming, and C. F. W. Roller.[107] Whereas several earlier efforts to found a professional journal had floundered, these editors managed to solicit the state's financial support and turn the *AZP* into a viable publication.[108] Damerow hoped the *AZP* would become a semi-official vehicle of ministerial policy.[109] He did not believe that close affiliation with the state compromised the journal's professional integrity. Nor did he view it as symptomatic of what one critic described as the editors' hankering (*"captatio benevolentiae"*) for state recognition; indeed, precisely because it was subordinated to the "organism" of the state, psychiatry had at its disposal "ways and means to prosper and achieve its truly free and independent existence."[110] In typically Hegelian fashion, professional autonomy was achieved through and within, but not against the state. Damerow envisioned the relationship not as a one-way street, but in terms of cooperation and mutual recognition, with the state calling on and heeding the expertise of psychiatrists. As he saw it, the *Allgemeine Zeitschrift* was not the instrument of the state, but rather an intermediary between the state and alienist practitioners.

In fact, evidence suggests that especially after 1848 the *AZP* was not simply a mute conduit of state influence and policy. The journal's—and indeed the profession's—affiliation with the state was not defined by abject submission or dumb instrumentalization. It actively sought to influence government policy. For example, in 1858 the editors relinquished their responsibilities to Heinrich Laehr's in hopes that, from his station near Berlin, he could make the profession's voice heard in government circles.[111] And in 1864 the same editors spearheaded the creation of the *Verein deutscher Irrenärzte*, because they felt that the views of psychiatrists were not being taken into account in the formulation of state policy. Such strategic maneuvering is a reminder that what most often characterized relations with the state and what especially frustrated liberal-minded professionals after 1850 was the state's deaf ear and persistent apathy toward things psychiatric.[112]

Klaus Dörner has described the founding of the *Allgemeine Zeitschrift für Psychiatrie* in 1844, in a clear reference to Helmut Plessner, as "belated".[113] For Dörner, Heinrich Damerow's programmatic article in the inaugural volume was a requiem to the passing tradition of psychiatry as natural philosophy.[114] In terms of its theoretical content in relation to England and France,

Dörner certainly has a point. However, if one assesses the *Allgemeine Zeitschrift* in terms of its significance in the consolidation of the psychiatric profession across particularist German borders, its appearance seems more timely and indeed marks symbolically the very historical origins of that profession. The *Allgemeine Zeitschrift* helped create and give voice to a community of practitioners engaged in like work. That inclusive, community-building function was emphasized time and again by its editors. Damerow went to great lengths to stress that the journal was published in the name of *all* German alienists.[115] He considered it to be a "general organ" which, rather than advocating a specific theory, was an open "forum of science" and a "construction site" accessible to all who wished to contribute to the betterment of psychiatry.[116] Likewise, Laehr spoke of the *Allgemeine Zeitschrift* as a "common undertaking" of all alienists and a "meeting place of different forces and theories."[117] The collective character was also reiterated by Roller, who spoke in the first person plural of "our journal."[118] From its inception, the *Allgemeine Zeitschrift* was intended to serve as a forum uniting all alienists.

In keeping with this aim, the *Allgemeine Zeitschrift* tried to accommodate the divergent interests of psychiatric practitioners beneath an anthropological umbrella. For Heinrich Damerow the journal embodied an anthropological view of the individual as a natural psychophysical unity of body, spirit, and intellect. The journal itself was taken as tangible evidence of an anthropological root running deeper than "all the artificial theories" that divided psychiatrists.[119] However, showing the influence of German historicist thought on his ideas, Damerow drew the evidence of this anthropological psychiatry not from idealistic speculation on the nature of humankind, but rather from the actual existence and objective practice of psychiatry as it had evolved "naturally" in history. He believed that no theory that had evolved over time could be true if it failed in real-life practice. Although not discounting theory, it was the reality of psychiatric practice, i.e. of specific tasks performed by psychiatrists, which united the profession and guided its progress.[120] To illuminate this position, it is worth quoting Damerow's programmatic introduction to the *Allgemeine Zeitschrift* at some length:

> More than anything else the practical, factual, real, *objective* psychiatry, extending from the treatment of the individual patient to the consideration of all manner of public issues relevant to psychiatry, proves that anthropology is the latent root of all theories and systems in the tree of psychiatry. Everywhere that psychiatry is applied in daily life, it frees itself from the narrow confines of theory and adopts a freer, anthropological, and at the same time humane standpoint. The theories of blood, of ganglions, of nerve fibers, of passions, of sin and so forth do not suffice when it comes to healing and caring for the mentally ill in private practices or public asylums, when it comes to assessing the rights and accountability of the mad, or when it comes to making decisions concerning the organic, administrative, and legal status of psychiatric care.[121]

The anthropological foundation to psychiatry was intended to overcome the bitter theoretical disputes of the 1820s and 1830s by refocusing on the practical work and the professional responsibilities common to all alienists. The *Allgemeine Zeitschrift* was an attempt to "remove all theoretical and intellectual barriers" dividing the young profession and cultivate the common ground of "energetic action and work."[122] The professional community which the editors of the *Allgemeine Zeitschrift* sought to build was one galvanized not by psychiatric theory, but by common tasks, by expert labor.

As much as they may have wished to impose it, however, the unity they sought was hard to come by. Although its editors spared no opportunity to reiterate the need for professional consensus and coalescence, the *Allgemeine Zeitschrift* had to overcome numerous obstacles standing in the way of that goal.[123] In 1858 Flemming, for example, rebuked his colleagues at the *Naturforscherversammlung* in Karlsruhe for their tepid support of the *Allgemeine Zeitschrift*. He called on them to hold the line and resist publishing their psychiatric writings in other journals.[124] And in taking stock of the development of his discipline in the same year, there was more wishful thinking than tangible evidence for Laehr's contention that the "discipline knows what it wants and the paths it needs to travel to attain its goals."[125]

One serious impediment to the preeminance of the *Allgemeine Zeitschrift* was the appearance of another journal, the *Correspondenzblatt der Deutschen Gesellschaft für Psychiatrie und gerichtliche Psychologie* (1854–77).[126] Its two chief editors, Gottlob Heinrich Bergmann and David Mansfeld, had been longtime contributors to the *Allgemeine Zeitschrift*, and their secession threatened to split professional loyalties. Like the *Allgemeine Zeitschrift,* it also claimed to represent the entire spectrum of issues from psychiatry and forensic psychology to internal diseases of the brain and the nervous system. But the *Correspondenzblatt* aimed specifically to attract readers among physicians who were *not* psychiatric specialists. To this end, the editors published only very brief articles, convinced that the longer, more technical contributions to the *Allgemeine Zeitschrift* went "wholly unread" in the ranks of time-strapped general practitioners.[127] The editors also hoped that by publishing twice a month rather than quarterly they might provide a "more frequent and lively" exchange of views among physicians.[128] Hence, more so than the *Allgemeine Zeitschrift,* the *Correspondenzblatt* was a vehicle serving to enhance psychiatry's standing within the medical profession itself.

Der Irrenfreund (1859–1902) was a third important psychiatric journal.[129] It was edited by the alienists Friedrich Koster, director of the provincial asylum in Marsberg in Westphalia, and Max Brosius, owner of two private asylums near Koblenz. *Der Irrenfreund* drew on contributions largely from the ranks of the German physicians and alienists.[130] However, its intended readership was the wider general public, patients' families, local bureaucrats, and town practitioners. Unlike both the *Allgemeine Zeitschrift* and the *Correspon-*

denzblatt, it sought to extend debate on psychiatric issues beyond the medical profession and reach out to the general, educated public. The goal of its editors was openly pedagogical, designed to dispel deeply harbored myths and lay prejudices about madness and to counter sensationalist accounts of asylum life. They worked to promote "correct notions about the mad, madness, madhouses, and mad care."[131] Consistent with these edifying intentions, they also had hygienic aims and tried to enlighten local officials and physicians about the causes, symptoms, and prevention of madness. In their advice to families, however, the editors' aims were far more sedative, designed to assuage their fear and shame and to encourage them to have their relatives committed to an asylum as soon as possible. Although *Der Irrenfreund* also advised families on the proper care of their relatives at home, that advice aimed more at recognizing the proper moment for institutionalization than at supporting care outside of the institution.[132] In other words, the journal tried to deflate the negative image of asylums and remove familial and communal barriers to admission. It was forthright in attacking the reluctance of family members and town officials to deliver their charges up to the good offices of the alienist.[133] Whereas the *Correspondenzblatt* had endeavored to improve the image of alienists within the medical profession, *Der Irrenfreund* sought to do the same in a wider social context.

All three of these psychiatric journals expressed different interests and concerns among alienist in the 1850s. The state-sanctioned *Allgemeine Zeitschrift,* edited and likely read exclusively by experts, provided a common forum for the promotion of scientific research and debate among alienists. Seeking to promote the harmonious development of the profession, it tended to play down divisive theoretical issues and focus its attention instead on the practical tasks common to all alienists. The *Centralblatt* aimed more broadly at attracting the participation and interest of general practitioners. It tried to expand psychiatric discourse within medical spheres in order to stabilize and exploit psychiatry's new-found territory and to enhance its *professional* image. By contrast, *Der Irrenfreund* set its sights not just on the medical profession, but on the educated public at large in the hope of dismantling prejudice and improving the *public* image of asylums and their directors.

Professional Associations

Professional societies represented integral components of educated middle class society and culture in nineteenth-century Germany.[134] As free associations of individuals sharing common political, socio-economic, and cultural interests, they were expressions of the values of the rising German *Bildungsburgertum.* Consequently, to the degree that they flourished, they can be taken as a measure of the strength of those values in German society as a whole. Insofar as political influence and legislative representation had been denied to those middle classes, as-

sociations often became forums of semi-public debate and, potentially, plat-
forms for nascent political organization. And to the varying degree that those
middle classes were the driving force behind German liberalism, associations
also stood for the ideals of individual autonomy, rationalism, and progres-
sivism.[135] They also brought together individuals of common social rank with
like economic interests. They therefore served as pivotal components of professional middle-class culture in Germany and as important local and regional
clearing houses for all manner of private and professional business. Finally, beyond their immediate political and economic import, they were also essential
components of middle class cultural identity and lifestyle. As instruments of predominantly male acculturation and socialization, associations became for the
middle class what the hunt was to the nobility and what the pub became to the
working classes. They provided important channels of social exchange and opportunities for increasingly secularized fellowship.

Aside from these political, socio-economic, and cultural aspects, professional societies also played a decisive role in the development of German psychiatry. Unlike many other groups of professionals, alienists plied their trade
in a rural environment. Due to their geographic isolation, many alienists
placed special value on regular meetings of professional societies. There they
enjoyed the rare opportunity of congregation in otherwise rather barren social
lives. Perhaps more so than in other professions, the sense of solidarity created
by such meetings carried alienists through busy, but lonely and month-long
stints in distant institutions.[136] That solidarity was all the more important
given their poor public image. At their meetings alienists could seek and find
solace in the face of public criticism or rally in defense of colleagues in distress.
Furthermore, there were concrete medical and scientific benefits to such professional organizations. As many contemporaries were quick to point out, in
bringing widely scattered psychiatrists together on a regular basis, professional
associations helped alleviate problems that had long hampered intellectual exchange. They created an important forum in which ideas and experiences
could be exchanged, consensus reached, and deviancy within their ranks cen-
sored.[137] As such they were also responses to the stigma of "excessive individuality and a certain one-sidedness"[138] that had so tarnished the profession's
medical and scientific image.

The *Gesellschaft Deutscher Naturforscher und Ärzte* (GDNÄ) represented
the first broad forum in which practicing alienists could congregate and air
their views.[139] The society was founded in 1822 by the biologist, natural
philosopher, and pantheist Lorenz Oken, whose romantic convictions found
expression in the broad, inclusive base of the society's membership. As a self-
organized and self-governing association which distanced itself from official
patronage and from the state academies, the GDNÄ embodied middle class
confidence and liberal values. It aimed to unify all branches of knowledge
under the common roof of the natural sciences. Although from its inception

papers on psychiatry had been read at its meetings, it was not until 1846 that psychiatry was represented in a special section of the program.[140] In the following years of revolutionary turmoil and political reaction, however, psychiatrists' attendance in these sections was dismal.

Nevertheless, in the latter half of the nineteenth century, the GDNÄ had an important role to play as psychiatrists sought the approbation of medical colleagues and natural scientists. Of course, that high sanction was forthcoming only if psychiatry participated in basic research in anatomy and physiology and adopted the methodological precepts of scientific medicine.[141] As a result, the psychiatric sections of the GDNÄ were dominated by papers on nosological and anatomical issues. In effect, the GDNÄ served as a transmission belt between psychiatry and the natural sciences and as a bellwether for the profession's medicalization.

But as important as the GDNÄ was for the early professional formation of psychiatry, it could neither supply a unifying platform nor act as a springboard for reforms.[142] While its emphasis on pure science could lend psychiatry much needed prestige, it also hampered discussion of the more mundane, yet pressing administrative, economic, and legal problems faced by alienists in their day-to-day work.[143] Furthermore, the GDNÄ was conceived as a society for all scientists and physicians and could therefore hardly provide auspicious surroundings for the consolidation of narrower psychiatric interests.[144] This point was driven home in a plenary address to the GDNÄ in Bonn in 1857 where Oscar Schwartz appealed to his colleagues to help overcome the "unnatural divisions" fracturing medicine into specialized disciplines. According to Schwartz, doctors needed to treat "the entire person, his body and soul indivisibly united, just as God had made him." Whereas alienists needed to be cognizant of the somatic afflictions of their patients, general practitioners had to pay greater attention to mental conditions.[145] As much as alienists might have been prone to agree with Schwartz, their small numbers at the GDNÄ made them simultaneously fearful of the implications of his message. Schwartz's call to dismantle the barriers separating psychiatry from internal medicine may have heralded long sought recognition in medical circles, but it also threatened to eclipse narrower alienist interests.[146]

Such concerns began to expose rifts within the psychiatric section itself. The question of whether psychiatry should have its own section or meet jointly with other sections (such as *Staatsarzneikunde*) was a matter of heated debate. On the one hand, generalists such as Adolf Erlenmeyer warned of the dangers of fragmentation; on the other hand, specialists like Heinrich Damerow were concerned that the sections were too heavily frequented by general physicians and that they produced resolutions at odds with the views of most psychiatric practitioners.[147] Increasingly, he and his alienist allies felt constrained within the framework of the GDNÄ and began urging the formation of an autonomous professional association.

Damerow's concerns were made all the more urgent in 1854 by the formation and rapid expansion of the *Deutsche Gesellschaft für Psychiatrie und gerichtliche Psychologie*. This society has been virtually erased from the historical memory of the profession and very little is known about it. It would appear that the driving force behind its formation was the aforementioned Erlenmeyer in alliance with Hermann Eulenberg and two Hannoverian alienists, Gottlob H. Bergmann and David Mansfeld, all of whom were editors of the *Correspondenzblatt*. The society met annually during conferences of the GDNÄ and was instrumental in organizing the GDNÄ's psychiatric sections. After 1856 those sections were held jointly with *Staatsarzneikunde*, reinforcing the decidedly forensic bent of the society's membership.[148] However, in keeping with the GDNÄ's aversion to specialization, the society was founded with the expressed intent of overcoming the "one-sided cultivation of the art and science of psychiatry in the asylums" and of promoting closer contacts between alienists and practicing physicians.[149] Consequently, it admitted not only dyed-in-the-wool alienists, but also non-alienist physicians. It did so in the hope of enlisting their cooperation in prophylactic endeavors and of improving their skills in diagnosing early symptoms of mental disease.[150] A mere two years after its formation, the *Gesellschaft* already had over two hundred members and by 1865 its rolls tallied well over four hundred.[151] With such impressive numbers and under the auspices of the GDNÄ, the *Gesellschaft* became the most important forum of professional debate in the decade from 1854 to 1864.

Damerow and the supporters of the *Allgemeine Zeitschrift* did everything they could to thwart the formation of the *Gesellschaft* and the publication of its organ, the *Correspondenzblatt*. Seeing their authority and the unity of the profession threatened, they accused members of the *Gesellschaft* of splitting the profession and succumbing to biased partiality.[152] At the same time, they also appealed to the national and professional loyalties of all alienists and called on them to boycott the new society.[153] But these efforts proved ineffective, and the number of members in the society continued to rise ominously. Indeed, so disconcerted were the editors of the *Allgemeine Zeitschrift* that they began laying the groundwork for a rival professional association.[154] In a well planned and deft strategy to wean members from the *Gesellschaft*, organizers grasped the distant venue of the GDNÄ conference in Königsberg in 1860 as an opportunity to undercut support for the *Gesellschaft*. Because the statutes of the *Gesellschaft* linked its meetings to those of the GDNÄ, the editors of the *Allgemeine Zeitschrift* hoped that by calling a rival meeting of alienists in the heart of Germany they could siphon off support and retake the initiative in the nascent process of professional development.

This they in fact did, calling their colleagues together at that most evocative of German national monuments, the Wartburg near Eisenach. Eisenach became the first of a series of meetings to follow in Landau (1861), Dresden

(1862) and Berlin (1863), which laid the ground-work for the founding of the *Verein deutscher Irrenärzte* in 1864.[155] At the inaugural meeting of the *Verein* in Frankfurt, C. F. W. Roller promptly advanced a motion to dissolve the psychiatric section of the GDNÄ. Although the motion failed to find majority support among the thirty alienists in attendance, it was consistent with the implicit aims of the *Verein*'s initiators, and it effectively laid down the gauntlet in the struggle with the *Gesellschaft* over supremacy within the profession. As an organization that later also met in the wings of the GDNÄ, yet as one which was *closed* to non-alienists, the *Verein* began successfully to court the favor of German psychiatrists, quickly eclipsing its rival and ultimately becoming the most influential professional psychiatric association in Germany for the next seventy years.

The initiators of the *Verein* all hailed from the editorial staff of the *Allgemeine Zeitschrift,* and its members were drawn largely from the ranks of its subscribers and contributors. Accordingly, the *Verein* was an association of alienist practitioners that focused on their day-to-day problems, while theoretical issues tended to be left to the sections of the GDNÄ. The *Verein*'s agenda encompassed many of the core professional concerns in the 1860s that included a compilation and homogenization of government regulations; a statistical survey of all German asylums; full academic chairs, clinical courses, and inclusion in the academic curricula; a consensus on forensic psychiatry; and discussion of admissions policy.

Initially, alienists described the *Verein* as the organizational embodiment of the collegiality and friendship, which had informally bonded the alienist community together in the first half of the century. However, no sooner had the *Verein* been constituted than it threatened to self-destruct. At the annual meeting in Heppenheim in 1867, its reputed harmony appeared to shatter after the association neglected, in the words of Roller, to "restrict the admission of members in order to keep out foreign elements," by which he meant the election of Wilhelm Griesinger to the executive committee.[156] Within a year, the animosities in the executive committee had moved the association's most influential leaders (Flemming, Roller, Jessen, and Laehr) to threaten their resignation, taking most members with them and leaving Griesinger with a rump association.

In addition to this inner turmoil, the summer of 1867 saw the rapid proliferation of other associations and regional branches of the *Verein*. Three such branches were the *Versammlung der südwestdeutschen Irrenärzte,* called to order by Roller in March 1867, the *Psychiatrischer Verein zu Berlin,*[157] a gathering of alienists from Berlin and Brandenburg from June 1867 and under the leadership of Laehr, Ideler, and Kahlbaum, and the *Psychiatrischer Verein der Rheinprovinz,* founded in July 1867 by Werner Nasse, Franz Richarz, and Carl Pelman, among others.[158] Although such regional associations had been a topic of discussion since 1862, their emergence in 1867 was at least in part a reaction to a new rival association in Berlin, the *Berliner medizinisch-psychologische Gesellschaft* under the auspices of Wilhelm Griesinger and Carl Westphal.[159] Following the lead of these larger associations, over the next several decades numerous other regional societies were also founded.

Psychiatric Training

In the first half of the nineteenth century views differed widely on the question of where and how to train psychiatrists. One of the most hotly disputed issues concerned the impact which clinical demonstration could have on patients and their therapeutic regimes. It was generally accepted that the clinical visit was a delicate affair, demanding the practitioner's tactful composure and deportment. However, some alienists argued that students did not possess such composure and that their immature bearing would have a detrimental impact on the patient's condition and that, as outsiders, they would upset the putative familial harmony of the asylum.[160] These alienists placed a premium on the asylum's therapeutic environment and resisted any suggestion that patients could be removed from it with impunity. Academicians countered these arguments by stressing that under the direction of an experienced teacher, who was able to select suitable patients and impress upon students the delicacy of the situation, such dangers could easily be avoided. In well organized wards outside of the asylum, they argued, clinical courses could be held without fear of compromising patient health.

The effects of demonstration on patients was certainly an important strand of professional discourse. But more was at stake in these disputes than simply therapeutic efficacy. Intertwined in expressly therapeutic concerns were also other, perhaps less visible but still deeply contentious issues of professional jurisdiction over the task of professional training. In a rough classification, three different schools of thought can be distinguished in these debates.[161] For some, small wards or 'filial' asylums attached directly to the university clinics were deemed most appropriate. A second point of view altogether rejected clinical education as practiced at the universities and advocated instead postgraduate internships in the asylums. Finally, a third group had no objection to clinical training, but believed that it should be conducted in the asylums rather than the university. Before turning explicitly to the debates of the 1860s, it's helpful to assess each of these positions in some detail.

The most prominent advocate of the first standpoint, that is, of filial asylums, was Christian Friedrich Nasse. He was among the earliest to lay out in detail the argument in support of academicians' claims to psychiatric education.[162] Himself a professor of medicine in Bonn, Nasse was eager to expand the didactic reach of medical faculties to include psychiatric training. Therefore, deeply convinced of the intimate relationship between body and soul, he insisted that every student needed to study mental diseases: "the cultivation of medical skills [*das ärztliche Geschäft*] in the treatment of the insane must comprise a necessary and indispensable part of the cultivation of each and every physician."[163] In Nasse's opinion, the university was the most appropriate place for this nascent branch of medicine to be taught. At the same time, however, he was deeply dissatisfied with the existing state of psychiatric education at German universities. In the 1820s and 1830s, he surveyed a barren landscape in which course offerings were seldom, largely theoretical, and rarely involved clinical demonstration.[164] Most debilitating of all was the schism dividing theory and practice. "Words alone and mere listening and learning will not suffice for the education of the young physician; it is necessary that he also act, observe, and practice for himself; and just as one has long since had to recognize this in other branches of medicine, one will likewise have to recognize it for the field of mental disease."[165] Whatever the usefulness of lecture courses, they had to be augmented by clinical demonstration.

The clinical institutions available to medical faculties—polyclinics and regular academic hospitals—provided neither the kind of patients that academicians wanted to see, nor the basic didactic prerequisites for effective instruction. Polyclinical demonstration, such as visiting patients in their homes, was restricted to the same urban population, year in and year out; educators were hostage to the whims of patients and their families; they lacked the means to ensure appropriate patient supervision and obedience; and they could not draw on the therapeutic arsenal of the asylum. Furthermore, the polyclinical setting itself, in the "huts of the poor" with family and relatives waiting in the wings, made it impossible to conduct "exact observations" of the patient.[166] Nor were academic hospitals any better outfitted to accommodate Nasse's vision of clinical instruction. In such hospitals, the cohabitation of patients, the inability to isolate them, inadequate architectural facilities, a lack of opportunity for therapeutic work, inadequate nursing staff, and an insufficient number of patients all posed daunting obstacles on the path toward effective clinical teaching. This state of affairs prompted Nasse to conclude that "no part of medicine is more neglected by our educational institutions than mental diseases."[167]

Rather than moving him to support asylum training, such deficits prompted Nasse to call for the construction of small academic clinics.[168] He envisioned institutions, each equipped with six to eight beds, that worked closely with a nearby asylum. At ten week intervals patients would rotate in and out of the clinic. This supply of patients would also be supplemented by polyclinical courses. Although Nasse did not think that special chairs in psychiatry were necessary, he did believe that the needs of academic clinicians and students demanded that these filial asylums should be constructed near universities.

Advocates of the second standpoint were opposed to clinical instruction altogether.[169] They believed that it could no more be removed entirely from the environment of the asylum and placed in the hands of academicians, than it could be reconciled with the asylum's therapeutic mission. They wanted essentially nothing to do with university students and believed that Nasse's vision was irreconcilable with the therapeutic goals of isolation. C. F. W. Roller was certainly the most prominent advocate of this position, which he defended in an acrimonious dispute with the medical faculty in Heidelberg.[170] He was convinced that students would adversely affect his patients' prognoses and violate their privacy. Furthermore, the distraction of having to hold theoretical lectures represented an irresponsible neglect of the alienist's other, all-consuming responsibilities. Voicing a conviction that he would carry to his grave, Roller insisted that "an asylum may never be used as a psychiatric clinic."[171]

But Roller did propose an alternative. In his opinion a few beds in special rooms in or near other university clinics would entirely suffice for the purposes of clinical instruction and for the practical demonstration of theoretical lectures. In addition, he suggested that a few recent university graduates should be allowed to practice in the asylums as so-called "*élèves internes*" (internal students). With the distractions of academic life behind them, these graduates would be assigned to a ward for several months to study individual cases. The subtle art of alienist practice could be learned only by working in the asylum and never by simply participating in weekly university lectures or in a mere semester of clinical visits. While theoretical training at the universities was an important first step, it had to be backed up by practical experience. And as long as asylums provided such essential practical experience, then, far from holding the young science of psychiatry in bondage, they would provide the very precondition for truly rational observation and expert training.

The impact of the decades-long dispute between Roller and the Heidelberg medical faculty was enormous in Baden and influenced discussions in other German localities as well. But in spite of this visceral conflict, alienists in other parts of Germany were more willing to entertain the idea of clinical courses within asylum walls. They comprised a third body of opinion. For this majority, clinical training was best disposed of in the asylums.[172] One early advocate of this view was Johann Michael Leupoldt, professor of medicine in Erlangen. Leupoldt believed that clinical education in psychiatry could never simply adopt the methods used in general clinical courses; instead, it had to be organized in its own special way. As long as only as small number of advanced students who were fully acquainted with asylum life were involved, clinical instruction posed no threat to the orderly functioning of the institution. Students could write up cases, examine new admissions, participate in autopsies, and converse with patients "as between rational individuals."[173] Because of the exceptionally long duration of mental illness, Leupoldt also recommended that clinical courses last an entire year, although he did not believe that students needed to reside in the asylum.

Many of these sentiments were also expressed by Heinrich Damerow. However, Damerow insisted that teachers could never be professors of medicine and that only the asylum director was qualified to conduct such courses.

There was no place in Damerow's clinical courses for "comprehensively developed, systematic lectures on general and specific pathology and therapy." His was an expressly empirical undertaking designed not to illustrate nosological types, but rather to take nature as a guide, to let theory be "enlivened by natural truths and to teach using the example of life itself."[174] At best, the clinical teacher would provide his students with general concepts and theoretical principles, but never with a closed theoretical system. In addition, Damerow integrated professional training into his larger program of architecturally combining curative and custodial institutions into so-called *relativ verbundene Heil- und Pflegeanstalten*. He recommended using chronic patients in custodial institutions for pedagogic purposes. Having learned the fundamental principles of patient examination and treatment there, students could then graduate to the hospital for curable patients.

The degree to which these three models of clinical education were actually realized varied from institution to institution and from state to state. Although very little is known about just how these clinical courses were conducted, it is clear that a group of asylums enjoyed pedagogical reputations extending beyond their immediate regions. Being among the very first medical hospitals for the curably insane, the asylum Sonnenstein in Saxony held a "monopoly" on psychiatric training in the 1810s and counted among its early assistants many of the most influential alienists of the century, including P. Jessen, C. F. Roller, Carl Flemming, and Moritz Gustav Martini.[175] That preeminence then passed to the Prussian asylum in Siegburg in the 1820s and 30s, where under the direction of Maximilian Jacobi it became an "alienist Mecca"; few were the alienists of that period who had not either visited or been assistants under Jacobi.[176] The southern German state of Baden then assumed pedagogical leadership once the asylum Illenau opened its doors to patients in 1842. A prototype for asylums linking medical and custodial care, Illenau retained a "de facto monopoly on training" in psychiatry well into the 1860s.[177] On the wards in Illenau and under the authoritarian direction of Roller, such young and ambitious psychiatrists as Bernhard von Gudden, Richard von Krafft-Ebing, and Heinrich Schüle were trained in their craft.[178] While Sonnenstein, Siegburg, and Illenau were not the only institutions teaching young psychiatrists in the first half of the century, they did become standard-bearers in clinical instruction.

At universities, however, facilities for clinical training in psychiatry were a patchwork of widely varying and, in part, provisional arrangements that were often subject to the individual proclivities and whims of academicians and asylum directors.[179] Even at Prussia's first university in Berlin, clinical training had all but ceased under the auspices of Carl Wilhelm Ideler.[180] This had enormous impact, because, well into the 1850s, Prussian medical students were required to take their state exams in Berlin. Consequently, many medical students chose to prepare for them by studying in the Prussian capital. Elsewhere, at Breslau, where Heinrich Neumann was adjunct professor, courses had been purely theoretical, and it was not until 1876 that an agreement was signed between the university and the city providing for the clinical use of patients on the psychiatric wards of the city hospital. In Greifswald, the professor for internal medicine, Friedrich August Gottlob Berndt, established a "clinic" in the local asylum in the 1830s, but it was not—or if so, only very rarely—used for clinical instruction. And at other universities there were for all intents and purposes no standard clinical courses on offer; even in university towns with large asylums nearby, either courses were not offered at all (as in Halle), or attendance was very poor (as in Bonn).

The situation at universities outside of Prussia was little better. In Hannover, although an asylum designed to provide clinical training was being constructed, university students in Göttingen had theretofore heard only theoretical lectures. In the kingdom of Württemberg things were still worse: in Tübingen there was neither a physical clinic, nor courses or practica in the asylums, nor even theoretical lectures in psychiatry. In the kingdom of Saxony the state of clinical education was likewise bad: neither at the university in Leipzig nor in the asylums were courses being offered. In Sachsen-Weimar clinical instruction was offered, but the director of the asylum in Jena, Franz Xaver Schömann, was a surgeon and orthopaedist with apparently little enthusiasm for his psychiatric responsibilities. In the Grand Duchy of Hessen after 1854, interest in advancing the cause of psychiatric education was dormant. And not surprisingly in light of Roller's influence in Baden, the medical faculties in Freiburg and Heidelberg had little opportunity to expose students to psychiatric patients.

Similarly, a ministerial inquiry into clinical education at Bavaria's three state universities in 1859 produced discouraging results.[181] In Würzburg, where, in the Julius-Spital, Karl Friedrich Marcus had given public lectures on psychiatry nearly every year since 1847–8, the academic senate reported attendance of between one quarter and one third of all enrolled medical students. It should, however, be added that after 1850 Marcus was blind and that his assistant and successor, Franz von Rinecker, denied that the lectures could in any sense be called clinical. Rinecker's assessment was also shared by his assistant and later professor of psychiatry in Berlin, Friedrich Jolly, who described Marcus's courses as little more than popular demonstrations that had often given rise to protest and scandal. Worst of all, in Munich the annual courses in psychiatry offered by Oskar Mahir over the past fifteen years had never had participants. Only at the university in Erlangen, which unlike Würzburg entertained rudimentary relations to its local asylum, was the situation somewhat better. Solbrig, who held an honorary professorship at the university, was able to count on average thirteen or fourteen participants in the clinical courses he offered and was full of praise for the mutual benefits which the patients, students, and the asylum derived from the classes. Thus, in the 1850s clinical training at universities in Bavaria and other non-Prussian lands had been, at best, uneven.

But in Bavaria the situation was rapidly changing, as alienists began laying claim to the tasks of clinical education. Having long been a relative backwater of psychiatric care, Bavaria had embarked on an extensive building program in the 1840s and 1850s and had coupled it with a commitment to academic training.[182] As a result, in the opinion of many contemporary observers, clinical training was nowhere as advanced by the early 1860s as in that southern German state.[183] Unlike prospective doctors elsewhere, Bavarian students were certain to face psychiatric topics in their state exams after two psychiatrists— Bernhard von Gudden and Franz von Rinecker—were appointed to the state examination commission in 1858.[184] And when in 1859 a new asylum was built in Munich, August Solbrig proceeded systematically to reorganize psychiatric training and to argue forcefully that this training was essential to every physician's education and that it needed to be conducted in asylums by alienists.[185]

What makes Solbrig's position on clinical training so important is that he managed to line up the members of the nascent *Verein deutscher Irrenärzte* behind him. Initially, the emerging *Verein* had balked at the idea of clinical courses in asylums. Although general agreement had existed on the desirability of psychiatric chairs and clinics, "the proper path [leading to them] had yet to be ascertained."[186] But Solbrig succeeded in convincing the majority of his colleagues to accept clinical training in asylums. He argued that there existed no fundamental conflict of interest between alienists' therapeutic goals and professional education. Indeed, the alienist was the "most natural and legitimate representative of clinical psychiatric teaching" and patients would profit greatly from the asylum's enhanced image as a "center of scientific research."[187]

These preliminary debates culminated at the inaugural meeting of the *Verein* in Frankfurt in 1864. There, in a seven-point resolution, alienists laid down their position on clinical instruction:

> (1) Every university must offer a clinical lecture course in psychiatry; without it, medical education is fragmentary. (2) Wherever feasible, the instructor of the clinical lecture in psychiatry should also be the director of a modern asylum. (3) The clinical instructor's asylum should have at least 150 to 200 patients. (4) The clinical instructor must be a member of the medical faculty and a full professor. (5) If necessary, the clinical instructor should be provided with a few rooms for teaching purposes in one of the other clinical facilities. (6) Instruction in psychiatry must attain parity with other fields. (7) Students must attend clinical lectures in general medicine [*medicinische Klinik*] before receiving instruction in psychiatry.[188]

The resolution adopted in Frankfurt was clearly tailored to the interests of asylum psychiatrists and was premised on the assumption that there need be no jurisdictional conflict between alienists' responsibilities as directors of state asylums and as academic instructors. The prerequisite that clinical instructors simultaneously head large asylums was a condition that academic professors patently could not fulfil; nor was there much prospect of them being able to do so. In fact, it was even recognized by some university professors that the task of educating students in psychiatry had slipped from the general academician and was increasingly passing to the specialized alienist.[189] In the early 1860s, and with Solbrig's Bavarian model in the back of their minds, alienists had thus at least outwardly overcome their differences and positioned themselves to consolidate their jurisdiction over clinical education.

CHAPTER 3

Wilhelm Griesinger's Reform Program: The Professional Politics of the Urban Asylum

Griesinger Contested

In an otherwise sharply fragmented discipline, Wilhelm Griesinger has become for contemporary German psychiatry a kind of fixed star on the horizon of historical memory, serving to orient both biological and psycho-social paradigms. Advocates of the former tend to downplay the idealistic content of his theories while hailing his maxim that "mental disease is brain disease."[1] The latter emphasize his vision of community and rehabilitative care and see him as a historical precursor to the reform psychiatry of the 1970s.[2] That one can read Griesinger in such apparently divergent ways is symptomatic of the sense that he today represents the lost unity, coherence, and putative historical innocence of a profession that had escaped the throws of theology and romantic philosophy, but that had not yet been caught up in the inexorable gravitational pull of specialized, "rational", "scientific" medicine. He has come to be situated in an historical eye of psychiatry's stormy past, and it is not the least a consequence of this historical locale's distance from both the "irrational" strains of romantic psychiatry and the systematic, mechanized destruction of the mentally ill under National Socialism, that Griesinger has been put into service as a potentially unifying figure within the discipline.[3]

Yet, back in the late 1860s, Griesinger was the single most controversial figure in German psychiatric circles. Although not necessarily intending to fracture his profession, Griesinger became embroiled in a series of acerbic and polemical exchanges with his alienist opponents.[4] One of his most prolific critics, Heinrich Laehr, penned an uncompromising assault on his professional integrity, accusing him of betraying his colleagues and of appropriating the same language and arguments that amateurs and dilettantes had used to vilify alienists.[5] Others, such as Max Brosius, found Griesinger to be "grossly ignorant" of historical developments in German psychiatry and accused him of behaving "as though he didn't belong" in their midst.[6] Hermann Dick and August Solbrig thought so little of his reforms that they did not even bother to critique them, while Roller belittled them as pontifications ("*Katheder Weisheit*").[7]

Thus Griesinger was pilloried in 1867–68 for soiling the good name and reputation of his profession.

The final act of Griesinger's fall from alienist grace was staged in Dresden in September of 1868 at the annual meeting of Germany's most prestigious gathering of scientists and physicians, the *Gesellschaft Deutscher Naturforscher und Ärtze*. In a well choreographed assault, he was removed from the executive committee of the *Verein* and his reform program was publicly denounced in a special supplemental section of the conference.[8] The core tenets of his reform program were rebuked, with almost no one rising in their defense and under circumstances that smacked of a professional ambush.[9] Nor did the attacks entirely subside even after Griesinger's death a month later: in an obituary, his opponents sarcastically dispatched his views, remarking that he had had many "new and good ideas, but that the good ones were not new and the new ones not good."[10]

Many factors contributed to Griesinger's contested standing in alienist circles. His personality was an amalgam of extreme irritability, directness, arrogance, and a bitingly polemical literary style.[11] Furthermore, his life-long affiliation with internal medicine hardly recommended him as head of the Charité's psychiatric wards. Alienists were highly skeptical of his professional qualifications as an administrator of a large institution, and the fact that he had no experience as director of a Prussian provincial asylum was particularly irksome. They could not help but view it as a bitter setback that a foreign academic with conspicuously shallow alienist qualifications had been chosen at a time when they were actively lobbying for greater control over clinical education.[12] This was resented all the more because one of their own, Heinrich Laehr, had been passed over in favor of Griesinger.[13]

Another bone of contention between Griesinger and leading alienists was his new journal, the *Archiv für Psychiatrie und Nervenkrankheiten* (*AfPN*), which he had founded shortly after arriving in Berlin. From its inception the *Archiv* had distanced itself forthrightly from alienist psychiatry, criticizing it (and by association the *Allgemeine Zeitschrift*) for its philosophical predilections and preoccupation with institutional concerns.[14] True to Griesinger's conviction that mental disease was brain disease, the *Archiv* attempted to redefine psychiatry in neuropathological terms and thereby anchor it firmly alongside internal medicine. However, because alienists believed that neuropathological principles already permeated their own thought and practice, they took Griesinger's proclamation that the *Archiv* represented the dawn of a new psychiatric age to be an arrogant rebuff.[15] And indeed, the *Archiv* was an integral part of an aggressive campaign to co-opt the older, more prestigious *Allgemeine Zeitschrift* and, when this failed, to rob it of its publisher.[16] It is therefore little wonder that Griesinger's harshest critics all hailed from the editorial board of that rival journal.

As important as all of these considerations are in explaining the animosities that Griesinger aroused in alienist circles, they do not suffice as historical explanations for the vehemence of the debates.[17] One can understand their intensity only by recognizing that Griesinger's reform program of 1867 touched on far deeper professional concerns. His reforms advanced alternative claims to solving many of the fundamental problems facing German psychiatry in the 1860s and in doing so challenged nothing less than the central tenets, interests, and authority of the profession itself.[18] Griesinger was a controversial figure because his reform program shook the very foundations on which the profession had been constructed.

After reviewing the substance of Griesinger's reforms, the remainder of this chapter will consider some of the deeper conflicts from which psychiatric clinics ultimately emerged. With an eye toward the different professional tasks described in the introduction, four important *discursive fields* bearing decisively on the development of university clinics will be investigated:[19] first, Griesinger's psychiatric theory; second, the debate on non-restraint in the 1860s and Griesinger's advocacy of "free treatment;" third, the urban asylum's role in clinical teaching; and fourth, questions of socio-economic class, nationalism, and the beleaguered state of the profession's public image. Each of these overlapping discourses touched intimately on core professional problems. First, Griesinger's psychiatric theory was closely intertwined with psychiatry's adoption of the medical model of mental illness and its ongoing struggle for recognition among more established fields of medicine, as well as with the delineation of its boundary with neurology and the mastery of laboratory technologies. Second, the charged therapeutic debate on non-restraint contained an important subplot concerning the conditions of possibility of accurate clinical observation, research, and diagnosis. Third, Griesinger's conception of the urban asylum as a clinical institution challenged established practices of professional training. Fourth, and finally, the urban asylum represented a new kind of elite institution, situated outside of the traditional spheres of alienist influence, where it staked a claim to and siphoned off the more desirable, affluent, and acutely afflicted patients, while leaving the mass of less agreeable, indigent, and chronic cases to alienist care. In laying claim to these patients, urban asylums undercut the traditional therapeutic and prophylactic responsibilities of the asylum. Closely associated with this socio-prophylactic task, and as an effective means of undergirding their battered public image, psychiatrists showed increasing willingness to identify their work with larger social issues.

Each of these levels of discourse bore on specific professional tasks and contained competing claims to perform those tasks in the resolution of pressing scientific, didactic, and socio-medical problems. What made Griesinger's reform program so controversial among his colleagues was that it implied a thoroughgoing reorganization of psychiatric work. Some, especially medical faculties, stood to profit from that reorganization, while others, like Germany's entrenched alienist elite, rightly saw their hard-won privileges endangered and their professional standing jeopardized. At stake in these debates was the division of expert labor in psychiatry and the power to speak with authority on a wide range of theoretical, diagnostic, and therapeutic issues.

Griesinger's Reform Program

Griesinger published his ideas on asylum reform in a programmatic article in the first issue of his *Archiv* in 1868.[20] Under the title "On Asylums and Their Further Development in Germany" Griesinger confirmed the crisis of overcrowding, which Damerow and others had already diagnosed, and lamented the lethargic transmission of scientific knowledge into institutional practice. At the root of the problems plaguing the system lay the ineffective criterion of curability. Over the past half-century curability had become an important medico-administrative principle guiding the construction of many new institutions and the distribution of patients and resources to the asylums. Yet, as Griesinger argued, that criterion lacked any viable medical basis and could be applied at best only to a very small proportion of patients; for the vast majority, no reliable and definitive demarcation between curable and incurable was possible. He concluded, therefore, that a different standard was needed, one based not on the therapeutic prospects of the patients, but rather on strictly pragmatic considerations of the duration of treatment. Although psychiatrists were not in a position to determine whether a disease was curable or not, they could establish with far greater reliability whether a patient required long-term care, or whether only brief institutionalization (such as during the acute phase of an otherwise perhaps incurable illness) was necessary. On the basis of this assessment, he proposed that two primary modes of patient care be established, one for long-term patients, and another for short-term, transitory patients; and because in Griesinger's mind these two modes of care dictated wholly different physical environments, therapeutic equipment, and administrative organizations, it was essential that they be institutionally segregated from one another. To accommodate these two modes of care, Griesinger therefore envisioned two kinds of mental institutions.

The first kind, designed to accommodate long-term patients, Griesinger termed rural asylums (*ländliche Asyle*).[21] As their name implied, they would be located away from urban centers on large tracts of comparatively inexpensive land and accommodate upwards of 400–600 patients of both sexes. Agricultural labor would be one of their core organizational principles and help to offset their operating costs. In therapeutic terms these asylums were expressions of Griesinger's convictions that idleness was a debilitating force in the lives of "robust lunatics" and that physicians were duty-bound to do "everything possible to protect [chronic patients] from further decline."[22] Those whose affliction made them unable to work in the rural asylum were to be transferred immediately to nursing homes. But at the same time, rural asylums were not to degenerate into spartan work-houses. They required parks and other elaborate facilities to distract and entertain residents who might well find themselves spending the remainder of their lives in the institution.

Dating from the first decades of the nineteenth century, large asylums located in the countryside had become the backbone of psychiatric care in Germany and elsewhere in Europe. These institutions framed Griesinger's reform vision, and he was sharply critical of them. He was especially disturbed by their barrack-like mass-incarceration (*Casernirung*) of chronic patients. Though paying tribute to the humane intentions of their planners and under no illusions about the occasional need for patient restraint, such forms of treatment had seen their day and now held no promise for the future. At the core of Griesinger's critique lay his belief that asylums failed sufficiently to differentiate between categories of patients and had therefore effectively become carceral institutions. Many patients neither required nor benefitted from the costly, often unimaginative forms of treatment that asylums provided. Other patients, while benefitting from some form of institutionalization, hardly needed the kind of tight security that had evolved in the asylums over the years. In fact, the blanket application of mechanical restraint as practiced in some asylums often created precisely the kind of dangerous patients that it had been intended to bridle. Furthermore, many chronic patients suffered unnecessarily because of the physical proximity of acutely ill ward-mates and needed to be freed of this psychological burden. And in general, many patients could and indeed needed to be granted more "well regulated freedom."[23] Hence, central to Griesinger's critique of existing asylums was an emancipatory logic intended to free patients from unnecessary incarceration, from arbitrary mechanical restraint, and from the potentially detrimental influence of their fellow inmates. Thus liberated, they could be placed in more therapeutically effective and economically productive environments.

Griesinger envisioned two such environments for chronic patients, both adjunct to the main rural asylum. First, Griesinger proposed building agricultural colonies for patients to live outside the main asylum and engage in agricultural labor. The colonies would accommodate only more robust patients of peasant origin (rather than educated city-dwellers) and provide a framework in which their labor could be put to productive use. In doing so, colonies would generate a beneficial "atmosphere of contentment, work, community, and freedom." The second form of emancipated environment was the family itself. Taking the Belgian town of Gheel as his point of departure, Griesinger's family care (*Familienpflege*) sought to place quiet, non-violent, and especially female patients in the homes of nearby residents or asylum personnel. There they would share in all aspects of their hosts' daily lives, while doctors from the main asylum would occasionally visit the family to inspect conditions and guide therapy.

More important for the purposes of this study than the rural asylum is its urban counterpart, Griesinger's second kind of mental institution. Griesinger's urban asylums (*Stadtasyle*) were institutions for short-term, so-called transitory patients, and would be situated near large population centers. The urban asylum was intended to admit not only members of the lower and lower-middle classes, but also the educated urban middle class that could neither financially afford the expensive care of private institutions nor socially cope with the specter of admission to the rural asylums. It differed from rural asylums in that the short duration of patients' stays, as well as their acute condition, obviated the need for large grounds, agricultural plots, workshops, chapels and recreation facilities. Instead, Griesinger argued that a pleasant, protected garden and a veranda adjoining a structure situated on the quiet periphery of the city would entirely suffice to ensure the well-being of patients. Furthermore, the urban asylum was to be so amply stocked with well qualified medical personnel that Griesinger believed it unnecessary for the director physically to reside on the asylum grounds as alienist patriarchs did. The admissions criteria likewise differed from those of the rural asylum: whereas it was vital that admission to rural asylums be made as difficult as possible in order to prevent them from "silting up" with patients who belonged in nursing homes, restrictive bureaucratic barriers on admission to and evacuation from urban asylums would be reduced to an absolute minimum wherever possible, so that acute and emergency cases could receive immediate medical attention. To these ends, Griesinger insisted that assurances regarding the rapid transfer of patients out of the urban asylum be secured from other institutions in order to prevent the asylum from degenerating into a stigmatized "*Irrenhaus*" for long-term, chronic patients. The urban asylum would be relatively small, with between sixty and one hundred and fifty beds for patients whose stay was restricted to twelve or, in exceptional cases, eighteen months. The inner atmosphere of the urban asylum was designed to avoid any hint of a madhouse and to project instead the image of a hospital, including "incessant, round-the-clock observation and care."[24] Upon admission patients would immediately be placed on observation wards, which Griesinger saw as the most important wards in the entire institution.[25] And finally, Griesinger's urban asylum ensured that directors could regulate the interaction between patients and their families. On the one hand, Griesinger was adamant that the family not be granted the right to remove their relatives from the urban asylum without the expressed consent of the director; on the other hand, he grasped the physical proximity of patients' families as a therapeutic opportunity to reassure and comfort patients and to ease their transition back into society.

Of further key importance for the purposes of this study is the fact that Griesinger linked the construction of urban asylums to the interests of psychiatric education.[26] Griesinger believed that—with some noted exceptions—those interests had been thwarted by the same entrenched forces of opposition that had so rigorously objected to other progressive psychiatric ideas. "The ifs, ands and buts that are brought up *ad nauseam* over and over again, the rhetoric of the incredible difficulties of teaching psychiatric courses, the agitated fear of the enormous costs of huge clinical institutions, the groundless claim that clinical demonstration harms patients, as well as the *vis inertiae* adhering to all things human—they have all delayed and undermined the beneficent and, for the purposes of the state, so very important cause [of psychiatric education]."[27] Griesinger refuted each of these objections. Accusations that clinical demonstration had a detrimental impact on patients were nothing but idle talk; in fact, clinical demonstration often had a surprisingly favorable impact on the patient's state of mind.

After putting his critics to heel, Griesinger proceeded to lay down five key preconditions that would ensure the vibrancy of psychiatric clinics. First, students had to have easy access to clinical instruction. Courses offered at institutions far from the gates of the city or remote from the other university clinics would from the outset doom the cause of clinical education in psychiatry. Second, every psychiatric clinic required an ample and rich supply of acute cases, since it was necessary to instruct students in the subtle beginnings, complex course, and remission of psychiatric disease as exhibited only in acute cases. Third, it was essential that there be a rapid turnover of patients, and hence, while a good clinic need not be a large one, it did need to discharge patients once their pedagogical usefulness had expired. Fourth, only a small number of chronic and incurable patients were required for the clinic to fulfill its didactic responsibilities. And finally, all other requirements of a psychiatric clinic corresponded fully with the those of the urban asylum: "If one furnishes the urban asylum in a university town with the resources necessary to make it a true scientific observatory and then adds a lecture hall—then the urban asylum . . . becomes a clinical asylum."[28] In the mind of Wilhelm Griesinger, the urban asylum was a proto-university psychiatric clinic.

Griesinger expanded the didactic reach of his ideas still further by insisting that psychiatric clinics be granted parity in all respects with other academic clinics.[29] Lecture courses in psychiatry needed to become an obligatory part of the curriculum. As in other academic hospitals, administrative provisions were needed to ensure ready access to patients and corpses. Furthermore, clinicians had to be both teachers and "men of science" freed as much as possible from burdensome administrative duties so as to pursue their academic responsibilities. And in keeping with the practice of other clinics, if to the consternation of all patriarchal alienists, Griesinger also proposed (at least for small urban asylums) that distinctions of class be done away with.

This, in summary, was Griesinger's reform proposal. Instead of constructing separate asylums for the curable (*Heilanstalt*) and incurable (*Pflegeanstalt*) or some hybrid combining the two, Griesinger advocated the construction of small urban asylums for acute, short-term care and larger rural asylums for long-term, usually chronic cases. He thus sought to shift the criteria governing the distribution of patients and resources *from curability to duration of treatment.* Alienists understood this institutional reorganization to entail a degradation of their asylums to mere convalescent homes and their work to mere custodial management.[30] But the reform proposal represented more than just a shift in the administration of psychiatric care. It implied also a radical realignment of professional jurisdictions and the redistribution of professional labor. It is to the contests over these issues that I now turn.

Griesinger's Theory: A Gateway to Laboratory Research

Griesinger laid the foundation of his psychiatric theory in the early 1840s during his years as an assistant to Ernst Albert von Zeller at Winnenthal in the kingdom of Württemberg. In 1845 he published *Pathologie und Therapie der psychischen Krankheiten,* a textbook that secured his reputation as one of the leading figures in modern, "scientific psychiatry."[31] The book reflected the inductive methods, hierarchical ordering, and mechanistic models of other mid-century physiologists and psychologists, such as Johannes Müller, Ernst Heinrich Weber, and Gustav Fechner. Like them, Griesinger was seeking to explain the relationship between physical and psychological processes. He drew an analogy between the physiological reflex action of the nervous system in response to external sensory stimuli and the "mental reflex" (*psychische Reflexaktion*) of the brain.[32] He believed that these two kinds of reflex action (spinal and mental) were governed by the same physical laws and that they functioned in much the same manner. Just as centripetal sensory input into the central nervous system produced motor activity in the corporal periphery, so too did the brain react to representations (*Vorstellungen*) to effect human drive or action. In their aggregate and their dynamic interaction, these representations comprised the "psychological tonus" or character of the individual. Furthermore, depending on their intensity and in accordance with an Hegelian dialectical process, those representations either remained subconscious or were qualitatively transformed into consciousness. Psychiatric disorders arose, analogous to their neurological counterparts, when the mechanisms governing "mental reflex" broke down, that is, when the mental reflex was either retarded, as in melancholy, or excessively active, as in mania. Thus, by way of an analogy in which sensation and reflex action in the spinal cord found their counterparts in the representation and drive in the brain, Griesinger applied a mechanistic model of physiological reflex action to psychopathology. Indeed, the brain became the focal point of his entire psychiatric theory and resulted in his name becoming nearly synonymous with the somatic battle cry: mental disease is brain disease.

This emphasis on the brain points to an important distinction between Griesinger and the so-called *Somatiker,* with whom his name is so often associated. *Somatiker* such as Maximilian Jacobi, Friedrich Nasse, and Christian

Friedrich Flemming had argued that the physical symptoms and diseases attending madness were not caused by psychological deviance, moral turpitude, and sin, i.e. by a so-called disease of the soul or *Seelenkrankheit*, as their adversaries the *Psychiker* had argued. Instead, they reversed this causal chain, contending that madness was not a cause but an effect of other somatic diseases afflicting the patient's wider body. Although, like the *Somatiker*, Griesinger was convinced of the organic root of madness, he differed from them in viewing it chiefly as a disease of the brain and less a secondary manifestation of other, extra-cerebral bodily diseases. Indeed, he went even further, arguing, well into the 1860s, that madness was a consequence of one single disease of the brain, namely of a "unitary psychosis" (*Einheitspsychose*),[33] and that the obviously manifold symptoms of madness were not the result of different diseases, but instead simply different stages of a single disease process.

Griesinger had adopted this concept of unitary psychosis from his mentor Ernst Albert von Zeller, but he understood it an altogether different context, abandoning the independence and unity of the soul (*Seele*) that for Zeller had secured its coherence.[34] Strongly influenced by natural philosophy and the anthropological currents of German psychiatry from the 1820s to the 1840s, Zeller had believed that it was this unified human soul or character (*Gemüt*) that was afflicted in madness. For Griesinger, however, that character was nothing more than the psychological tonus produced (by mental reflex) through the accumulation of representations over the lifetime of the individual. He did not so much deny the existence of a soul, as he grounded it in the material tissue of the brain and associated it with individual development, thereby subordinating it to historical process and contributing to its further secularization. The soul became a mere function of the brain, a product of its anatomical and physiological attributes.

Since madness was an affliction of the brain's mental reflex, within the logic of Griesinger's theory it was a legitimate object of medical inquiry. To be precise, it fell within the jurisdiction of internists who were appropriately versed in the workings of the central nervous system. As such, Griesinger's theory posed no great threat to an emerging professional consensus, which by mid-century had come to define insanity in medical terms.[35] In fact, by 1845 the association of madness with diseases of the brain was hardly controversial at all: the *Somatiker* had always made similar claims, although with less fervently materialist arguments than Griesinger.[36] Nor did the analogies which he drew with physiology cause much consternation among psychiatrists who were increasingly struggling to establish their sense of medical identity. On the contrary, Griesinger's localization of madness at the physical organ of the brain paralleled contemporary trends in general medicine, in particular Rudolf Virchow's cellular pathology, which conceived of disease in terms of a physiological disorder, with a local, clearly definable, anatomic seat.

Aside from its medical underpinnings,[37] the attraction of Griesinger's theory was enhanced by a series of parallel scientific and technological innovations. As Werner Leibbrand and Annemarie Wettley have pointed out, Griesinger's theory of "mental reflex" was deeply embedded in the energetic vocabulary and mechanistic concepts so fashionable by the middle of the century; the decidedly modern, scientific flavor of these ideas only enhanced the attractiveness of his theory. The rise of experimental physiology, in particular the work of Hermann Helmholtz, Johannes Müller, and Gustav Fechner, all seemed to lend added authority to Griesinger's theoretical picture of centripetal signals traveling to the brain, being processed, and then reacted upon with centrifugal signals moving to peripheral organs. In the imaginations of many contemporaries, his theory paralleled the exciting new images and possibilities of the telegraph. Indeed, the comparison drawn between the central nervous system and the telegraph by Helmholtz represents one of the more persistent and recurrent images in German psychiatry in the latter half of the nineteenth century.[38]

Beyond its scientific and cultural plausibility, Griesinger's theory also held out a number of professional advantages. For one, it could serve as an integrative bracket designed to stabilize psychiatry's status in the face of public criticism. It could reinforce efforts to secure psychiatry's recognition as a legitimate branch of medical science and thus open the way for academic posts and funding. Within medicine itself it could back up calls for a union of psychiatry and neurology, thereby responding to those diehard critics who saw no place for psychiatry in the medical sciences. By the same token, it could help the profession stake its claim not just to psychiatric patients, but to neurological ones as well. In short, psychiatrists had much to gain and little to loose by aligning themselves with Griesinger's vision of a neurological psychiatry.

Thus, perhaps somewhat surprisingly, what did *not* contribute to Griesinger's contested professional standing in the latter half of the 1860s were the core somatic assumptions of his psychiatric theory. There existed increasingly a general consensus among psychiatrists that mental disorder was the result of organically based diseases of the brain.[39] In working to align psychiatry with the somatic tenets of internal medicine and pathological anatomy, Griesinger helped provide the profession with the medical credentials its practioners so eagerly sought. He blazed a trail from internal medicine to psychiatry and pointed the way for laboratory research to explore the anatomical and histological structures of the brain.

At the same time, however, Griesinger's theory placed alienists in a very awkward position. They were geographically and intellectually isolated from the university and its specialists in internal medicine. They were also overburdened by the administrative responsibilities of large asylums that were often bursting at the seams with patients. Alienists were therefore at a distinct disadvantage when it came to mimicking the scientific techniques and models of academic medicine.[40] They found themselves in the difficult position of desiring, on the one hand, closer association with university medical faculties, while, on the other hand, insisting upon psychiatry's alienist traditions and upon the imperative of their asylums' rural locale. If they recognized the "indisputable truth" of Griesinger's central tenets, they were nevertheless loath to see alienist psychiatry reduced to neuropathology. As important as a bridge to academic medical science was, alienists were sympathetic to Roller's adamant contention that asylums "were not indebted to any theoretical doctrine of pathology. Nor [would] such a doctrine alone help them fulfill their destiny."[41] Either way, alienists clearly recognized that the paramount challenge confronting their profession in the early 1860s was "the transition from its exclusive situation to the sphere of general medicine."[42]

The contribution of Griesinger's psychiatric theory to the professional development of German psychiatry was therefore of a decidedly ambivalent nature: on the one hand, it was a gateway expediting psychiatry's entry into general medicine; on the other hand, it deepened an ominous and widening rift in the profession between those engaged in the work of "scientific" research and those responsible for the administration of psychiatric care. Griesinger had called into question the professional identity of alienists as scientists. And, more fundamentally, he had explicitly disputed their jurisdiction over the crucial professional task of basic scientific research. He insisted that academic clinicians and asylum directors differed markedly from one another. The former was a "man of science" who had dedicated his life to discovering the truth, while the latter was a "mere alienist."[43]

The Debate on Non-Restraint and Clinical Research

In 1861 Griesinger republished his textbook *Die Pathologie und Therapie der psychischen Krankheiten*. The republication did not correspond with any substantial change in his theoretical position. Yet in one significant practical respect it differed radically from the earlier version: in its outspoken advocacy of *non-restraint*—that is, of the abstention from mechanical restraint in the treatment of psychiatric patients.[44] Griesinger had become convinced that the bedlamic din of many asylums was largely a product of alienists' own therapeutic policies and that if they applied the principles of non-restraint, then their asylums could become quieter, more orderly, and be more therapeutically effective institutions.

The mid-century debate on the question of restraint had been given new impetus by the publication of John Conolly's *The Treatment of the Insane without Mechanical Restraints* in 1856. In Germany the debate intensified after Conolly's work was translated into German in 1860.[45] Alongside Ludwig Meyer,[46] director of the Hamburg asylum Friedrichsberg and later professor in Göttingen, Griesinger numbered among the earliest German supporters of Conolly's program. Following his first-hand encounter with non-restraint on a visit to England, France, and the Belgian colony of Gheel in 1861, Griesinger quickly articulated that support in the revised edition of his *Pathologie und Therapie*.[47] In the late 1860s he then redefined non-restraint in broader terms, giving it both an emancipatory as well as a stronger therapeutic connotation in the rhetorically more effective lexical construction of "free treatment" (*freie Behandlung*).[48] As early as 1864 Griesinger had sought to introduce "free treatment" in Zurich, and after arriving at the Charité in Berlin in 1865 its implementation became one of his most urgent priorities.

There is no doubt that Griesinger's advocacy of non-restraint was nourished by powerful humanitarian impulses. He steadfastly insisted that it was the responsibility of those charged with the care of mental patients to ensure their lives be as dignified and humane as possible. In an appeal to this sentiment, he argued eloquently that patients were "not living machines" and that their feelings and interests needed to be protected and cultivated like "precious sparks beneath the ashes."[49] He insisted that their day-to-day lives not be reduced to monotonous routine and idleness and that they not have to forego modest amenities and simple pleasures. An intact, humane "second world"[50] needed to be constructed for patients who could not longer exist in the first one. Such a world was incompatible with the application of mechanical restraint.

Of course opponents were indignant at the charge that restraint, as applied in their asylums, might in any sense be considered inhumane. For them the entire system of asylums in Germany had been built upon high moral and humanitarian principles.[51] And they were more indignant still that now, from the halls of the university and in the name of medical science, their therapeutic practices should be subjected to such harsh criticism. For, in their view, it was not "science, but humanitarianism that [had] provided the driving principle behind the . . . asylums in civilized Europe and soon throughout the entire world." Asylums had not been born the child of "psychiatric knowledge," but instead of an "unshakable belief in *future* knowledge, which could germinate only in the soil of the asylum."[52] That academicians such as Griesinger could now, in the name of progress and humanity, denounce the very institutions that had made their science possible was considered more than an outrage: it was deemed malevolent and hypocritical as well.[53]

Important as these moral, humanitarian, and patient-centered dimensions of the non-restraint debate are, focusing exclusively on them easily obscures other deep-seated professional issues which were likewise being contested. The debate, though certainly not void of moral principles, *also* reflected conflicting professional claims and therefore needs to be assessed not simply in terms of the benefits accruing to patients, but also in terms of those accruing to psychiatric professionals. Griesinger's advocacy of non-restraint was part of a strategy that entailed both a radical realignment of professional jurisdictions as well as a reorganization of the way in which professional knowledge would be generated.

To appreciate the professional advantages which non-restraint could have, it is crucial to recognize the great rhetorical force that it exerted in tandem with the growing influence of the natural sciences in psychiatry. Non-restraint provided Griesinger's reform program with a powerful *emancipatory theme* that he skillfully exploited in his confrontations with alienists. As Heinrich Laehr noted, Griesinger appealed to the broader climate and political rhetoric of his day in order to advance his convictions and improve the public image of the profession. For example, Griesinger's vocabulary was spiked with "words of the New Era" such as "humanity, freedom, and justice" that he juxtaposed with "prison, coercion, and costliness."[54] Furthermore, Griesinger lent his voice in support of the patients' families who protested alienist use of mechanical restraint.[55] In the heated debates of the 1860s, in which liberal aspirations of 1848 were revived and fused with hopes of far-reaching medical reforms, the emancipatory rhetoric of non-restraint did not fail its mark.

The emancipatory thrust implicit in the doctrine of non-restraint moved well beyond Griesinger's direct concerns for patients to encompass the profession as a whole. He believed psychiatry itself to be laboring under its own "guild-like isolation" in the asylums.[56] For him, non-restraint was a highly effective rhetorical instrument which undercut established alienist practice. In other words, Griesinger employed it not just to liberate the patients from mechanical bondage, but also to extricate his own profession (and academic psychiatrists in particular) from the burdens of the alienists' practice and their sinking public image. That he did so at a time when alienists themselves were working hard to distance themselves from their historical and institutional proximity to penitentiaries, and at a time when many were eager to recast their image from quasi-prison wardens to academics and scientists, only added to the virulence of the debates. His rhetoric of "free treatment" effectively branded alienist practice as a carceral undertaking and their asylums as penal institutions. While alienists were accustomed to such attacks from outside their ranks, to be confronted with them from within the professional fold was deeply disconcerting.[57]

Of course, rhetoric alone was not enough to change the profession. Old carceral habits had to be discarded and an entirely new kind of psychiatrist had to be cultivated. For this reason non-restraint also served important pedagogical aims. According to his successor in Berlin, Carl Westphal, Griesinger "spared no opportunity" in his lectures to explain and demonstrate how the "old method of treatment" had employed mechanical restraints.[58] In his account of the implementation of non-restraint on the psychiatric wards of the Charité, Westphal also reported that in the 1860s all of the instruments of mechanical restraint had been banished from the clinic—with one exception: for purposes of instruction and demonstration, one strait-jacket was carefully preserved as a relic of bygone therapeutic benightedness.[59] The demonstration of such artifacts and the ubiquitous stories of maltreatment they evoked were important components in the construction and ritual reaffirmation the profession's new legitimacy. As a symbol of mechanical restraint, the strait-jacket was a powerful pedagogical tool that at once damned the fathers and exonerated the sons on the threshold of a new psychiatric age. Non-restraint, therefore, served the interests of psychiatrists wishing to emplot the history of their profession as a narrative of heroic struggle against the dark past of mechanical restraint. Non-restraint became an "article of faith," a touchstone of professional enlightenment and progressiveness to a new generation of students.[60]

If non-restraint helped produce a new kind of psychiatrist, it also had potentially far-reaching consequences for the daily routines of hospital personnel and for life on the wards. Implementing non-restraint required that the "spirit of the nursing personnel be trained and fostered in the proper aversion to restraint."[61] A successfully implemented system of non-restraint called for "numerous, intelligent, active, and good-natured attendants."[62] However, weaning staff from the traditional ward practice of restraint was difficult and regularly met with opposition. Griesinger himself, for example, encountered stiff resistance to his introduction of non-restraint in Berlin, making necessary the "wholesale replacement" of the personnel.[63] Similarly, after Otto Binswanger was appointed director in Jena and moved to introduce non-restraint, the majority of the personal refused to cooperate and his lone assistant quit his position.[64] In conjunction with his introduction of non-restraint in Munich, Bernhard von Gudden subjected ward personnel to a particularly relentless disciplinary regime, including control clocks and spot checks that one observer characterized as "nothing short of gruesome."[65] Thus, the practical implementation of non-restraint usually meant the replacement of a significant portion of the personnel, its reeducation in the maxims of non-restraint, and generally the reorganization of the ward's entire disciplinary matrix.

Griesinger was also convinced that restraint led to neglect.[66] For him and his supporters, restraint and neglect were two sides of the same coin, and alienists had been all too willing to employ mechanical restraint on overcrowded and understaffed wards. In place of this disciplinary pattern of restraint and neglect, Griesinger proposed an alternative mechanism that joined non-restraint with "uninterrupted medical attention."[67] Ensuring order and effective therapeutic care required that staff and physicians engage in diligent and incessant observation of the patients. The challenge of non-restraint was, in Griesinger's mind, to replace "mechanical surveillance with live observation" and thereby to transform the entire manner of institutional treatment and care.[68] The focal point of this concentrated observation was the observation ward or *Wachabteilung*. Drawing on Parchappe's idea of continual observation (*"surveillance continue"*), Griesinger envisioned the *Wachabteilung* as a "uniquely organized" and the most important of all wards in his urban asylum.[69] It was there that not just new admissions but also the most difficult and protracted cases in the institution were placed under the closest possible scrutiny. The observation wards were to be staffed by the most experienced personnel and visited by the physicians at every available opportunity. While in the 1860s, at least according to Max Brosius, such wards existed only in the Charité, by the 1870s *Wachabteilungen* came into vogue among advocates of non-restraint.[70]

Such wards and the shift in disciplinary patterns that they represented had obvious advantages for the young profession. In therapeutic terms, close observation could prevent patients from harming themselves and counteract the unpalatable image of the strait-jacket. The practice of "silent observation" helped recast the institution's image into that of a disciplined and well-run general hospital.[71] Most important in the present context were the advantages which non-restraint provided in the dispute over jurisdictional claims to clinical science. Advocates of non-restraint, such as the future director of the clinic in Göttingen, Ludwig Meyer, were adamant that mechanical means of coercion hindered the empirical observation of the "natural course of psychiatric symptoms."[72] Without the ability to observe the so-called natural state and course of an illness, psychiatrists could neither be sure that their observations were valid, nor that the patients which they demonstrated to students were true exemplars of reified psychiatric states. For Griesinger, Meyer, and other like-minded psychiatrists, non-restraint was more than simply a program of therapeutic reform: it was a precondition of scientific clinical observation itself and of the pedagogical demonstration of psychiatric symptoms.[73]

Thus, the dispute over non-restraint was linked directly to debates on clinical observation and demonstration, and more generally on the empirical methodology of mid-century alienism. Alienists had long cherished the opportunities which their asylums provided for "pure experience" and for "careful, continuous, frequent, extensive, and uninterrupted observation."[74] But Griesinger's urban asylum and his doctrine of non-restraint challenged this assumption and indeed implicitly called into question the very reliability of clinical science as practiced in the asylums. If restraint had distorted the symptoms of patients, then the clinical observations of alienists, already under attack by Kahlbaum for their often arcane and blinkered subjectivity, were further exposed to the debilitating charge that they had captured not "objective natural facts," but simply pseudo-facts arising from the institutional practice of restraint. Here again, insofar as the empirical rigor of alienists was called into question, alienist claims to jurisdiction over psychiatric research were challenged in a fundamental way. Just as the scientific cast of Griesinger's theories had isolated alienists and undercut their claims to jurisdiction over laboratory research within the discipline, so his advocacy of non-restraint undermined alienist claims to clinical expertise by questioning the reliability of their empirical methodology.

The Politics of Clinical Instruction

THE CHARITÉ ADMINISTRATION AND GRIESINGER'S CALL TO BERLIN

Griesinger's arrival in Berlin in 1865 had been proceeded by a number of events that set the stage for debates on the nature of clinical instruction in psychiatry. On 22 September 1860 the Prussian ministry of education issued an edict to provincial presidents on the acute shortage of qualified alienists.[75] The rescript encouraged them to increase the number of assistants serving in provincial hospitals for the insane. The fact that the rescript was directed at the provincial governments and not at medical faculties confirms that as late as 1860 the Prussian state considered the asylums to be the only means available for the recruitment and specialized practical training of young psychiatrists. Since medical faculties across Germany had thrown up stiff resistance to any expansion of the psychiatric curriculum, the state focused its efforts on postgraduate training in the asylums.[76]

This appeal to the provinces also came against the backdrop of a languishing and intractable situation at the Charité hospital in Berlin. Indeed, the above rescript was distributed on the very same occasion that the ministry inquired about the position left vacant by the recent death of Carl Wilhelm Ideler. Ideler's passage had sparked a resurgence of the long standing trench warfare between the administration and academic clinicians within the Charité. The Charité had been designed and built by the Prussian government as a hospital for the instruction of military surgeons, and not as a university institution. However, over the course of the 19th century clinicians from the university of Berlin had acquired increasing access to its wards.[77] Ideler himself had been both a member of the medical faculty and head of the hospital psychiatric ward. A fragile balance between civilian and military interests permeated the entire institution and was a source of recurrent friction and conflict. The powerful influence of the ministry of war, the presence of university clinicians, and the administration's own statutory responsibilities made the task of administering the Charité a most unwieldy assignment, taxing to the limit the diplomatic skills of its chief administrator Carl Heinrich Esse.

It was this very delicate institutional matrix that was undoubtedly in Esse's mind when, just five weeks after Ideler's death, he successfully petitioned the ministry of education to abstain from replacing Ideler and to appoint Esse's co-administrator, Ernst Horn, as interim head of the psychiatric ward.[78] Although Esse advanced a variety of arguments in support of his petition, his chief aim was to curtail the power of the medical faculty within the Charité and preempt any efforts to replace Ideler by an academic clinician.[79] In Esse's view the most appropriate place for psychiatric training was not the Charité, but Prussia's provincial asylums.[80] And judging by the favorable response to the petition, the Prussian ministry of education generally agreed. Although the ministry did query Esse and Horn on better ways of utilizing the Charité's "considerable [patient] material"[81] for educational purposes, over the next three-and-a-half years it stonewalled all efforts of the medical faculty to fill the position left vacant upon Ideler's death.[82] Due in part to Esse's tactical success in outmaneuvering the medical faculty, relations between the two parties dipped to a relative nadir over the next few years. It was not until early 1864 that the ministry solicited suggestions for the first full academic chair in psychiatry at a Prussian university.[83]

Finding an experienced alienist who was willing to accept the position at the Charité proved to be highly contentious. In fact, drawing up a list of potential successors to Ideler exposed deep divisions within the medical faculty along disciplinary and generational lines. The majority of the faculty approved a list of experienced alienists including (in order of preference) August Solbrig, Heinrich Neumann, and Heinrich Laehr.[84] However, two of the faculty, Moritz Heinrich Romberg, a neurological specialist and director of the medical polyclinic, and Bernhard Langenbeck, director of the university's surgical clinic, wanted Westphal chosen in the event that the other candidates declined. More forcefully still, in his vote Rudolf Virchow expressed wholehearted support for Westphal, arguing that the choice of an "old alienist" would hamper the future development of psychiatric science. In view of Westphal's research work, his teaching experience, and his practical familiarity with the difficult circumstances of the Charité, Virchow saw no grounds for passing him over in favor of an "outside competitor" unproven as both a research scientist and a teacher.[85] Yet in spite of Virchow's dissenting voice and the ministry's own initial reservations, August Solbrig received the call to Berlin.[86]

But Solbrig placed stiff conditions upon his acceptance. In a memorandum on clinical instruction that he presented to the Prussian Minister of Education, Solbrig laid out three prerequisites on which he believed the success of clinical psychiatry depended.[87] First, sufficient "clinical material" had to be at the disposal of the instructor. Only an institution with two hundred and fifty to three hundred beds could supply an adequate pool of patients and thus enable most forms of disease, their different stages, as well as the manifold social, educational, and professional backgrounds of the patients to be demonstrated. Second, the instructor had to "fully permeate and control" the clinical material by way of "social cohabitation" with the patients. Without actually residing in the institution itself, no such mastery was possible. And finally, the success of clinical teaching in psychiatry depended on a third condition: the instructor's work had to be buttressed by a well organized asylum. Clinical psychiatry would flourish only if it could draw on the entire register of administrative and therapeutic means available to an asylum. In closing his memorandum, Solbrig found the Charité severely wanting in all three of these areas and therefore foresaw no chance that it might serve to advance the study of psychiatry. Thus, in spite of subsequent negotiations and probably swayed by an inspection visit in the Charité itself, Solbrig declined the call to Berlin in May of 1864.[88]

Solbrig's memorandum had clearly been an alienist agenda for clinical education. But his rejection of the prestigious position in Berlin unexpectedly reshuffled the clinico-political cards. Westphal's prospects, although certainly improved, continued to be clouded by the medical faculty's antipathy toward the interim director of the psychiatric ward, Westphal's uncle Ernst Horn.[89] Rudolf Virchow undoubtedly took satisfaction in seeing his reservations confirmed, while Esse restated his support for Westphal.[90] For its part, the ministry of education temporarily put the search on ice and abandoned the faculty's list of candidates altogether.[91]

Then, in the fall of 1864 the ministry seized the initiative and entered into negotiations with Wilhelm Griesinger.[92] The negotiations again opened up rifts within the medical faculty.[93] This time the disagreements focused not on the prospective candidate himself—Griesinger appears to have enjoyed widespread support—, but rather on the looming prospect of a ministerial *fait-accompli*. Blaming the ministry's initiative on his own colleagues' passivity, Rudolf Virchow insisted that the medical faculty now take action in defense of its own autonomy. Seconded by Emil Du-Bois Reymond, Virchow urged his colleagues to preempt the ministerial decision by adopting Griesinger as its own candidate. However, most of the members of the medical faculty were more worried that Griesinger's appointment would jeopardize the chair in *Staatsarzneikunde* that Johann Ludwig Caspar's recent death had left vacant. Rather than provoke the wrath of the ministry by intervening in its ongoing negotiations, the majority of faculty members thought it wiser to refrain from action. As Virchow sarcastically put it, the faculty resolved "to do nothing" and thereby "abdicate" its own rights and responsibilities. As a result, Griesinger's appointment to the first full chair of psychiatry in Prussia came not as the product of the recommendations of the Berlin medical faculty, but rather as a decree from the ministry of education.[94]

Griesinger's appointment resulted in an ambiguous mixture of self-congratulation and concern within the wider psychiatric community. The editors of the *Allgemeine Zeitschrift* saw the Berlin chair as swift fulfillment of the goal set at Eisenach just four years earlier. As Prussia's first university, the decision to establish a chair in Berlin held out the prospect of further academic posts throughout the country and indeed in other German states as well. However, that August Solbrig had found conditions in the Charité wholly unsuited for clinical training was certainly not forgotten. And Heinrich Laehr lost no time in reiterating that professors needed experience as asylum directors.[95] With Griesinger's arrival in Berlin, alienists were therefore confronted with a fundamental dilemma in pressing their claims to jurisdiction over clinical education. On the one hand, they were eager to reinforce their medical credentials through close cooperation with universities. On the other hand, they were loath to jeopardize their monopoly on access to patients, their practical therapeutic experience, and the traditional order and routine of asylum life. They found themselves at once reiterating psychiatry's status as a legitimate branch of medicine, while at the same time insisting that psychiatric science required asylum-based knowledge and wholly different diagnostic skills from those learned at the university.[96]

In spite of these reservations, alienists moved to close ranks and demonstrate in practical terms psychiatry's legitimacy as an academic specialty. Psychiatrists had now to prove that psychiatric clinics were just as important as other clinics and that their discipline had "its own techniques of diagnosis and treatment and that it could be taught in a manner compatible with the contemporary standards in the other medical disciplines."[97] It had to demonstrate its scientific mettle and produce results; it faced the pressing tasks of establishing a commonly agreed upon nosology, a pathology of mental disease, and rational therapeutic directives.[98] These were the immediate goals which alienists set for their profession upon Griesinger's arrival in Berlin.

THE CONDITIONS OF DIDACTIC EFFICACY

If alienists had hoped to harness Griesinger to their cause, those hopes were soon sorely disappointed. Griesinger did not support the pedagogical model advanced by Solbrig and sanctioned by the *Verein*. Calling on his experience as a clinician, Griesinger disputed alienist claims to jurisdiction over clinical instruction and insisted forcefully on his own "right to speak to these issues."[99] His urban asylum represented nothing less than a blueprint for wresting away jurisdiction of this work from alienists; it was the strategic tool by which the "rich observation material" languishing in rural asylums could be captured for clinical instruction and placed at the disposal of university professors.[100]

As no one knew better than Griesinger himself, in order to secure this jurisdiction, a number of fundamental preconditions had to be fulfilled. In particular, academicians first needed reliable access to not only patients, but, second, to the right kind of patients, and, third, to a broad spectrum of the right kind of patients. Griesinger's reform program was superbly tailored to these preconditions and warrants closer inspection in this regard. In achieving the first of these three aims—access to patients—Griesinger developed a strategy with two interwoven goals: to improve the profession's public image and lower barriers to admission at urban asylums. The profession's public image clearly stood to benefit from the association of Griesinger's somatic theories with the aura of mid-nineteenth-century medicine and the natural sciences. Furthermore, his advocacy of non-restraint helped to diffuse the profession's carceral image and held great public relations potential. In short, harnessing psychiatry to the natural sciences, as well as to a program of non-restraint, held out the prospect of psychiatry jettisoning the ballast of the alienists' sinking public image.

But simply dismantling public apprehension toward psychiatric institutions was not enough to secure access to more patients. The institutions themselves had to have the statutory capacity and flexibility to accept these patients. Griesinger therefore insisted in his reform program that the *statutes* of urban asylums in no way hamper admission. Because admission to public asylums had long been an arduous undertaking—involving time consuming bureaucratic procedures and often delayed by overcrowding[101]—Griesinger wanted to lower barriers to admission in order to enable patients to be institutionalized as early and as rapidly as possible. Consequently, he proposed using free admissions or reduced fees to attract more patients.[102] If the institutionalization of patients could be expedited, not only were the chances of cure much improved, but the dangers of degeneration into chronic states, of life-long institutionalization, and hence of institutional overcrowding could be avoided.

In voicing these opinions on institutional statutes, Griesinger entered a highly contentious and on-going debate among alienists on admission policy. Central to that debate—touched on briefly in chapter 2—were the issues of public trust and overcrowding. The debate had arisen in the wake of the public scandal enveloping Peter Jessen's Hornheim asylum in 1861/2 and conflicting viewpoints on the state's role in supervising private asylums. These debates were reinvigorated by an order of the provincial Ministry of the Interior in the Rheinland in 1864 which reminded public officials of the exact administrative procedures governing psychiatric admissions.[103] Many alienists objected to the order, reading into its provisions an implicit accusation that patients could be or had been incarcerated in asylums against their will. They considered the procedures outlined in the order to be unnecessary and argued that they prevented rapid admission, thereby undermining the therapeutic effectiveness and the good name of their institutions.[104] Though agreeing that the order undermined the reputation of asylums, differences of opinion surfaced on the issue of institutional statutes. These debates—which were not laid to rest until 1868—concerned the question of whether admission should be regulated by formal procedures and subject to police registration or whether it should be left entirely at the discretion of the asylum director.[105]

At stake in these debates was the very nature of the asylums themselves. In particular, the question was whether they were carceral institutions in which individuals were detained against their will (in which case legal statutes were necessary to protect against unjustified detention) or whether they were essentially identical to any other hospital and hence at liberty to admit patients as they saw fit (in which case no legal statutes were necessary). Roller defended the former position, arguing that asylums, though certainly medical institutions, necessarily also detained their patients against their will and that exacting statutes and admission procedures served to protect alienists from charges of misconduct and helped to distribute the burden of responsibility across the shoulders of other state authorities. The latter position was defended by Peter Jessen, who wanted nothing to do with formal admission procedures and police registration. Voicing the concerns and interests of other private asylum owners, Jessen feared losing the discretion which was so important to his wealthy clientele and warned that tighter state regulation would jeopardize public trust and thereby undermine the confidentiality of the doctor-patient relationship.[106] He therefore advocated that patients arriving at asylums of their own volition be admitted "without any [bureaucratic] formalities."[107] For Jessen, a psychiatric asylum was nothing other than a special kind of hospital.

Griesinger's program of reform was written against the backdrop of these debates, but with very different objectives in mind. As an advocate of non-restraint and convinced that madness was a disease like any other malady, he clearly had little sympathy for Roller's contention that asylums should be coercive institutions that differed fundamentally from other hospitals.[108] But nor was he prepared to support Jessen's position of wholly unrestricted admission. Instead, Griesinger came down between these two stances; or perhaps, more accurately stated, he drew the debate, which had pitted the owner-directors of private asylums against the civil-servant directors of large public asylums, entirely into the realm of public institutions. Griesinger called explicitly for different standards of admission for different public institutions: in urban asylums admission needed to be made as easy as possible, while in rural asylums it had to be made more difficult.[109]

This strategy of statutory differentiation aimed to solve the problem of overcrowding, while at the same time facilitating clinical access to patients. Easing the statutory conditions of admission in urban asylums would reduce overcrowding by institutionalizing patients earlier and hence preventing degeneration into chronic states, whereas stiffening admissions policy in the rural asylums would hold at bay those patients who did not actually belong in a psychiatric institution (i.e. invalids and patients capable of being cared for in their homes). Moreover, Griesinger's admissions strategy also undercut alienist control of psychiatric patients in public institutions. Raising the barriers to admission in rural asylums, while keeping those same barriers low for urban asylums, would effectively ensure the academic clinicians' access to the patients they so dearly sought for their clinical lectures. Together, the improved public image, as well as more liberal and expedient admissions criteria in urban asylums, had the potential to lower both the socio-familial and statutory threshold of resistance to admission. In this way, Griesinger, and after him many academic clinicians, sought to usurp the alienist monopoly of control over psychiatric patients. That such a strategy might also alleviate the problem of overcrowding only strengthened its argumentative force.

The second precondition of clinical education concerned the *right kind of patients*. Unlike Damerow, who in 1833 had contended that chronic patients in custodial institutions were ideally suited for clinical instruction,[110] Griesinger argued just the opposite: chronic patients were of little use in clinical teaching. Students needed to be shown acute cases in which the true course of a disease, its progress and remission, the full panoply of symptoms, and the efficacy of therapeutic measures could be demonstrated; that is, students needed to see patients before the confusing and ambiguous complications of chronic states had set in.[111] Griesinger had in mind those patients needing only brief institutionalization at critical, exacerbated periods of their illnesses. His program therefore proposed to open the urban asylum (and with it psychiatry in general) to a new category of transitory, short-term patient.

Such patients had traditionally fallen outside the purview of alienists.[112] Long waiting lists, the reservations of financially strapped communities, and the generally poor image of asylums all helped to ensure that patients in the early stages of their affliction were seldom seen in asylums. At times, the symptoms that had originally motivated applications for admission had subsided when space finally opened up in an asylum. Even if such patients had been maneuvered through the bureaucracy of admission, in the face of overcrowded conditions they tended to be among the first to be dismissed once the acute phase of their illness had passed. Such cases were far more likely to be found in treatment either in general hospitals or in private homes. Hence, while asylums may have controlled most institutionalized patients, for the immediate purposes of clinical research and education they had, in Griesinger's view, the wrong kind of patients, namely chronic ones. Only an asylum able to demonstrate acute cases of madness could fulfill the requirements for effective clinical training.

Moreover, Griesinger sought to attract not just acute cases, but also all nascent or so-called "fresh cases." This distinction is important in understanding the vehemence of the debate between Griesinger and his opponents. He took pains to emphasize that acute cases were not synonymous with "fresh" curable patients and that chronic patients also exhibited exacerbated symptoms.[113] Yet elsewhere in his reform writings he expressed himself in ambiguous and contradictory terms. In particular, with reference to psychiatric clinics, he explicitly lumped "fresh cases and acute states" together, viewing both as necessary for the purposes of clinical education.[114] Crucially, Griesinger was concerned that, after taking up private practice, students become medical sentinels to the onset of their patients' madness. If these would-be general practitioners did not have experience in recognizing the early stages of mental illness, then the imperative of early and rapid institutionalization could never be realized. Therefore, students had to be trained to recognize the subtle, yet still unadulterated signs of nascent madness; their diagnostic skills had to be primed toward identifying these early states on the borderline between health and disease. Development of those skills, which for Griesinger and later academic psychiatrists became one of the primary tasks of the university clinic,[115] demanded clinical instruction in the early stages of mental illness. Thus, behind Griesinger's reforms and their aim of replacing early nineteenth-century criteria of curability (curable vs. incurable) with that of institutional duration (long-term vs. short-term), lay an attempt to capture a specific group of patients for clinical psychiatry.

Implicit in the criteria of transitory patients was the third precondition which Griesinger believed crucial to the success of clinical education: the idea of a *higher patient frequency*. The question of the frequency or volume of patients passing through the urban asylum was intimately linked with the number of beds in the institution. Because of financial and geographic constraints, urban asylums would have to be relatively small in size, ranging from between sixty and one hundred and twenty beds.[116] Contrary to larger state asylums in the countryside with several hundred beds, urban clinics were never envisioned as contributing more than a small fraction of the total number of beds required to satisfy the needs of psychiatric care. This difference in size placed urban asylums at a potential disadvantage in their claims to the task of professional training. Whereas the asylums could draw on a very large reservoir of patients for the purposes of clinical demonstration, smaller urban asylums ran the risk of not being able to present to students the full spectrum of psychiatric disorders.[117] For Griesinger it was not enough that students be exposed to a small number of acute cases; they needed to receive clinical instruction across the entire spectrum of psychopathology. Therefore, in order to ensure this spectrum of patients was available over the course of a semester, he insisted that there be a rapid turnover of patients in the clinical asylum. In this manner, what the urban asylum could not guarantee in terms of sheer numbers of patients, Griesinger hoped to compensate for by expanding the volume of patients passing through his institution. Raising the frequency of admission could effectively enlarge his reservoir of demonstrable patients.

Needless to say, alienists were dismayed at Griesinger's intentions, which ran counter to their institutional ideals of rural seclusion and patriarchal beneficence. They criticized the idea of small urban asylums for not providing students the opportunity to observe the "well ordered organism"[118] of the asylum. Some alienists did not believe it possible to teach students the subtle complexities of insanity in a few short hours of clinical instruction over one or two semesters. Others were quick to point out that only larger institutions could provide the number of patients needed to ensure adequate clinical training. And while Griesinger's reform program was designed to close the gap in the clinical observation of early phases of mental disease, the shift in the admissions criteria from curability to duration hampered the demonstration of illnesses over time. Because of the shortened amount of time patients spent in the institution, psychiatrists could often demonstrate only individual phases and not the entire course of an illness. The resulting "discontinuity of observation" would have a detrimental impact on both the educational and research objectives of the clinic.[119]

The Politics of Prophylaxis

POOR RELIEF AND PSYCHIATRIC ADMINISTRATION IN BERLIN

While statutory restraints and psychiatry's tattered image were certainly significant hurdles standing in the way of the acquisition of adequate clinical "material," professional debates were also interwoven with other very powerful socio-economic and hygienic issues of urbanization. It was in the context of metropolitan health and welfare systems that Griesinger formulated his reform program; and it was ultimately in just such wider civic surroundings that psychiatric clinics in general would come to be situated. In other words, the construction of urban asylums with their implicit claim to the treatment of transitory cases involved not only their justification vis-à-vis alienist professionals in the countryside, but also vis-à-vis the city's own health and welfare administration.

Traditionally, city hospitals had been responsible for treating the indigent poor, including mental patients.[120] Prior to the 1880s, civic hospitals were financed in part by patient fees, state subsidies, and hospital insurance subscriptions for journeymen, domestic servants and workers. Most of their income, however, came from public welfare receipts.[121] As a result, these hospitals were burdened with the stigma of indigence. While wealthier families could more easily afford to place their relatives in private institutions or have them cared for at home, early nineteenth-century hospitals housed mostly poverty stricken patients. From their inception (and like mental asylums), city hospitals were first and foremost institutions of public assistance and only secondarily medical institutions. While this changed gradually over the course of the century, even after 1900 city hospitals retained an air of their origins as welfare institutions.

As the nineteenth century progressed, responsibility for providing medical care to indigent citizens passed increasingly to local communities.[122] In the early 1840s, a series of laws were promulgated in Prussia that sought to demarcate the extent of communal and provincial responsibilities for public welfare.[123] The laws would later become the foundation for the *Reichs-Gesetz über den Unterstützungswohnsitze*,[124] which, after German unification in 1871, effectively extended the Prussian system of welfare administration across the entire Empire. In essence, the laws were an attempt to address and defuse the growing problem of pauperism in the 1830s and 1840s. At the same time, they were well calibrated in support of broader liberal economic reforms. They sought to deregulate residency requirements and thereby to 'liberate' the productive potential of the rural labor force and to subject it to the market forces of a nascent industrial economy. In particular, the laws placed the responsibility for public assistance (*Fürsorgepflicht*) in the hands of the local community and stipulated the conditions (*Wohnsitzrecht, Ortsansässigkeit*) upon which that assistance depended. According to the laws, home towns were obliged to provide public support to their needy residents. Furthermore, the laws provided for the citizens to retain their rights of residency even long after they had migrated to another part of the country. In fact, local communities were responsible for providing welfare support for up to three years after residents had physically left their home town. In this system of community based assistance the provinces acted as safety nets: for those cases in which either an individual's residency status was unclear or the local community lacked the wherewithal to pay the cost, the responsibility for providing public support fell to the respective province in which the individual lived. Hence, responsibility for public assistance (and with it the costs of care in mental asylums) was shared between local communities and the Prussian provinces.

This system of public welfare came under tremendous financial pressures as the German economy faltered in the mid-1840s, as pauperism spread, and as migration to the cities began to rise rapidly. Many communities found themselves either unable or unwilling to support the growing financial burden of their impoverished residents. Faced with the prospect of such expenses, communities went to great (and devious) lengths to prevent the poor from establishing local residency and to saddle others with the financial burdens of public assistance.[125] Public assistance in Germany became an administrative battleground on which communities and provinces were pitted against one another in a protracted struggle to avoid welfare costs through the exportation of their poverty and, with it, of their financial liability.

The city of Berlin was no exception in being severely tested by mid-century domestic migration, poverty, and the growing costs of poor relief.[126] In an effort to address these problems, the city's welfare administration (*Armendirektion*) moved to reign in the exploding costs of public assistance and enhance the efficiency of the welfare bureaucracy.[127] While the full extent of these cost-cutting measures needn't be considered here, with specific regard to the mentally ill there was one potentially very lucrative source of savings for the city: the Charité hospital. What made the Charité such an attractive target of civic administrators was the fact that it was precisely *not* an integral part of the wider system of public assistance and hence not specifically obliged to care for Berlin's indigent sick. The Charité was neither a civic nor a provincial welfare hospital, but rather an institution run by the Prussian government with the explicit aim of training military physicians. Most significant for the calculations of the city government of Berlin, the Charité was funded mainly by the Prussian crown. As a consequence, having more patients admitted to the Charité, or having them admitted for longer periods of time, held out the prospect of reducing the city's public assistance budget at royal expense. To these ends the city sought to exploit to the fullest its relationship with the Charité.

That relationship was shaped by a complex web of institutional statutes, administrative orders, judicial rulings and royal decrees.[128] Undoubtedly the most important of these regulations was a Prussian cabinet order dating from

1835, according to which the Charité was obliged to admit and care for at its expense all mental patients who were both residents of Berlin and poor.[129] In addition to this explicit provision for mental patients, the order obliged the Charité to provide Berlin with an account of 100,000 days of free care for other patients who, for whatever reasons, had become charges of the welfare administration or subjects of police detention. Furthermore, on several occasions, earlier ordinances had reiterated that the Charité was a hospital for curable patients (*Heilanstalt*) and that incurable patients were "not tolerated" on its wards.[130] Put succinctly, there existed three chief criteria determining whether the costs of treatment would be covered by the Charité: (1) residency, (2) indigence, and (3) curability. The Charité was not legally obliged to admit and treat individuals who did not satisfy these criteria. Although ineligible individuals *could* still be admitted, they had either to be tallied to Berlin's account of 100,000 days of free care or the city had to pay the full hospital rate for their treatment. Ensuring that as many patients as possible satisfied the above three criteria comprised part of the fiscal belt-tightening undertaken by the *Armendirektion* in the 1850s and 1860s.

Efforts to exploit these formal criteria severely strained the relationship between the city of Berlin and the Charité. Because the regulations governing the relationship predated the enactment of the public assistance laws of the early 1840s, differences of opinion arose as to precisely what constituted the Charité's responsibilities. One of the most contentious issues of dispute in the early 1860s concerned the residency status of recent migrants to Berlin.[131] In particular, what definition of residency applied with respect to the specific obligations of the Charité to care for the indigent sick? Was the Charité required to pay the hospital expenses of only those psychiatric patients who were legal residents of the city (*juristischer Wohnsitz*), as the Charité maintained? Or was it required to admit and pay the costs of all patients who meet the residency criteria set down in the laws on public assistance (*Unterstützungswohnsitz*), as the city of Berlin contended? Furthermore, who was responsible for the costs of treatment prior to a determination on the issue of curability? If, after several weeks of observation, Charité doctors concluded that a patient was incurably insane, was the city obliged to pay the higher Charité rates retroactively from the date of admission? Or had the city simply to cover the costs accruing after incurability had been diagnosed? Answers to all of these questions were pivotal in allocating the costs of care for the indigent sick.[132]

Debates on these issues occupied administrators throughout the 1850s and finally came to a head in the early 1860s. In order to throttle the rising number of admissions coming from the *Armendirektion* and the police, the Charité director Carl Heinrich Esse began in April of 1862 to insist unilaterally that, prior to admission and contrary to established practice, the city provide full and detailed documentation of patients' residency status, their impoverishment, as well as their curability.[133] By insisting upon this documentation, Esse was not only trying to reduce costs and cut admissions to the psychiatric ward, but also refusing to perform the time-consuming administrative work required to establish the patient's admissibility to the Charité. Against the backdrop of rising migration to Berlin, establishing a perhaps uncooperative patient's indigence and residency status involved troublesome investigations and often inconclusive correspondence with distant communities. Definitive verification of the patient's status usually took between three to four and, in some cases, as many as six weeks.[134] Esse's actions were intended to relieve his administration of all such burdensome tasks.

Both the *Armendirektion* and the police complained vociferously about the tightening of admission procedures. The *Armendirektion* protested that because establishing the admissibility criteria was so time-consuming, Esse's stipulations had made it necessary to first admit patients to the city's custodial facility (*städtische Irrenverpflegungsanstalt*), an annex to the work-house.[135] The city believed that many patients would suffer extremely detrimental effects from being admitted to the *Verpflegungsanstalt*.[136] For one thing, it jeopardized the patients' curability, because it delayed their admission to the Charité and thereby prevented them from benefitting immediately from the therapeutic arsenal of a *Heilanstalt*. Also, the city's facility was ill-equipped to accommodate acute and dangerous cases. The city considered these issues so important that it even took the Prussian crown to court, albeit only to have a series of rulings in favor of Esse's policies handed down to them.[137] Likewise, the police also complained about the Charité's reluctance to accept dangerous patients. For the police, Esse's measures posed a real threat to public security. In fact, one of the direct consequences of Esse's restrictions was a formal agreement between the police and the *Armendirektion* that, at the initiative of the chief of police, laid down precise guidelines for the transfer of patients from police custody to city hospitals.[138]

Esse's administrative decision drew the Charité back from the "front line" of psychiatric care and forced the city of Berlin to take greater responsibility for its mentally ill.[139] Rather than situating the Charité's psychiatric ward at the forefront of medical care for the insane, Esse turned it de facto into a subsidiary of the *Verpflegungsanstalt*. By placing administrative obstacles in the path of admission to the Charité and insisting that administrative procedures be followed to the letter, Esse effectively procured the redirection of admissions through the *Verpflegungsanstalt*. This shift in admission policy had two far-reaching consequences. First, admissions to the psychiatric ward at the Charité began to fall off after 1862 and plummeted after a court ruling against the city in 1864.[140] It was not until after Esse's departure in the early 1870s that the psychiatric ward began to recover from this setback. Second, the city's skeletal network of custodial institutions came under severe pressures as the police began regularly to deposit patients there. Over seven years, patient numbers rose by one hundred and fifty percent, resulting in a severe crisis of overcrowding in civic facilities that lasted into the 1870s.[141] In sum, Esse's policies both undermined the clinical interests of the Charité's psychiatric ward and forced the hand of city administrators.

Faced with Esse's unilateral restrictions, in April of 1863 the Berlin city council resolved to construct an asylum for some 600 patients.[142] After canvassing the advice of numerous experts, including Damerow, Flemming, Laehr, Esse, Meyer, and the son of the deceased Ideler, a deputation was formed in April of 1865 (just prior to Griesinger's arrival in Berlin) in order to work out plans for an asylum. However, when the magistrate proposed to install the newly arrived Griesinger as the chief psychiatric advisor to the project, the city counsel rejected this proposal and insisted that the existing deputation remain in charge of the building project. In the spring of 1866, after a further conference of alienists recommended a closed asylum on a large piece of land, a protracted search for an adequate construction site began.[143] It was in the midst of this drawn out frustrating search and also against the backdrop of the above administrative and welfare policies that Griesinger formulated and published his reform program.

THE LOCAL IMPLICATIONS OF GRIESINGER'S REFORM PROGRAM

Griesinger's opponents sought to undermine the far reaching implications of his program by suggesting that it was a child of a unique constellation of circumstances found only in the Prussian capital. As such, not only was its practical applicability as a blueprint for other Prussian institutions called into questions, but Griesinger was also accused of subordinating the wider interests of psychiatric care to the specific interests of his own academic position in Berlin. His reforms were criticized for their unjustified "preference for city dwellers and an unfair disregard for rural residents."[144] Griesinger, of course, denied that his project was in anyway hostage to local conditions.[145] But he could certainly not have been unaware of the potentially enormous local ramifications of his program. Deny as he might any local medico-political motives, Griesinger knew only too well that his program implied a radical reorganization of Berlin's system of psychiatric care. Thus, the fuller impact and historical meanings of Griesinger's reform project only become evident when viewed as an attempt to redress many of the deficiencies of the institutional configuration as it existed in Berlin in the 1860s.

Griesinger's reform project took aim at the aforementioned three admissions criteria of the Charité: residency, curability, and indigence. First, the imperative that Griesinger placed upon early and rapid admission would have circumvented the bureaucratic obstacles erected by Esse. Rapid admission meant, in effect, decoupling the admission procedure from the administrative task of establishing residency status. Griesinger's program marshaled therapeutic, financial, and pedagogic arguments intended to establish a definitive priority of admission over administrative verification. Although this had been common practice in emergency cases, and especially for patients brought to the Charité by the Berlin police, the logic behind non-bureaucratic admission implied that that practice should be extended to all classes of patients.

Second, Griesinger altogether rejected the criteria of curability as inadequate and ill-defined. As Griesinger straightforwardly put it, "The criteria of curability, insofar as they apply to asylum admissions, are extremely detrimental." As a medical and scientific prognosis, curability stood on "feet of clay" and was quite simply an "official fiction" of psychiatric administrators.[146] In advocating that the criteria of curability should be abandoned in favor of duration, Griesinger was effectively upsetting the entire apple cart of psychiatric care in Berlin. His proposals were tantamount to a repeal of the cabinet order of 1835 and a wholesale reorganization of the relationship between the Charité's psychiatric facilities and metropolitan government.

Thirdly, Griesinger's urban asylum was a bid to extricate the psychiatric clinic from the wider system of public welfare or *Armenfürsorge*. I have shown above how alienist reputations were undercut by public perceptions that their asylums were carceral institutions. Those same public perceptions were also compromised by the image of asylums as welfare institutions—as poor houses. Griesinger hoped to escape not just the carceral stigma associated with asylums, but also the stigma of poverty derived from the Charité's close association with public welfare.[147] In this regard, Griesinger's reform project envisioned the very reversal in the existing flow of patients from the *Verpflegungsanstalt* to the Charité. The urban asylum was not to be some branch or auxiliary facility of a civic hospital, no mere appendage of the public welfare system. On the contrary, the urban asylum was envisioned as being situated *prior* to the public welfare system. It would serve as a forward institution that could potentially relieve the system by ensuring early diagnosis, treatment, and the efficient distribution of patients to subordinate facilities behind it. Griesinger's reform proposals laid a claim to perform this preliminary work at the outer gates of the public welfare system.

CLASS AND CLINICAL PSYCHIATRY

Griesinger's attempt to fashion the psychiatric clinic as a portal to the public welfare system makes an assessment of clinical psychiatry in relation to socio-economic class worth more careful and detailed consideration. Issues relating to socio-economic class touched on the emergence of psychiatric clinics in numerous and very complex ways. Certainly, one of Griesinger's most contentious class-related propositions was his call for smaller urban institutions and the challenge they posed to the traditional spatial distribution of the patients within the asylum. Whereas large asylums allowed for the segregation of patients into different groups, any such partitioning of the patient population

posed considerable obstacles for smaller urban asylums.[148] Insofar as this segregation of the patients was characteristic of asylum psychiatry and insofar as
it represented an instrument of both therapy and control, Griesinger's urban
asylums implied a restructuring of traditional modes of institutional organization, new therapeutic practices, and different mechanisms of control: in short,
a new disciplinary matrix of power.

This reapportionment of institutional space sparked alienist fears of a break-
down in class distinctions. In asylums, as institutions of public welfare, it had
traditionally been understood that "the poor must be received first, the rich last;
and as such the latter really [did] not belong there."[149] However, governments
and directors had long made provisions for middle and upper class patients.[150]
Asylums continued to care predominantly for the poor, but as their number increased they came to serve ever wider spectrums of the population, including patients for whom admission to an expensive private asylum threatened their families or themselves with financial ruin. The result was a multi-class system of care
in which the asylum's function as an institution for the poor slowly receded over
the years. Alienists continued to employ familial and patriarchal metaphors to
project an image of harmonious institutional unity. But as the century progressed and class divisions within German society sharpened, those divisions
came to be reproduced in the spatial hierarchy of the asylum as well.[151]

In the eyes of his alienist critics, Griesinger's urban asylum did not make sufficient provision for class segregation. Alienists worried that the surveillance
ward (*Wachabteilung*) in particular, to which all newly admitted patients would
be assigned, posed a danger to the health of the well-to-do. Although they con-
curred that the urban asylum should provide a refuge for patients of the educated classes, they found it objectionable that those patients might be confronted
with their social inferiors on the surveillance ward. There, "a scholar might well
encounter his shoemaker, a merchant a laborer, a public official his office personnel, a lady her wash maid—honorable, but ill-suited company since for some
it is a source of disquiet, discomfort, shyness, and embarrassment, and hence a
source of detrimental stimuli to the acutely afflicted brain."[152]

Griesinger was certainly conscious of these bourgeois sensibilities. For this
reason, in his earliest remarks on the construction of clinical asylums in 1865,
he had been careful to exclude alcoholics and "vagabonds."[153] He also tried to
attract bourgeois patients by advertising his clinic as an elite institution, infused with the high ideals of medical science.[154] And he was certainly aware
that allowing patients and relatives to enter and depart the urban asylum more
easily would be attractive to self-conscious members of the middle classes who
feared forfeiting their freedom of movement and rights of suffrage if they entered public institutions.[155]

Class also touched on issues of clinical research and instruction. Increasingly, as public mental hospitals came to care for the middle classes, concern
arose over the exploitation of wealthier patients for purposes of research and

education. For one thing, students might violate the privacy and compromise the social standing of patients by gossiping about what they had seen on the wards. Clinical demonstrations might also be perceived as degrading for upper-class patients, especially for daughters and wives exposed to the undisciplined gaze of young male students. Early advocates of clinical education had therefore sought to defuse the issue of class by excluding wealthy patients from the pool of potential objects of demonstration. In Heidelberg, for example, Georg Heermann insisted that only lower class patients be admitted to the clinic because there was no great need to respect their privacy or social rank.[156] In Erlangen, Solbrig had likewise been careful to limit demonstration to patients from the lower classes.[157]

But middle and upper class patients also harbored a number of advantages for clinical research and training. It was easier for physicians to communicate with members of the upper classes. Consequently a fuller anamnestic assessment of their condition was possible and the procedures of examination and diagnosis simplified. Westphal believed that better educated patients improved the prospects of diagnosis, because they allowed for "better insight" into mental processes.[158] And later August Cramer would argue that educated patients were ideally suited for clinical demonstration, because they could better express themselves and articulate their experiences.[159] They could even contribute to the general education of young physicians.[160] And, of course, both the institution and the director stood to benefit financially from wealthy patients.

The question of whether public institutions should accommodate wealthier middle-class patients occupied Berlin civic deputies debating the merits of a new mental asylum in the mid-1860s. The city government believed that its responsibilities extended only to public assistance and safety: Berlin was under no obligation to provide psychiatric facilities for the middle classes.[161] However, many deputies in the council chambers disagreed and wished to see wards for middle class patients in the new asylum. In their view, under no circumstances should "the middle classes have to rely on private institutions for [the care of] of their sick."[162] In the debates of the finance committee, Rudolf Virchow, in particular, had insisted that middle-class patients should also be admitted to the asylum and ultimately his position found majority support on the chamber floor. Later, the same issue of care for the non-poor arose in debates on the construction of Berlin's large asylums in Dalldorf in 1881 and Herzberge in 1892, by which time a consensus had been reached that those institutions not confine admission to poverty stricken patients.[163]

CLINICAL PSYCHIATRY BETWEEN 'ARMENFÜRSORGE' AND 'SOCIALE FÜRSORGE'

Debates such as these point to both the great potentials and the considerable limitations confronting psychiatrists in their dealings with city magistrates.

University psychiatric clinics emerged in the context of cities confronted with both growing responsibilities for the urban poor and vocal demands of an emergent, self-confident middle class pressing for more affordable psychiatric care. How cities met these challenges had a direct impact on the prospects for and ultimately the character of psychiatric clinics. Griesinger's urban asylum was a bid to help solve these urgent civic problems. Griesinger sought to exploit what he saw as a natural alliance between the research and pedagogical interests of academic psychiatrists, on the one hand, and the pressing financial, public health and security interests of civic magistrates, on the other. As one disciple of Griesinger put it, in constructing urban asylums "the needs of the city and the interests of education meet in complete agreement. . . . The larger the city, the more the need for urban asylums."[164]

But city administrators did not necessarily agree. One of the more common responses of cities to their public health problems was to build their own general hospitals. These hospitals potentially stood in direct competition with university psychiatric clinics. Consequently, Griesinger was reluctant to support their construction. He did not deny that patients could be admitted to the wards of larger general hospitals and that a significant portion of mental patients could be treated there. But he was convinced that urban asylums were still necessary and far preferable to city run general hospitals. Urban asylums could far more effectively attend to the special needs of mental patients, especially those from bourgeois classes.[165] In the face of competition from civic hospitals, Griesinger was inclined to apply economic levers to capture the patients he wanted. He pressed for low hospital fees and, wherever possible, free care for patients of modest means.[166] Given the relatively high cost of urban asylums, Griesinger was thus implicitly demanding a hike in state subsidies in order to attract middle-class patients and undercut the competition of other hospitals. In this Griesinger was effectively doing the city's own bidding: if university clinics needed patients for educational purposes, then the Prussian state would have to assume some of the costs of public assistance to the relief of municipal coffers.

In spite of the potentially competitive relationship between clinics and civic hospitals, common interests also drew universities and cities into negotiation with one another and often resulted in contractual agreements. For their part, university clinics and the ministries of education stood to benefit from a ready supply of lucrative middle-class patients, which asylums had had great difficulty attracting. Cooperation with cities also held out the prospect of not having to carry the full burden of hospital costs for the mere sake of research and education. Cities could also provide land grants for the construction of urban asylums, an advantage of no small importance in urban centers where prices were relatively high. Of particular significance in Prussia was the fact that agreements with cities also circumvented the authority of unpredictable and recalcitrant provincial governments: on more than one occasion early efforts to organize clinical education in psychiatry had run up against the resistance of provinces that were reluctant to fund facilities for educational purposes.[167] Alliances with city magistrates could help relieve the state of its dependence on provincial governments.

Cities could also benefit from cooperation with universities. In exchange for property grants or other subsidies, they could demand medical services for their citizens.[168] There were also public security dimensions behind decisions to construct psychiatric institutions in a metropolitan setting. Rather than negotiating the transfer of violent mental patients to distant asylums and rather than holding them in inadequate police facilities or in city hospitals, Griesinger's urban asylums could provide a convenient receptacle for disruptive individuals. Urban asylums were potentially far more effective instruments of crisis management and "triage" in socially charged and rapidly growing metropolitan centers. And finally, self-confident civic bureaucrats could point to urban asylums and boast the existence of modern, scientific, elite psychiatric institutions. Hence as objects of great prestige, university clinics became symbols of civic prowess and of progressive medical science.

In light of what Griesinger's urban asylum had to offer city officials, rural asylums were left at a distinct disadvantage. Alienists were burdened by their hermetic seclusion, their cumbersome administrative apparatus, their overcrowded facilities, their dismal public image, their inability to train the medical students needed for an effective policy of mental hygiene, and finally by the unwieldy provincial powers which governed their situation. All of these burdens made it very difficult for asylum psychiatry to advance plausible sociohygienic and prophylactic arguments and solutions that would alleviate the problems spawned by rapid urbanization. The traditional solution that alienists had long advocated, namely, the construction of new asylums and the wider institutionalization of the mad, was losing its persuasive force. The intensification of prophylactic efforts was becoming an increasingly attractive alternative to the construction of ever more expensive and apparently less therapeutically effective asylums.

Yet for all of these disadvantages, alienists were not left entirely bereft of other, very powerful moral arguments. Heinrich Laehr's ideas about how psychiatric clinics could be built in urban environments are a case in point. Laehr coupled moral injunctions of the 1840s and 1850s with vested institutional interests of alienist psychiatry. For him, clinics were but "missionary stations of the state hospitals"[169] and their doctors peregrine "apostles" in the struggle against public prejudice.[170] Urban doctors were to wander among the city-dwellers, all the while braving the evils of urban civilization—that "malicious source of moral impropriety"—and spreading the light of psychiatric science. As alienist outposts in urban environs, urban clinics could at best hope to attract promising doctors and prepare them to join their alienist brethren in the hermetic seclusion of rural asylums.

Laehr and others considered Griesinger's urban asylum an attack on the moral sensibilities and architecture of mid-nineteenth century asylums.[171] He believed that the asylum's quietude and isolation would be compromised by its proximity to the hustle and bustle of urban life. He expressed deep apprehension with respect to the commingling of the sexes, which would inevitably follow in cramped urban quarters.[172] The paucity or complete lack of therapeutic labor and recreational distractions conjured up images of idleness and therefore jeopardized one of the asylum's core therapeutic pillars. Furthermore, the absence of a constant physical presence on the part of the director would compromise the rational administration of the institution, disrupt the patriarchal hierarchy and familial character of the asylum and thereby subvert the very moral bedrock on which it had been constructed. Thus, the potential that Griesinger's urban asylum held for pandemonium (sexual congregation, idleness, administrative disorder, and familial disjunction) made it an affront to the moral sensibilities of Laehr and other like-minded alienists.[173]

There was more to these views than simple moral rhetoric. The pauperism of the second quarter of the nineteenth century, in addition to being a catalyst for new welfare laws, had also fed a religious awakening in the 1830s and 1840s. First gripping Catholic and, later with much less force, Protestant regions of Germany, this awakening was associated with reorganization of church influence in the fields of nursing, convalescent, and psychiatric care. While the new welfare laws had transferred responsibility for public welfare into the hands of civic officials, they not so much eliminated church-based poor relief as displaced it into the private sphere. The *Caritas* movement, Johann Heinrich Wichern's *Innere Mission*, and several other religious orders spearheaded the foundation of church-run asylums, encouraged the formation of local aid associations, established networks of ambulatory care, and even began opening nursing schools.[174] By the mid-1860s these efforts seemed to be bearing tangible fruit in the field of psychiatry. In Westphalia the protestant asylum in Lengrich had recently opened its doors to receive patients from the acutely overcrowded asylum in Marsberg. And in Berlin, where the protestant church exercised considerable influence in royal circles, disputes over the quality of nursing staff at the Charité quickly took on religious overtones.[175] These and other developments reflected the efforts of Heinrich Laehr, Johann Wichern, and Friedrich von Bodelschwingh to expand the influence of the church over psychiatric care.[176]

Alienist support for church based hospitals overlapped happily with their support of private mental institutions. Many alienists eagerly argued that private institutions—not university clinics—had a key role to play in solving urban problems. They appealed for the transfer of wealthy patients to private asylums to relieve overcrowding. Then, they argued, state institutions would be placed in a position to admit more patients during the crucial early phases of their illness. Damerow had spoken in this vein when he called for the "emancipation of the public asylums" from the "excess of distinguished and well-to-do pensioners."[177] Furthermore, private asylums could serve as intermediate receptacles for patients whose admissions applications were being processed and residency status corroborated.[178] Far from being mere wishful thinking on the part of alienists, such ideas were actively debated and at times implemented. Indeed, so severe was the shortage of space in civic institutions in the late 1860s that Berlin began placing patients in privately owned facilities—at prices, it might be noted, far lower than the regular rates charged by the Charité.[179] Private facilities thus represented a further threat to the clinical livelihood of the Charité's psychiatric ward. Were the city to begin systematic exploitation of private asylums, the effects of Esse's restrictive admissions policies would be compounded. Griesinger's urban asylum thus faced competition from not only civic hospitals, but also church sponsored and private institutions as well.

It is therefore hardly surprising that an owner of a private asylum formulated one of the early attempts at a coherent alienist position on prophylaxis. The director of a private asylum for nervous disorders in Bremen, Friedrich Engelken, believed himself to be among the first to have addressed the question of prophylaxis in detail.[180] As a sign of the urgency and importance of prophylactic endeavors, Engelken pointed to an increase in mental disorders, which he attributed to two primary causes. First, he diagnosed a predisposing, organically based "nervous constitution" that since the mid-eighteenth-century had come to afflict ever more individuals. Second, "false civilization" had taken its toll on the mental life of the population. True civilization was based upon humans striving toward perfection and intellectual freedom through self-discipline and adherence to the word of God. False civilization, on the other hand, was identified with "luxury, effeminacy, and demoralization." Egotism, greed, and materialism had all contributed to the "centrifugal direction" of human lives of late; people struggling up the "ladder to fame and fortune" and trying to "emancipate themselves" had generated emotional disquiet that threatened to unleash full blown madness. In order to preempt such dangers, Engelken looked to the family as the source of a child's "moral and religious consciousness" and recommended pedagogical means designed to instill obedience (corporal punishment) and promote physical fitness (gymnastics). His advice on marriage, onanism, and drink focused on individual self-control, measure and "mastery over lawless volition." Engelken's was chiefly a program of Protestant moral prophylaxis designed to counteract the evils of modern life and erect moral breakwaters against the vulnerabilities of the body.

Like Engelken, Griesinger too believed that prophylaxis was "rarely the object of medical discourse."[181] But his solutions placed less confidence in the power of moral and religious persuasion than in that of natural science operating in a material world.[182] For him the key to prophylactic undertakings was to counteract the causes of excessive "cerebral irritation."

A general increase in cerebral activity is a precondition of the growth of industry, of the arts, and of the sciences; the ever growing distance from simple moral values and the cultivation of finer mental and physical pleasures introduces previously unknown inclinations and passions; general liberal education wakens aspiring ambition in the masses, which only a very few can satisfy and which bitterly disappoints most; industrial, political and social trickery unsettle the individual and the totality. Everything is quicker; a feverish hunt for possessions and pleasure and the extraordinarily expansive discussion of all political and social issues holds the world in constant agitation. As Guislain has said: these conditions in modern American and European society sustain a general, quasi-delirious condition of cerebral irritation which is very far from natural and normal behavior and must predispose one to mental disorders.[183]

This assessment of the vicissitudes of German society emphasizes that the construction of university clinics as urban asylums also needs to be seen as representing part of a larger socio-political commitment and claim on the part of academic psychiatrists to do battle with madness and other "diseases of civilization" in an urban setting.[184] Urban asylums were the flagships of a new scientifically based, social psychiatry;[185] they represented the psychiatric side of Virchow's medical reforms and his call to arms of a hygiene movement that would supplant the religious and moral foundations of traditional forms of welfare and organize them instead around principles of positivist medical science and community-based social services. Griesinger's urban asylum was an attempt to confront, outmaneuver, and overtake alienists in these endeavors. With his own faith in the progress of medical science, and with the emancipatory rhetoric of non-restraint, Griesinger attacked Laehr and his Lutheran associates as "Samaritans with the strait-jacket."[186]

Griesinger's reform initiative needs, therefore, to be read as an expression of resurgent anti-clerical, liberal, and scientific influence in German civic politics of the 1860s. In the wake of the death of Friedrich Wilhelm IV and the ensuing New Era in Prussia, the powerful influence of conservative protestant interests which had entrenched themselves in the 1850s suffered a severe setback. Over the course of the 1860s, the Protestant Church's influence was checked and conservative church leaders removed. Griesinger's initiative was part of the larger emergence in the 1860s of a public hygiene movement in Germany which, operating at the communal level and self-consciously distinct from the church as well as from state and provincial government, became a field for the unfolding liberal values of autonomous civic administration, socio-economic rationalization, and non-partisan politics based on objective scientific truths.[187] The organizational impetus of that public hygiene movement was provided by numerous civic associations that grew rapidly in the following decades and that often succeeded in attracting members well beyond the pale of the medical profession.[188] The aspirations of this movement were embodied in the person of Rudolph Virchow, who, in a speech to the Prussian parliament in 1868, renewed his call for a program of medical and public health reform, which he had first advanced in 1848.[189]

Griesinger's concept of the urban asylum situated him in the midst of these debates. His reform program was a well calculated professional and political strategy. It was a bid to displace competing civic, confessional, and private hospitals in providing psychiatric care and prophylactic services. It juggled the complex and conflicting interests of German cities, of the state, and of the psychiatric profession. In the area of mental health and prophylaxis, it addressed the problems of both poor relief (*Armenfürsorge*) and of general social welfare for all citizens (*soziale Fürsorge*).

CHAPTER 4

Laboratory Science: Psychiatric Research in the 1870s and 1880s

Introduction

Alienist science was essentially empirical, experiential, and asylum-based. It was in good part a product of institutions and the disciplinary regimes that governed their populations. For the first time, within the walls of the asylum large numbers of mental patients could be easily observed and compared at frequent intervals and over extended periods of time. The experience derived from these observations was the bedrock of alienist science. As Heinrich Laehr remarked, "Every natural science is based on experience that cannot be derived from the observation of a few individual cases . . . Ample experience in mental science—and it can never be ample enough—can only be obtained in asylums where numerous patients are concentrated. And only here can *pure* experience be obtained, away from the multitude of influences in the family which, often unbeknownst to the physician, affect the patients and disturb their symptoms."[1] The asylum was one of the fundamental conditions of possibility of alienist research: it held a population of scientific "objects" and constituted the appropriate observational environment. Scientific expertise was defined in terms of accumulated institutional experience studying patients—an expertise which, of course, only alienists were in a position to acquire.

Alienist science was also an administrative and therapeutic science. Alienists emphasized the practical orientation of their research and juxtaposed it to the theoretical constructions and cerebral hypotheses of schoolmen. The focal point of their work was the construction and maintenance of a therapeutic environment within an institutional setting. They spent an enormous amount of time working up, implementing, and fine-tuning institutional rules governing space, time, movement, diet, discipline, and hygiene.[2] These administrative skills were, at the same time, an integral part of a subtle art of healing or *Heilkunst*. The therapeutic task of the alienist *qua* artist was to mobilize his medical and paternal authority as well as the resources of the institution, and then bring these factors to bear on the patients. Alienists were in many senses therapeutic choreographers for whom the asylum's efficient organization and their own medical skills comprised the dramaturgical stuff of therapeutic prac-

tice.[3] Managerial and therapeutic skills were harnessed in tandem, each forti-
fying the other as component parts in the alienist's science and the institution's
disciplinary regime. As such, alienist science was an applied and practical science of hospital administration.

Academic psychiatrists in the 1870s and 1880s likewise viewed their science
as an empirical and experiential science. But most of them observed different
things and drew on different experiences. For a growing number of them, the
asylum was *not* the sine qua non of their science. Their observations were directed not so much at institutionalized patients, as at histological specimens
and vivisected animals. They drew less upon skills derived from years of asylum experience and more upon practices and techniques learned as students
and honed in rudimentary laboratory facilities. Their ideal was not the practicing alienist, but rather the diligent researcher who spent long hours in front
of the microscope and at the autopsy table. The psychiatric knowledge that
they extracted from their objects of study was the product of disciplined laboratory conduct in handling microscopes and specimens, in opening the cra-
nium, in applying electrodes. For them, psychiatry was a natural science with
its own rigorous techniques and modes of observation.

Perhaps no figure did more to reorient psychiatric science away from its
alienist moorings and toward the natural sciences than Wilhelm Griesinger.
He had undermined the exclusive therapeutic jurisdiction of alienists by un-
masking the administrative criteria of curability as scientifically untenable. His
reform project had suggested that the empirical basis of alienist science had
been distorted by its practice of mechanical restraint. He maintained that because alienists did not wholeheartedly embrace the tenets of a new medicine
based on the natural sciences, they could not cultivate and instill the scientific
ethos in students and prospective psychiatrists; and without that ethos, the
psychiatric challenges facing modern German society could not be met.

In his critique of alienist psychiatry, Griesinger was speaking from the vantage point of a group of young Turks within academic medicine.[4] These physicians, converging around figures such as Johannes Müller, Carl Ludwig, or
Rudolf Virchow, had from the 1840s begun to recast German medicine in a
natural scientific mold. The rise of pathological anatomy and experimental
physiology, as well as the growth of mechanistic ideas and the influx of natural scientific methods, had by the 1860s purged medicine of many remnants of
romanticism and natural philosophy. These developments also found expression in Griesinger's own work. The mechanistic and somatic analogies in his
theory of mental reflex, his consequent conviction that psychiatry and neuropathology[5] needed to be largely overlapping medical specialties,[6] and his belief that the brain and the nervous system were the local seat of mental disease—all of these characteristics of Griesinger's thought reflected his affinity
with the scientific medicine of his day. And it was this new scientific medicine
which, with his call to Berlin, was given institutional legitimacy on the wards

of the Charité. There, as the head of both the neurological and the psychiatric wards, Griesinger was instrumental in "placing psychiatry within the field of neurology."[7] His post in Berlin symbolized his efforts to disassociate the work of academic psychiatrists from alienist practice and simultaneously draw the psychiatric profession into the orbit of the natural sciences.[8]

Griesinger, however, was a transitional figure. He was himself neither a pathological anatomist nor an experimental physiologist. He facilitated, but did not confirm through anatomic studies or experimental research, psychiatry's association with neurology. During the 1850s and 1860s his textbook had served as a powerful catalyst to an entire generation of students, including Carl Westphal, Theodor Meynert, Eduard Hitzig, Paul Flechsig, and Karl Wernicke.[9] It was these younger contemporaries who wholeheartedly adopted Griesinger's conviction that "mental diseases were brain diseases" and who went about applying anatomic and physiological methods of inquiry. This same cohort comprised the core of the first generation of university clinic directors: they had pursued careers almost entirely within academia and had little or no experience with the asylum culture of the early nineteenth century. To them, alienists were "fossils from a distant past."[10] Griesinger's textbook, together with far more general developments in medicine, had helped focus their professional energies on the mastery of new natural scientific methods and their application toward the investigation of the anatomic structure of the brain and the map of its physiological attributes. This younger generation of psychiatrists also proceeded to shift the focus of professional research away from the patient toward the local organ of the brain and central nervous system. They considered themselves no longer alienist artisans (*Irrenheilkünstler*) as Damerow had labeled himself, but rather cerebral pathologists.

For the professional development of psychiatry, the implications of Griesinger's efforts to move psychiatry closer to neuropathology went beyond a critique of alienist practice. Within the context of academic medicine, it was simultaneously a claim to jurisdiction over patients who suffered from diseases of the brain and central nervous system. In fact, the great professional utility of Griesinger's belief that mental disease was brain disease lay in its dual functionality. It helped define the status of academic psychiatry in relation to *both* alienist science and general medicine. On the one hand, Griesinger was committed to the somatic precepts for which alienists had fought so hard in the first half of the century; but he did not fear that the therapeutic culture of alienism was being reduced to a branch of pathological anatomy or experimental physiology. On the other hand, Griesinger shared the interests of some university medical faculties to extend natural scientific methods to mental disorders and gain greater access to psychiatric patients and corpses; but he disagreed with those medical faculties that disputed his psychiatry's claim to all patients afflicted by disorders of the brain and the central nervous system. The claim "mental disease is brain disease" was therefore a professional strategy of overlapping somatic localization and natural scientific methods, of psychiatry's medicalization and its academic specialization.

The success of this strategy depended ultimately on how effectively natural scientific methods could be brought to bear on madness. Could psychiatry succeed in mimicking the successes of anatomy and physiology? Would it, on this basis, be able to claim parity with other medical disciplines? The following chapter explores the extent to which Griesinger's heirs were able to merge neuropathology and psychiatry. It will first survey the neighboring fields of pathological anatomy and experimental physiology and show how new research techniques served to create a new kind of psychiatric observer. It will then assess the application of these methods to psychiatry and treat the work done by laboratory psychiatrists in the 1870s and 1880s. The chapter will then turn to the competing claims of alienists, academic psychiatrists, and internists to perform this type of work, considering first the alienist critique of so-called scientific medicine and then the jurisdictional disputes over psychiatric cadavers. In doing so, I will pay special attention to two prominent German neuropathologists, the director of the psychiatric clinic in Halle, Eduard Hitzig, and Griesinger's successor at the Charité in Berlin, Carl Westphal. An investigation of their efforts to optimize the conditions of psychiatric research will shed light on the character of the clinic's economy of power and knowledge.

Scientific Medicine: Developments in Physiology and Anatomy

General histories of medicine have commonly ascribed to the middle decades of the nineteenth century an era of scientific medicine.[11] The era was characterized by attempts on the part of physicians to introduce the methods and techniques of the natural sciences into medicine. Physicians used new kinds of research instruments (microscope, air pump, microtome) in specially designed institutes and laboratories; they employed methods of physical examination (auscultation, percussion) and chemical analysis (blood, urine, spinal fluid); they were attracted by numerical methods (statistics, graphs) and relied increasingly on a number of new measuring techniques and devices (thermometry, sphygmography, kymography, spirometry, pneumatometry); in clinical examinations they employed new kinds of endoscopic instruments (ophthalmoscope, laryngoscope) and turned to new therapeutic technologies (electrotherapy, hypodermic syringes, anesthesia, antiseptic surgery).

The influence of the natural sciences was felt most strongly in experimental physiology and pathological anatomy.[12] In physiology, Carl Voit in Munich and Carl Ludwig in Leipzig confidently espoused their loyalties to the natural sciences. According to Ludwig, the function of any given organ would not be understood until "an analogy of its machinery in non-organic nature has been understood."[13] His institute was a monument to the technological innovations of his age: it evoked the amazement of many of his colleagues at home and abroad for its factory-like laboratory rooms equipped with water, gas, and mechanical power.[14] Perhaps the most prominent representatives of a new generation of young research physiologists gathered around Johannes Müller; it comprised the so-called "Berlin School" of physiology.[15] Ernst Brücke, Hermann Helmholtz, Emil Du Bois-Reymond and others had all sworn their allegiance to the natural sciences and were instrumental in incorporating microscopy, vivisection, as well as rigorous empirical and experimental methods into physiology. For Du Bois-Reymond there was "no other method of inquiry than the mechanical one, no other mode of scientific thought than the mathematical and physical one."[16] Physiology was truly an amalgam of mechanics, mathematics, applied chemistry and physics. Of no less significance was Rudolf Virchow and his work in pathology.[17] For Virchow natural philosophy and natural history had been but incomplete stages on the path toward the true science of pathological physiology and toward those ultimate arbiters of truth: clinical observation and, above all, experimentation. For him the basis of disease lay in the physical and chemical disruption of cellular activity or function.

The influence of Virchow and the Berlin school of physiology was magnified many times over because of the great influence of Berlin on medical education. According to regulations dating back to 1825, all Prussian medical students were required to take their state licensing exams in the Prussian capital at the Charité.[18] The examination board was by and large drawn from the Berlin faculty. In preparation for those exams it was, therefore, not uncommon that during the course of their studies students would spend time in Berlin familiarizing themselves with the work of their later examiners.[19] In 1856, physiology was made a special section of the state examinations in Prussia and shortly thereafter the same was done for pathological anatomy. Virchow and Du Bois-Reymond were the driving force behind efforts to reform intermediate examinations in 1861. The replacement of the *tentamen philosophicum* with the *tentamen physicum* saw anatomy and physiology ensconced into the examinations and greater emphasis placed on physics and chemistry.[20]

The expanding influence of the natural sciences in medicine also was reflected in changes in the curriculum, faculty, and medical examinations at other German universities.[21] In Bavaria in the 1840s, requirements in the natural sciences were stiffened, while courses in philosophy were gradually reduced to a minimum.[22] In Württemberg in 1859 new prerequisites for admission to state examinations included an intermediate examination in the natural sciences, anatomy, and physiology.[23]

These changes to the academic curriculum were testament to the contemporary conviction that for purposes of medical research and diagnosis, students needed knowledge of the basic sciences. The exchange of knowledge between medicine and the natural sciences made it important for students to be familiar with the terminology of physics, chemistry, and biology; they needed to know how an electric battery worked if they were going to conduct physiological experiments; and they had to have at least an inkling of the physics behind such instruments as the thermometer, ophthalmoscope, or, later, the X-ray.[24] Exposure to the laboratory and to exact instrumental measurement would instill a scientific ethos in students that would serve them in their day-to-day diagnostic work. For it was in the realm of medical diagnostics rather than therapeutics that the professional fruits of scientific medicine were envisioned to be most bountiful.[25] And last but not least, the ethos of the natural sciences would help to reinforce the physician's social and cultural standing vis-à-vis laymen and other professionals.[26]

Disciplining the Observer: Microscopy and Necroscopy

Much of the theory and practice of physiology and pathological anatomy revolved about the possibilities associated with the *microscope*.[27] Many of the technological difficulties in manufacturing microscopes had been overcome by the late 1830s, enabling manufacturers to produce inexpensive, high-quality achromatic instruments.[28] As the use of these microscopes spread, there emerged an intricate and constantly evolving culture and economy of microscopic practice. Instructions governing the use, maintenance, handling, care, and storage of the physical instrument itself were formulated and no doubt adhered to by budding microscopists. Microscopes became inseparably associated with an array of techniques which defined proper usage, including correct posture, optimal viewing conditions, proper magnification, and accurate measuring techniques. Similarly, the use of the microscope's various attachments and all of the accoutrements employed in the manipulation of specimens (glass slides, scalpels, pincettes, water and chemical baths, test-tubes, etc.) were accompanied by exacting guidelines. In other words, with the microscope came an intricate economy of labor and observation. Anyone who wished to claim to be doing serious research had to master the practices and techniques associated with the instrument. In this way, microscopes and the conventions of their proper usage inevitably framed the terms of psychiatric research, setting out the conditions and limits of possible inquiry and to a degree even prefiguring the concepts of madness and normality.

Microscopy also demanded a unique mode of scientific perception. Work with the microscope meant the user's acculturation to a new kind of "microscopic vision [*das mikroskopische Sehen*]."[29] Microscopic vision differed in critical ways from ordinary vision. The eye needed to be specially trained so that it could "correctly perceive what it viewed in this unaccustomed way."[30] One skeptical surgeon, wary of new instruments designed to extend the visual range of the physician, remarked that for many students microscopic viewing "was entirely fruitless because their own eyes were not organized for [the microscope]."[31] Prospective microscopists therefore had to learn to recognize corrupted specimens, foreign particles, impurities in their glass slides, and even variations in the secretion of their own tear ducts. Furthermore, microscopic vision was directed toward unique objects. As the microscope extended the range of the medical scientist's vision deeper into the human body, it exposed new objects of inquiry (nerve strands, cell tissue, etc.). Microscopic vision was, however, not directed at objects in a putatively "natural" state, but rather at specimens which had been manipulated and prepared by the laboratory scientist in such a way that a satisfactory image could be extracted from them in a microscopic environment. Special techniques and instruments for cutting specimens,[32] methods of hardening tissues, injection of dyes, chemical treatment of specimens were all crucial preparatory and enabling operations associated with microscopic vision.

But while the microscope and microscopic vision made it possible to explore the internal depths of the body, that vision remained ephemeral as long as it could not in some manner be preserved. Indeed, it was scientifically useless if it could not be fixed and reproduced, and it was therefore supplemented by "inscription devices"[33] such as written notes and physical measurements designed to capture ephemeral observations. Hand drawings also fixed visual impressions, allowing them to be recalled at a later date. Drawings also had the advantage of disciplining the observer's eye and of forcing it to explore the entire surface and depth of the object. From the 1840s photography was also beginning to be used in microscopy, allowing the visual image of objects to be reinscribed in a more durable medium.[34] Elaborate techniques were also developed to preserve fragile or perishable specimens. Such methods were crucial, because they made it possible "to compare different objects with one another, to investigate them repeatedly, and to renew one's impression of their proportions and forms."[35]

However, as loudly as many researchers extolled the virtues of this disciplined microscopic vision, it could never be taken for granted as a rote exercise in verification of objective fact. As one alienist pointed out, after years of "seeing" vascular dilation in infections, researchers had now thoroughly refuted this view, so that "for years a lot of 'observers' had seen something which did not exist."[36] Recalling his own years of instruction in Vienna, the psychiatrist August Forel complained that he had never seen what his teacher, the neuroanatomist Theodor Meynert, had seen.[37] And even if researchers saw the same things, agreement on just what it was that they saw and what it implied were by no means assured. Thus, as powerful as this new laboratory technology of microscopy became, it did not guarantee scientific consensus. On the contrary, it in turn generated fields of conflicting interpretation and renewed discourse. The microscope and its accoutrements, the entire economy of labor and observation which came with it, and the new images of madness that it produced all gave rise to a new and constantly mutating discourse on madness. Psychiatrists came to debate what they saw through microscopes, how they had prepared their specimen, and what they believed their observations meant.

Thus, there evolved a complex interaction of instruments, microscopic techniques, observing eyes, and disciplined bodies intended to generate and capture images of otherwise invisible objects. The ultimate goal of microscopic research was, as the eminent microscopist Johann Purkyně put it, "total transparency of all spatial objects and therewith full awareness of all visible things."[38] Reaching that goal, however, demanded that observers should be sufficiently acculturated to new modes of practice and perception. For the microscope to be employed as a scientific instrument, a well trained and disciplined observer was required in order to elicit useful images from the specimens under investigation. Training in microscopy therefore had both a pedagogical and a scientific function: microscopy at once disciplined both the observer and the object of investigation.[39]

Of course, microscopes were useful only if adequate specimens were available for observation. Aside from the myriad technical problems of simply producing useful and durable images, access to collections of microscopic slides and to the means of producing such slides was restricted. Regardless of whether such collections were maintained in hospitals, pathological institutes, or by private individuals, access to them was often a privilege reserved for the select few. Most important of all, however, the institutional availability of specimens depended ultimately upon the acquisition of jurisdiction over a body of patients and implicitly over cadavers and brains.

Up until the early nineteenth century, autopsies were relatively rare events in medicine. In the first half of the nineteenth century, however, they became increasingly common. The increase in their numbers was in good part a derivative of the growth of hospitals, since institutionalized corpses were more accessible to necroscopic inquiry. The hospital represented a "reservoir of chronic, usually incurable patients"[40] and thus evoked considerable interest among anatomists and pathologists alike. Indeed, medical faculties were eager to acquire hospital cadavers, and the fact that institutes of pathology could be called "cadaver clinics [*Leichenklinik*]"[41] was testimony to their success.

Acquisition of the corpses which medical scientists and teachers so valued varied widely, depending on legal restrictions and local circumstances. Traditionally, researchers had relied on cases of suicide, victims of capital punishment, and the death of prison inmates to satisfy their demand for cadavers.[42] In the late nineteenth century in Prussia and most other German states, access to corpses was eased by the fact that doctors required no explicit consent from patients or relatives before conducting an autopsy. As a result, at least in such large cities as Berlin, academics rarely faced a shortage of corpses for their anatomic research or instruction. In smaller university towns, however, access to adequate "material" was a recurrent problem.[43] No less problematic were the internal divisions within medicine itself, which pitted the interests of surgeons, anatomists, pathologists, clinicians, and members of various subdisciplines against one another.[44] The most obvious, but certainly not the only manifestation of these differences is witnessed in the fact that at almost all universities practical training in anatomy was restricted to the winter semesters, while in the summer corpses were left to surgeons for their courses.[45]

Beyond conditions governing the availability of so-called "educational material," the ability to "parade the facts of pathology in front of an audience" depended upon a number of different variables.[46] For one, the physical architecture was important in acquiring the necroscopic skills. Whether for purposes of research or for clinical demonstration, necroscopy was assigned to well defined and segregated spaces in hospitals. More so than other hospitals, university clinics segregated the work of post-mortem examination from other hospital routines: autopsies were usually performed in institutes of pathology by a prosector and specially designed lecture halls were constructed for purposes of demonstration.[47]

The anatomist's endoscopic intrusion into the body was furthermore conditional upon acquired skills of dissection. In order for students to be able to "observe successfully" they needed to acquire a collection of skills not the least of which was "manual dexterity."[48] Proficiency in these skills required in turn their demonstration in practical courses and laboratories, where the "catechism of the scientific age could be transmitted to the faithful."[49] And, indeed, in the middle decades of the nineteenth century these courses had become mainstays in the medical curriculum at most German universities.[50]

Psychiatric Autopsies

Autopsies were nothing new to psychiatry in the 1870s. In fact, there existed a long tradition of opening and inspecting the corpses of the mad.[51] However, in the first half of the nineteenth century autopsies were rarely conducted systematically and had usually been compiled as casuistic collections of experiences, the intent being more to gather (sometimes curious and monstrous) individual specimens. As such, they were used far more often as illustration or evidence of deduced theory than as an empirical basis of inductively oriented research.[52] Published autopsy reports were not preconditions of psychiatric theory, but rather supplemental resources and stores of knowledge on which to draw in support of psychiatric theory and clinical observation. As most alienists understood their practical use, autopsies could help illuminate somatic aspects associated with mental illness, but they could never disclose the root causes of insanity.

Damerow's views on autopsies are a case in point.[53] He valued them, because they could clarify the hotly contested and professionally divisive issue of the relationship between body and soul. They could illuminate which symptoms were of somatic origin, thereby separating clinical truth from error and exposing those symptoms that were expressions of the true causes of the illness as opposed to its mere effects. Furthermore, anatomic inquiry could reveal how the soul acted on the body and thereby indirectly assess the workings of the soul itself. Because in conjunction with insanity other somatic diseases exhibited unusually complex and unique symptoms, psychiatric practitioners could explore and compare the anatomic difference of known illnesses in both the sane and the insane. In this way the workings of the soul could be investigated by examining the different traces it left in bodies suffering from the same disease. Finally, autopsies might also serve as surrogates for patients' descriptions of their own illness, either because doctors were otherwise unable to extract information from patients or because patients may have been simulating or dissimulating an illness. In these cases, autopsies could supplement clinical observation and expose information which the patient had been unable or unwilling to supply.

In spite of these potential benefits, Damerow thought that ultimately the explanatory power of pathological anatomy was very limited. He believed that the examination of cadavers would never reveal "the substantial reason for or the essential cause of mental disease [*Seelenkrankheit*], because the corpse of a human is not a human, but simply the cadaver of a former human, in other words, not an animate being [*beseeltes Wesen*] in whom the unity of body and soul dissolves upon death with each element going its own separate way."[54] In other words, whereas post-mortem examinations might help in circumscribing somatic factors associated with insanity, they were useless when it came to addressing the role of the soul. Damerow also contended that the findings of pathological anatomists said very little about insanity itself. Anatomic abnormalities could be found in the sane and insane alike; they were nothing unique to psychiatric patients per se. And finally, most sweepingly of all, there existed no single pathological anomaly which in itself was a sufficient and necessary cause of insanity. Autopsies might help illuminate the somatic condition of the patients upon their death, but they could never explain the root cause of insanity itself. Crucially for Damerow, psychiatry was irreducible to pathological anatomy because it concerned animate human beings: it was an anthropological and not a veterinary science.

Wilhelm Griesinger attributed an entirely different purpose to autopsies. For him, pathological anatomy was an ultimate adjudicator, which would definitively reveal which disease had "really" caused clinically observed symptoms.[55] At the autopsy table, at last, the proper foundation of "true, i.e. anatomic diagnosis" could be established. Autopsies were no exercise in satisfying the curiosity of the physician or in collecting specimens, but rather important means of improving diagnosis of living patients and expanding medical knowledge of the "essence" of mental diseases. Griesinger admitted, of course, that many times no anatomic lesions could be detected in post-mortem examinations. But in large measure he attributed this failure to the carelessness of the observer. There were simply too few diligent observers qualified to conduct professional autopsies. To his mind, very many of the negative autopsy results came from alienists

> who, although perhaps excellent administrators and moralists, had had no time to become familiar with the structure and pathological changes of the brain and who only knew how to cut the brain using a knife and fork. Of course they never find anything. One must remember how easily some finer but nevertheless important alterations . . . escape the notice of mere common observation [*gewöhnliche Aufmerksamkeit*]. Reports on the normal or abnormal constitution of the organ can only be accepted from those who thoroughly demonstrate in their work that they are familiar with pathological anatomy, that they accept its tenets, and that they know what one needs to look for and to take into consideration.[56]

Scientific Psychiatry in a Neuropathological Key

The rise of physiology and pathological anatomy evoked considerable excitement within psychiatric circles. Many practitioners, although to varying degrees, were swept up in the enthusiasm of these wider developments in scientific medicine. The professor of psychiatry in Jena, Otto Binswanger, captured in retrospect the mood of scientific optimism and progress that molded an entire generation of psychiatrists in the 1870s and 1880s:

> Under the influence of the tremendous progress of medical science in anatomy and physiology, the improved aids for manual and physical patient examination, as well as the extraordinary increase in the use of the microscope and chemical analysis at the bedside, a degree of disdain for imponderable psychic influences became the norm. This [scientific] progress literally intoxicated the heads [*Gemüter*] of many; in heated efforts to derive the cause and manifestations of all normal and pathological life processes from the fundamental precepts of biological research, from chemical, physical, and mechanical processes, the old facts derived from observing nature [*Naturbeobachtung*] were jettisoned as irrelevant and unproven, and hence inexplicable ballast as soon as they could no longer be fitted into the framework of so-called exact research.[57]

Binswanger's assessment of the neuro-anatomic enthusiasm of 1870s and 1880s is borne out in numerous other contemporary remarks. The state of flux within the profession was noted by one observer who in 1877 saw developments in medicine enveloping the "entire field of psychiatry in a state of complete transition."[58] In 1878 August Erlenmeyer, the director of the private asylum in Bendorf near Coblenz, observed that "for the moment purely neurological and cerebral-spinal, anatomic work comprises the vast majority [of articles]" in professional journals.[59] Even for more clinically minded psychiatrists such as Ewald Hecker, the ultimate goal of psychiatry had become the "establishment of disease forms on a pathological and anatomic basis."[60]

Changes in professional associations also bore witness to the reorientation toward neuroanatomic work. Between 1876 and 1886 the psychiatric section of the GDNÄ changed its name twice to reflect the growing importance and ultimately the dominance of neurology in psychiatric research.[61] Likewise, the influential *Berliner medicinisch-psychologische Gesellschaft* altered its name to *Berliner Gesellschaft für Psychiatrie und Nervenkrankheiten* in 1879.[62] At the meeting of the *Südwestdeutscher psychiatrischer Verein* in Heppenheim in 1874, psychiatrists had eagerly embraced neuroanatomic and experimental approaches and methods.[63] Two years later, however, the regional professional organization fractured, leading to the founding a new, neurologically oriented society.[64]

These and other outward manifestations of a shift toward neurological research were grounded in the work of psychiatrists doing neuroanatomic and physiological research.[65] In the 1870s and 1880s, drawing on many of the new scientific methods and research techniques, psychiatrists supplied evidence backing up localization theories and solidifying the reputation of their profession as a medical science. Pierre Paul Broca and Jean-Baptiste Bouillaud had shown that patients, in whom a relatively small region of the brain (Broca's gyrus) had been damaged, lost their motor capacity to articulate speech (motor aphasia). In the early 1870s Eduard Hitzig distinguished and localized motor and sensory regions of the cerebral cortex.[66] These achievements were augmented by Carl Wernicke's discovery of a further speech center which, when damaged, compromised not the motor capacity, but rather the patients' ability to understand speech (sensory aphasia).[67] Hermann Munk's localization of optic and acoustic functions in the brain as well as his discovery of hemianopsia added to these findings. And in parallel studies both Karl Westphal and Wilhelm Erb described patellar reflex which became a standard part of psychiatric diagnostic procedure after the mid-1870s. All of these findings were further flanked by the detailed anatomic studies of the brain by Theodor Meynert, Bernhard von Gudden, and Paul Flechsig.[68] So pervasive did such research become that one observer was moved to note that many prominent psychiatrists virtually ignored their own discipline, preferring to devote their attention instead to neuropathology and cerebral anatomy.[69] In fact, it was as students and assistants in the laboratories of institutes for pathological anatomy or physiology that most first-generation clinic directors had worked and carried out their early research.[70]

Such training as neuropathologists had a profound impact not only on psychiatrists' conceptualization of madness, but also upon their understanding of their work as medical professionals. As more and more research was published, experts zeroed in on madness and attempted to circumscribe it in ever more narrowly defined cerebral regions and functional constituents. If Griesinger had described madness as a disease of the brain, then Theodor Meynert went still further to suggest that it was a "disease of the anterior brain [*Vorder-hirnkrankheit*]" and to draw heavily on Virchow's cellular pathology in his explanatory models.[71] Carl Westphal narrowed the scope of enquiry still further, suggesting that restructuring the madman's personality was analogous to the chemical restructuring of physical elements.[72] In as much as their instruments allowed them to do so, these and other psychiatrists moved through successively deeper layers of their patients' bodies in search of scientific explanations. The power of their own laboratory instruments and increasingly sophisticated skills in manipulating specimens made the diligent exploration of all levels of observation not only possible, but also scientifically imperative. As Carl Westphal noted, their science demanded that "if during life we have observed a series of symptoms which can only be attributed to a disease of the brain and if upon death we find no macroscopic sign of change, then we shall always consider it desirable, that the entire brain, slice for slice, be subject to systematic microscopic investigation. This is because, in spite of the integrity [*Intactheit*] of its mass, the most severe symptoms [*Erscheinungen*] can potentially be the result of very circumscribed alterations."[73] Such were the challenging tasks facing the psychiatric neuropathologist.

Pathological anatomy and experimental physiology came to psychiatry not by way of the asylums, but rather through academic medicine. Their highly specialized research methods were, and for a long time remained, foreign to asylum culture.[74] Instead, members of the Berlin school in particular, including the neurologist Moritz Heinrich Romberg[75] and his student Carl Westphal, played pivotal roles in extending these methods to psychiatric research.[76] Academic psychiatrists believed that clinics needed to be, in essence, nothing other than neurological clinics.[77] Similar views reaffirming the fusion of psychiatry and neurology were advanced time and again throughout the ensuing decades and effectively became Griesinger's legacy in the 1870s and 1880s.

Two of scientific psychiatry's most avid spokespersons, Paul Samt and Carl Wernicke, echoed the sentiments of many contemporaries. Paul Samt was an assistant to Carl Westphal in Berlin's Charité hospital in the 1870s. Samt is best known for a paper on "The natural scientific method in psychiatry," which he delivered to the *Berliner medicinisch-psychologische Gesellschaft* in 1873.[78] Samt was motivated to pen his article in part by Emil Du Bois-Reymond's address in 1872 to the meeting of the GDNÄ on the limits of scientific knowledge.[79] Following the leads of Du Bois-Reymond and Carl Voit, Samt adopted an extreme mechanistic and materialistic position. His prose was spiked with metaphors such as "speech apparatus," "signals," and "brain mechanics" and he insisted that the soul could not act without the brain: the soul was no "metaphysical constant" but rather a physical variable which depended upon the mechanics of the brain. Samt pictured subconscious psycho-motor processes performing all the functions of the conscious will, yet without the need for human volition. "We think and feel not as our consciousness wishes, but rather as the material of the brain allows us to think and feel. The mechanics in a given region of the brain determine mental individuality."[80] By the same token, any alteration in the physical material of the brain produced aberrations in mental functioning. According to Samt's model, mental disease would be understood when the mechanics governing a region of the subconscious had been fully understood and when laws explaining the form and development of "concrete pathological patterns" had been discovered.[81]

While Samt's writings on scientific psychiatry aroused interest, more prominent still were the views of Carl Wernicke, who had received his doctorate of medicine in 1870 and had worked on the wards of the Breslau city hospital. After spending a year in Vienna studying with Theodor Meynert, he moved to Berlin in 1875 and worked on the psychiatric ward of the Charité under Carl Westphal.[82] In his research in the 1870s, Wernicke attempted to apply Theodor Meynert's anatomic findings toward an understanding of speech disorders or aphasia. So important was Wernicke's work that some have considered it the very beginning of "exact cerebral physiology."[83]

In tribute to the importance of his work on aphasia, Wernicke was one of only a handful of psychiatrists ever to have been chosen to address a plenary session of the prestigious GDNÄ. At the annual meeting in Danzig in 1880, Wernicke juxtaposed physiology and alienist psychiatry in a lecture "On the Scientific Standpoint in Psychiatry." The diligent efforts and enormous amount of energy that alienists had invested in the collection of "empirical material" over the past one hundred years had, in Wernicke's eyes, been essentially for naught. Although considerable progress had been made in the treatment of patients, alienists had failed to establish "any sort of sound theory of mental disease." Wernicke then defined scientific psychiatry in explicit opposition to the empirical and therapeutic activities of his alienist predecessors:

> Let us confidently distinguish psychiatry's practical and scientific goals! As laudable as it is for psychiatric practitioners to fulfill their difficult therapeutic calling, psychiatry is also a branch of the natural sciences. As such, it has tasks to perform which are every bit as worthy as other great tasks of natural science. For it must observe and explain not only deviations from healthy mental life. It must also derive from these deviations useful information which the diseases, as natural experiments, tend to have for knowledge of the normal function of an organ. Only modern physiology of the brain will enable us to perform this task.[84]

Alienists now had the responsibility to conduct their clinical observations "with specific physiological assumptions" in mind. Only then could they penetrate more deeply into the mental world of patients, gain their trust, guide them according to the physician's will, and implement effective therapies.[85]

Wernicke's address was essentially a physiologist's challenge to alienist science. He drew on the results of Meynert's anatomic studies, on the animal experiments of Hitzig and Fritsch, and on his own work at the dissection table to stake a claim to explain and treat mental disorders. The research tasks of effective administration and therapy were counterposed to those of microscopy and necroscopy. The institutional economy of alienist science was countered by a new matrix of power and knowledge evolving from the disciplined use of new instruments and systematic techniques of dissection—research practices around which academic clinics were conceived and constructed. Wernicke's address was, in other words, an assault on alienist experiential science and on the professional claims that rested on that science.

Laboratory Work

Given the enthusiasm with which many psychiatrists greeted developments in scientific medicine, one might have expected to find them in charge of large laboratory facilities. Yet this was far from being the case. In fact, laboratories came relatively late to psychiatry, and where they did exist they were often quite rudimentary in their architecture and equipment.[86] Nevertheless, they became core sites of institutional research. Directors boasted of the spartan facilities at their disposal and eagerly mimicked the practices of scientific medicine. Even when limited to simple work-benches in director's offices, early psychiatric laboratories became sites of highly specialized and disciplined professional labor.

Among the most common form of work conducted in psychiatric laboratories was animal experimentation. Vivisection had long been generally accepted and commonplace practice in the emerging profession of psychiatry.[87] Little moved by the protests of anti-vivisectionists, psychiatrists such as August Forel, Eduard Hitzig, Julius Wagner-Jauregg, and Paul Flechsig were all eager experimenters on animals.[88] One of Germany's most avid experimenters was the director of the local asylum in Munich, Bernhard von Gudden. Gudden's experimental approach or "extirpation method"[89] involved the transection of neural strands and surgical excision of portions of the brains of young experimental animals. Following the operation, the immediate "symptoms" would be observed and their alteration over time studied. The experiment was ended with the dissection of the animals and histological analysis of the brain tissue. Over the course of his career, Gudden amassed more than 50,000 microscopic slides, each of which he had finely labeled and categorized.[90] Gudden's research was typical of the enormous distance that scientific psychiatry had traversed in moving away from the psychiatric patient whose disorder it proclaimed to study. For Gudden the laboratory became a haven and "refuge" from what he considered the more unsavory routine on the hospital wards of the Munich asylum.[91] In the words of one of his students, unlocking the "labyrinth" of psychiatric disease was solely a matter of "penetrating anatomic dissection," so much so that his "unflagging scientific zeal was entirely focused on the rabbit brain."[92]

The laboratory was not only the site of these intricate morphological mappings of the brain. It was also the environment in which psychiatrists sought to reproduce madness. In part because they sometimes lacked patients, but chiefly because they could not easily conduct experiments on those that they did have, they went to great lengths in trying to simulate various mental disorders in animals. In a paper delivered to the Berlin Medical-Psychological Society in 1868, Westphal demonstrated how he had experimentally produced a Brown-Séquard syndrome; and in experiments on guinea pigs involving the severance of their spinal cords, Westphal was similarly convinced that he had come close to recreating not just the symptoms of epilepsy, but an artificial form of the "disease" itself.[93] Addressing the Prussian Academy of Sciences, Emanuel Mendel described how he had employed a turntable in his experiments on dogs in order to evoke hyperemia and so artificially to reproduce the symptoms of paralysis.[94] In his anatomic experiments on rabbits, Bernhard Gudden contended that he produced "idiots," exhibiting the same symptoms of sleepiness and retarded development as their human counterparts. These "idiots" needed to be carefully watched over (especially as concerned their cleanliness) and held in isolation because, left alone among their peers, they would succumb in the "struggle for survival [*Kampfe um's Dasein*]."[95]

Where possible, however, psychiatrists also sought to extend their experimental studies to humans. Friedrich Jolly pronounced that he could reproduce acoustic hallucinations in his experimental subjects by applying electrical stimuli to the nerves in the ear.[96] In the 1880s, Emil Kraepelin conducted psychological experiments on himself, his wife, and his students in which through the ingestion of various drugs, coffee, tea, and alcohol he brought about so-called "artificial insanity."[97] In Würzburg, Konrad Rieger—inspired by a visit to Charcot in Paris—used hypnotism to induce "experimental insanity."[98] One of the bolder probings of the ethical boundaries of experimental physiology as it related to psychiatry was undertaken by Hermann Kuhnt, professor of ophthalmology in Jena. In the GDNÄ section on psychiatry and neurology in 1882—which in that year proudly hosted the Grand Duke of Saxony—Kuhnt reported on his examination of "two persons put to death by decapitation 25 and 27 seconds respectively after the sentence had been carried out. He found that, when electrical current was applied perpendicular to the spinal cord in the region of the sixth cervical vertebra, the pupils contracted."[99] All of these and other experiments represented attempts on the part of psychiatrists to reproduce in their laboratories the symptoms and diseases which they observed and sought to cure on their wards. In the controlled environment of their laboratories, they hoped to generate an artificial version of insanity that they could manipulate and ultimately subdue.

The professional implications of laboratory research were profound. One of the great advantages of such work was its relative autonomy from the institutional strictures of the asylum. Microscopy, dissections, autopsies, animal experimentation, etc. did not need the kind of elaborate institutional resources which alienist science did. Nor did they necessarily require access to large numbers of patients in the asylums. Contrary to the experiential work of alienists, these were kinds of research that were far less architecturally determined. They were not bound to conditions as found in the asylums in the way that alienist research had been. They liberated academic psychiatrists from alienist science and provided a platform from which to launch their own claims to professional jurisdiction over psychiatric research.

The research work of scientific psychiatrists also differed from that of their alienist counterparts in so far as it tended to privilege diagnosis over therapy. Alienists had usually emphasized just the opposite: they had subordinated diagnosis to therapeutic practice. Carl Wilhelm Ideler, for example, is said to have observed patients for months on end before making his diagnoses.[100] And when push came to shove in the busy daily routine of asylum life, Max Brosius made the priorities of his alienist colleagues clear: if mistakes were going to be made in the asylum, then "in the interests of its health as well as of ill residents [he] preferred that the diagnosis rather than the administration be neglected."[101] By contrast, psychiatrists who understood themselves to be natural scientists did not make therapeutic administration the object of their research. Indeed, therapy was a concept often foreign to their natural scientific ethos. Consequently, to the extent that psychiatry was recast as a natural science, it simultaneously lost touch with the therapeutic culture and practical orientation of alienist science. The introduction of natural scientific methods and concomitantly the specialization of academic psychiatry put greater distance between professional research work and therapeutic tasks. The new research culture privileged diagnostics (and nosology) at the expense of therapy. Alienists were as aware and critical of this development in 1855, when Friedrich Wilhelm Hagen maintained that the natural sciences had done "little or nothing at all for therapy,"[102] as they were in 1906, when Konrad Alt would remark in his critique of psychiatric clinics, that "too much emphasis was placed on diagnosis while therapy was far too neglected."[103]

Yet in spite of their distance from therapeutic labor, the positivist precepts of scientific psychiatry simultaneously undermined alienist jurisdictions over therapeutic and pedagogical work. For if mental disease was a natural, biological phenomenon unrelated to the patient's subjective environment, its cure might also be effected outside the institutional setting of the asylum itself. Thus, the therapeutic claims of alienists were compromised and patients might just as well be treated in the environs of a university clinic. And, by the same logic, if the symptoms exhibited by patients were not a function of the institutional setting in which they found themselves, but rather of an objective, natural state, then concerns could be discounted that clinical demonstration (as well as the transportation to such demonstrations) might somehow distort patient symptoms. Teacher and student alike could then proceed on the assumption that the observed symptoms were an objective reflection of a natural reality.

Just how far academic psychiatrists had distanced themselves from the mid-century alienist views of the asylum as a therapeutic instrument was poignantly illustrated by Adolf Dannemann, a psychiatrist at the clinic in Giessen. Dannemann, who at the turn of the century was one of the more vocal disciples of Griesinger's reform ideas, found in detractors' criticisms of clinical demonstration evidence "that even in psychiatric circles the conviction had not yet everywhere taken root, that the course of a mental disorder was really independent of external influences such as the patient's work or his transport from one asylum to another. The course of a mental disorder is alone governed by the laws of natural science."[104] Although this extreme position was not shared by all of Dannemann's colleagues, the issue was one which sparked heated debate and which tended to put alienists on the defensive.[105]

Finally, scientific psychiatry began to reshape the discipline's professional image. Laboratory work allowed academic psychiatrists to project an ethos of precision and efficiency which alienists could not match. In turn, that ethos helped to confer authority and legitimacy upon them. Laboratory work therefore also served as an intermediate conduit between psychiatrists and the various audiences to which they stated their professional claims to jurisdiction over psychiatric research.[106] The generous faith in science which characterized German public opinion from the 1850s onward, made it that much easier for the claims of neuropathologists to receive a favorable hearing among lay audiences.

Alienist Responses to Scientific Psychiatry

In spite of the growing strength of scientific psychiatry, entrenched resistance to it survived in alienist circles. As late as the mid-1860s, many psychiatrists still resisted seeing mental disorders as expressions of pathological processes in the brain.[107] The *Verein deutscher Irrenärzte* had even voted down a proposal to devote more attention to pathological anatomy at its meetings.[108] Others engaged in incisive critiques of the pretensions of scientific psychiatry. Karl Kahlbaum discounted the contemporary infatuation with pathological anatomy as simply one more historical fad alongside rationalism, empiricism, and speculation. Reliance on "necroscopy" had produced the "same heterogeneity, imprecision, and confusion" that had dominated earlier phenomenological terminology, so that "rummaging around" in still more cadavers was fruitless.[109] Similarly, the director of the Bavarian asylum in Irsee, Friedrich Wilhelm Hagen, believed that simply peering ever deeper into the "inner depths" of the organism—as "micro-anatomic research" did—would not help psychiatrists discover the cause or cure of madness. Instead, researchers needed to draw on psychological explanations and on their own rational faculties. Yet Hagen admitted that his appeal to rational thought was "anathema to the 'new age,' which views as sacrilegious every attempt to discover something which employs the faculties of thought rather than those of sight and hearing."[110] And finally, August Solbrig and C. F. W. Roller argued that pathological anatomy was all but useless to alienists in their forensic work. Called before a court of law to assess the mental state of living and breathing defendants, psychiatric experts had no recourse to knowledge derived from the autopsy. Especially for very difficult borderline cases, the psychiatrist's forensic report had to be based on psychological, not on pathological findings.[111]

Of course, some self-conscious alienists also conducted laboratory and autopsy work. The asylums had long been hubs of scientific inquiry into mental diseases and alienists often remained respected researchers even in academic circles. Heinrich Schüle's careful anatomic studies in Illenau were every bit as rigorously "scientific" for their day as those carried out at the universities.[112] Transitional figures such as Hubert Grashey and Richard von Krafft-Ebing were long-time advocates of closer relations between neurology and psychiatry.[113] The director of the Württemberg asylum Winnenthal, von Zeller, diligently took his microscope and dissection kit with him on vacations.[114] And even as late as 1907, August Cramer considered the research on metabolic disorders carried out in the asylum at Uchtspringe to be on par with that of the clinic in Munich.[115]

But such assessments clearly became rare by the early twentieth century. Instead, complaints about the state of research in the asylums became legion in alienist literature. Robert Wollenberg, one time director of the clinics in Straßburg and Breslau, complained in his memoirs that due to ward responsibilities his tenure of service at the asylum Nietleben in the 1880s had been "scientifically barren."[116] Another observer remarked that although often equipped with laboratories, alienists were not working in them as one might have hoped.[117] And while admiring the "splendidly equipped laboratory" at the Berlin asylum Buch, an American visitor nevertheless concluded that advanced pathological and psychological research was impossible there.[118]

The realization that asylums had become backwaters of scientific research prompted spasms of reflection. In the years immediately preceding World War One, alienists agonized over the causes and potential remedies for the desolate state of alienist research.[119] Concerned observers complained about the administrative burdens, shortage of personnel, overcrowded institutions, poor laboratory facilities, and the continuing physical isolation of the asylums, all of which had severely hampered their research efforts. The solutions that they advanced to alleviate the problem were as diverse as the assumed causes themselves, including the exchange of physicians between clinics and asylums,[120] the compulsory employment of pathological anatomists in asylums, and the reorganization of annual administrative reports to include scientific publications. Johannes Bresler went furthest in advocating scientific centers in the asylums which could compete on an equal footing with the university clinics.[121] But younger, equally strident colleagues had no desire to beat the clinics at their own game and wished instead to reframe the terms of the debate. They cast doubt on the therapeutic utility of laboratory research altogether and reemphasized the importance of the alienists' pivotal contribution to "social assistance [*sociale Fürsorge*]." Others were more resigned to their plight and conceded the priority of university clinics in scientific research. Yet whatever their position, it was clear by 1910 that asylum based research was in the doldrums and there was little prospect for improvement. On the eve of World War One, the work of laboratory research had been taken over almost entirely by university clinics.

Progressive Paralysis

While academic psychiatrists were able to capture from alienists the professional jurisdiction over laboratory research, their claims were also disputed by advocates of internal medicine.[122] In response to this opposition, progressive paralysis was a powerful professional weapon that helped advance the medicalization of psychiatry.[123] Progressive paralysis was a psychiatric disorder arising, it would soon be found, in the late stages of syphilis. Its early symptoms were characterized by memory and speech dysfunction. Prior to World War One, its prognosis was poor, usually ending in dementia and death within a few years of its diagnosis. Patients suffering from progressive paralysis comprised a significant contingent in the psychiatric wards of many hospitals, at times exceeding ten percent of all patients in treatment. For example, in the 1870s fully one third of all patients admitted to the *Verpflegungsanstalt* in Berlin were diagnosed with progressive paralysis.[124] No other disease so dominated the psychiatric literature of this period. Described by some as the "disease of the nineteenth century," it came to acquire paradigmatic status within the profession.[125]

It is difficult to overstate the importance that progressive paralysis played in strengthening the bond between psychiatry and neuropathology. Its significance can be attributed in good part to the fact that it happened to lend itself especially well to the investigative methods of scientific medicine. For no other form of mental disorder was there such a clear-cut correlation between mental symptoms and pathological anatomy. As Carl Wernicke remarked, each case of progressive paralysis was like a new variation on an experiment, which time and again generated lesions that psychiatrists could examine in great detail in post-mortem investigations.[126] Progressive paralysis fit the disease concepts of somatic medicine especially well and proved to be a most fruitful source of scientific investigation. It therefore came to comprise the new "hub of theoretical psychiatry."[127] Of seminal importance in this respect was the work of Griesinger's successor in Berlin, Carl Westphal, who was a neuropathological expert on tabes and progressive paralysis. Prior to his research, it was generally believed that paralysis was caused either by an infection of the brain or by an infection in combination with hyperaemia.[128] Westphal demonstrated, however, that the process of paralysis belonged essentially to the diseases of the spinal cord.[129] As a result of this and other research—which Westphal explicitly attributed to microscopic inquiry—he helped significantly to advance Griesinger's unity of psychiatry and neurology and his reflexive model of mental activity. As Otto Binswanger (Westphal's own son-in-law and professor of psychiatry in Jena) remarked, dementia paralytica was a brace that inseparably connected psychiatry to neuropathology.[130]

Furthermore, the very distinctiveness of the disorder undercut traditional psychiatric assumptions. Progressive paralysis was characterized by a unique course, a great number of clearly identifiable symptoms, and a well defined prognosis. In other words, it appeared to represent a disease entity in its own right. As such, it undercut the concept of a "unitary psychosis" that had characterized mid-century thinking on insanity and that had implied that the multitude of psychiatric symptoms were merely specific and individual manifestations of but one disease entity.[131] It appeared impossible to accommodate progressive paralysis within the nosological strictures of this unitary psychosis. Progressive paralysis therefore helped to reorient psychiatry away from the anthropological assumptions about individual specificity and toward a universalist, ontological concept of mental disease. The attention of psychiatrists was shifting from the individual patient to disease entities.

Valuable as it was for psychiatric theory, progressive paralysis also harbored other professional advantages. It was seen to be chiefly a disease of the upper and middle classes. Griesinger had found it to be more prevalent in the commercial and educated circles: businessmen, artists, scholars, officers, and public servants were all more likely than other groups to be afflicted.[132] These individuals comprised a relatively more accessible and financially solvent group of patients outside the asylum-dominated system of public care. Attracting them with appeals to scientific medicine could bring advantages to the clinic and potentially to the private practices of their directors as well. There were also clinical advantages to attracting such patients, because psychiatrists found it easier to extract anamnestic information. Since most were deemed to come from stable households, there were relatives at hand who could speak to the course of the illness and to the patient's hereditary disposition.[133] Psychiatrists could thus obtain a better overall clinical picture of the patient. Thus paralytics and their relatives became attractive targets of psychiatric intervention—targets to which academic psychiatrists could pitch their claims to expertise and anticipate that those claims would receive a sympathetic hearing.

Significantly, progressive paralysis also helped secure the approbation of the military and the state. For the disease was not only seen as the "disease of the century" afflicting the well-to-do, but also a predominantly male disorder associated with the sexual mores of the period and of great concern to the aristocratic military caste.[134] It was to these very concerns that Carl Westphal spoke in a survey of his discipline delivered to military physicians in 1880.[135] According to Westphal, among the ranks of military officers, progressive paralysis represented one of the most common forms of mental disease. While an officer's deep sense of duty might be able to withstand the buffets of the early phases of the disease and enable him to continue his work, ultimately, if the disease remained undiagnosed, mental collapse was inevitable. "It is an astonishing and incredibly sad spectacle the watch how an excellent man, mustering his last reserves, fulfills his duty to the very end before then collapsing and . . . falling precipitously into the depths of mental infirmity! Just how important the task of early recognition of such diseases by psychiatrically trained military doctors is for officers, for the army, and for the fatherland in times of peace and of war is self-evident. Fortunately, in this regard the army can place its full trust in its physicians."[136] Westphal thus spoke to some of the deepest fears of his audience: he painted a picture of physical collapse for men who placed a premium on self-discipline and composure. But he also assuaged those fears by casting psychiatrists as saviors of the officer corps, the army, and indeed the entire fatherland.

Against the backdrop of the Charité's responsibility for training military physicians, such arguments packed considerable persuasive force and did not go unheard in Prussian ministries. As early as 1872, the army medical office had taken steps to ensure that medical recruits in the Prussian army received instruction in psychiatry. According to an agreement between Westphal and the Friedrich-Wilhelm-Institute (or *Pepinière*), where military physicians were trained, recruits were required to visit lectures and clinical courses in psychiatry—long before civilian medical students in Prussia were required to do so.[137] And later, in a position paper of 1889, Friedrich Althoff singled out Westphal's work on progressive paralysis as justification for maintaining the linkage between the Charité's neurological and psychiatric clinics.[138] Thus, on the clinical wards of the university of Berlin, where so often trends for other Prussian universities were set, the potential military benefits of research in progressive paralysis seem to have helped stabilize the institutional linkage of psychiatry and neuropathology.

Psychiatrists also profited in various ways from closer relations with the military. The wars of German unification, especially the Franco-Prussian War of 1870/71, had been a windfall of some importance for the profession. The wars gave psychiatrists the opportunity to package their professional work in terms of a contribution to the task of nation-building. The wars reinforced perceptions of the profession's national utility among both the general public and state officials.[139] In particular, deficiencies in recruitment experienced during the war sparked efforts in the 1870s to improve the standing of psychiatry within the military's medical administration.[140] Sometimes military doctors were actively sought out by clinic directors, both because they provided some respite to overburdened medical staff and because they represented a relatively cheap source of otherwise scarce medical labor.[141] Psychiatrists also found therapeutic benefits accruing to their institutions thanks to the war effort. In assessing the impact of the lazarettes which had been erected in many psychiatric hospitals, one observer concluded that they had had no adverse effect on the patient population. On the contrary, the psychological impact of the lazarettes had "made some improvements possible, which would have been more difficult to achieve in peace time."[142] Finally, the war also advanced the interests of psychiatric science, for it had delivered up a wealth of clinical "material" which significantly "enriched" psychiatric research.[143]

Eduard Hitzig's Electrophysiology

One neuropathologist whose research profited directly from the German war effort was Eduard Hitzig. Hitzig was born in Berlin and studied medicine both there and in Würzburg.[144] In Berlin he heard the lectures of Romberg, Westphal, Du Bois-Reymond, Virchow and others before completing his medical degree in 1862 and his *Habilitation* in 1872. During the wars of 1866 and 1870 Hitzig served as a military physician in lazarettes in Berlin and Nancy. Following the wars, he worked in Berlin until 1875 when he was appointed full professor and director of the Swiss asylum Burghölzli near Zürich. In 1879 he accepted a professorship in Halle, where he was simultaneously director of the asylum of Nietleben until 1885. After the wholesale collapse of his relationship with the government of the Prussian province of Saxony, Hitzig spearheaded the construction of the first Prussian psychiatric clinic in Halle. The clinic was initially constructed in temporary quarters and after 1891 was housed in a newly built clinical edifice. Hitzig remained director of the clinic in Halle until blindness forced him into retirement in 1903.

Few psychiatrists were as well connected in the Berlin establishment as Hitzig was. His grandfather had been a prominent criminologist and publicist in Berlin. Hitzig's father had been a no less influential architect who had designed such evocative monuments to the prowess of the German middle classes as the Imperial Bank, the Stock Exchange, and the Technical University. His wife was the niece of the historian Leopold von Ranke and daughter of the theologian Ernst Ranke. Hitzig himself became one of a very small handful of German academics to enjoy a closer personal relationship with the powerful ministerial director Friedrich Althoff, becoming both his personal physician and confidant in psychiatric affairs.[145] Hitzig was a member and officer in numerous national and international professional organizations. Put succinctly, from the mid-1880s until his retirement in 1903 Hitzig was likely the most in-fluential and powerful psychiatrist in all of Germany.

Hitzig may have been well connected, but he was certainly not an especially well-liked man. He was variously described as having had an "abrasive and re-served character" and as being "an egotist and autocrat through and through," pugnacious with a bitingly sarcastic sense of humor.[146] He had few friends among his medical colleagues and his scientific enemies became the ob-jects of ruthless and unremitting attack.[147] His relations with hospital person-nel in Burghölzli in the late 1870s had been terrible, and when he left the asy-lum Nietleben in 1885 his departure was hailed by hospital staff as a "liberation."[148] Both his first and second assistants at the provisional clinic in Halle quit in unison, and he was unable to find anyone willing to fill the third position, thus leaving the clinic altogether bereft of medical personnel.[149] He was so feared by students in Halle that many of them fled to study at the neighboring University of Leipzig.[150] And finally, the careers of young aca-demics who didn't enjoy his favor were in acute peril; and anti-vivisectionists in Zürich can, without exaggeration, be said to have hated his guts.[151]

Disliked though he may have been, the work which Hitzig had conducted together with Gustav Fritsch in Berlin in the first half of the 1870s represented a revolution in cerebral physiology.[152] Prior to their research, physiologists such as Pierre Flourens had assumed that different mental functions were not localized in specific regions of the brain.[153] Rather, Flourens maintained that the work of the brain was distributed evenly throughout the cerebrum and that each portion of the brain contributed equally toward mental activities such as sensation, volition, or motor functions. In other words, the brain was not com-prised of a collection of different functional components, but instead was an equipotential physiological unity. During the 1860s this interpretation had been called into question by a number of clinical studies. Most prominent among these was the work of Pierre Paul Broca, who had linked motor apha-sia to the destruction of specific regions of the brain. In addition, Theodor Meynert's morphological studies had traced muscle activity to neural path-ways in the brain.

Hitzig and Fritsch had also begun seriously to question Flourens's findings. Their laboratory research on dogs and rabbits gave the still tentative research of their colleagues explicit and reproducible experimental verification. Their work involved the electrical stimulation and extirpation of different regions of the canine brain. They found that electrical stimuli applied to specific regions of the cerebral cortex produced movement in corresponding muscle groups, whereas stimulation of other regions produced no such movement. Further-more, they found that removing sections of the brain disrupted corresponding muscle function. From these experiments they concluded that, contrary to es-tablished scientific opinion, mental functions could be localized in well circumscribed anatomic regions of the brain.[154] Hitzig and Fritsch attributed the success of these experiments to their use of new scientific methods. As they saw it, their experimental approach and use of electrical stimulation had generated new results inaccessible to their predecessors.[155]

Their success also hinged on important medical and theoretical implications of their research for the psychiatric profession. The assertion that brain function was localized seemed to provide plausible explanations of a variety of disorders, including epilepsy as well as motor and speech dysfunctions. Hitzig's work paved the way for future brain research and marked the beginnings of neurosurgery in Berlin and Halle in the 1880s.[156] Coinciding roughly with Kahlbaum's nosological critique as well as his clinical work on catatonia and Hecker's work on hebephrenia, Hitzig's work also helped promote research into discrete disease entities.[157] Most importantly, however, his research seemed to provide the first strong and timely experimental verification of Griesinger's own assumptions about cerebral localization. His and other findings (especially Wernicke's work on aphasia) provided strong confirmation that mental disease was, in fact, as Griesinger had postulated, brain disease. It was hardly surprising, therefore, that Hitzig wasted no time in pointing out the correspondence between his and Griesinger's findings.[158]

Finally, their research had also profited directly from their electrotherapeutic practice on humans during the war. By their own account, Hitzig and Fritsch had come to question Flourens's findings based on their observation of muscular spasms produced in humans during electrotherapy.[159] Both Hitzig and Fritsch were only too aware of the limits of animal experimentation and of the need to extrapolate their findings to human patients.[160] To these ends, they took advantage of the German wars of unification to conduct experiments on wounded soldiers. In fact, the Austro-Prussian and Franco-German wars of 1866 and 1870/71 became most propitious events for their research. The soldiers lying on the wards of the lazarettes in Berlin and Nancy provided them the opportunity to extend and corroborate their experimental work.[161]

Hitzig drew on these wartime experiences for the publication of a major article in Emil Du Bois-Reymond's journal *Archiv für Anatomie, Physiologie und wissenschaftliche Medizin* in 1871.[162] There he investigated the influence of electrical stimuli to the head on motor activity and coordination. In his study, Hitzig found that applying electricity to certain areas of the head resulted in involuntary movement of the person's muscles and eyes. After observing this phenomenon in humans, Hitzig was eager to duplicate his finding in animals and to locate the exact site at which observed symptoms could be reproduced. This he did in a paper delivered to the Berlin Medical Society in a lecture on 3 July 1872 in which he found that his experiments with rabbits correlated exactly with his electrical stimulation of human patients. A few months after Hitzig's address in Berlin, he also delivered a paper to the GDNÄ in Leipzig on the value of electrical therapy.[163]

While Hitzig was presenting these results to his colleagues, he was also working to secure control over a group of patients in the Charité that he hoped would help him to advance his experimental research in physiology. In the summer of 1872, just after he had addressed the Berlin Medical Society, Hitzig petitioned the Ministry of Education to allow him to set up his own ward within Theodor Frerichs's Charité clinic for internal medicine.[164] On that ward, Hitzig proposed to engage in the electro-therapeutic treatment of patients. He took pains to justify his request by pointing to the great resonance that his recent research publications had enjoyed. Unfortunately, he remarked, it had been "utterly impossible" to draw on autopsies in order to verify his research findings.[165] Hitzig thus saw access to the patients on Frerichs's wards as an opportunity to confirm his research findings through post-mortem examinations. Initially, the Ministry of Education had no objection to Hitzig's proposal and granted it conditional approval.[166]

It was not until early 1873 that Westphal learned of Hitzig's intentions and that the ministry had approved them. This prompted him to submit a petition of his own that enjoyed the support of the dean of the medical faculty, Rudolf Virchow.[167] Westphal appealed to his superiors to rescind their approval of Hitzig's ward on the grounds that it "fundamentally called into question" the Charité's neurological clinic and would be tantamount to establishing a second neurological ward. He pointed out that a full complement of electro-therapeutic instruments already existed in his neurological clinic and that any new ward was therefore both unnecessary and a potential competitor to his own facilities. It would fragment the amount of "material" admitted to his ward and compromise both research and teaching. In Westphal's eyes electrotherapy was one useful instrument of therapeutic intervention, but it was not so important as to warrant the construction of a ward designed specifically to provide for it.

The ministerial response to this dispute favored Carl Westphal. In deference to Westphal's neurological ward, Hitzig's application was rescinded.[168] No record survives of Hitzig's response to this rebuff. Nevertheless, it was clear that if he wished to pursue his research in Berlin, he faced considerable opposition from Westphal's neurological clinic. Indeed, in 1874 Hitzig's research on aphasia came under sharp attack from Westphal, who cast doubt on his postulate of a speech center in the brain[169]. Such opposition dissipated any prospects that he may have had in Berlin and was most likely instrumental in prompting a shift in his career path in the mid-1870s. Hitzig had long striven for a position in internal medicine, yet he lacked the general training needed for him to assume such a post.[170] Hence, at a rather late stage in his academic career, this cerebral physiologist somewhat reluctantly turned his undivided attention to psychiatry where he hoped to continue his experimental work with relative impunity. Hitzig became a psychiatrist not because of any alienist inclinations on his part, but rather because it now held out greater career prospects for a young, overly specialized internist with research ambitions in experimental physiology. In his own career path, Hitzig mirrored the influx of experimental physiology into psychiatry in the 1870s and 1880s.

Following stints of service as the director of the asylums Burghölzli and Nietleben, Eduard Hitzig went on to found the first truly independent Prussian psychiatric clinic in Halle in 1891.[171] The clinic evolved out of acerbic disputes with the government of the Prussian province of Saxony in the early 1880s. The feuds centered on Hitzig's control over the admission and dismissal of patients in the Nietleben asylum. It began as a dispute over clinical training and ultimately led to the collapse of the contractual arrangement between the province and the university and the construction first of a provisional clinic in 1885 and then of a full-blown psychiatric clinic in 1891.[172] In orchestrating the construction of the new clinic, Hitzig had worked in close cooperation with Friedrich Althoff in the Ministry of Education. It was Althoff's industrious persistence over the better part of a decade and his skills in political horse-trading that ultimately overcame many of the political obstacles standing in the way of the new clinic.

Upon opening in 1891, Halle became the first psychiatric hospital in Prussia to be financed and built solely by the Prussian ministry of education for the express purpose of psychiatric research and education.[173] In other words, Halle represented a major shift in policy on the part of the Prussian government. Whereas prior to 1885 the Prussian government had relied chiefly on existing mental asylums to provide clinical instruction in psychiatry, the clinic in Halle was a bellwether signaling the government's ultimate intent to construct psychiatric clinics at all Prussian universities. In addition, the clinic in Halle was the first administratively autonomous psychiatric hospital in Prussia to combine psychiatric and neuropathological wards.[174] Consequently, the government's new policy held out not only the prospect of new clinics at other universities, but also the assurance that those clinics would be built (in the tradition of Griesinger) with a strong neuropathological orientation. As the expression of the Prussian government's new policy on psychiatric education, Halle therefore represented the academic institutionalization of psychiatry at the height of neuropathological influence within the profession.

The significance of this policy shift was not lost upon Eduard Hitzig. In his address at the clinic's opening ceremony on 29 April 1891, he noted that the clinic's construction had resolved a fundamental "question of principle" and ushered in a "new era of academic instruction in neuropathology."[175] Perhaps more so than other psychiatrists, Hitzig could appreciate the significance of the new clinic. For he had been witness to academic psychiatry's precarious footing not only in relation to provincial governments but also within the academic community itself. In fact, just as the clinic in Halle was being built another dispute erupted in Berlin pitting psychiatrists and internists against one another. In his address, Hitzig made oblique reference to this dispute, which had cast a dark shadow over the construction project in Halle.[176] But what had been the cause of renewed tensions between internists and neuropathologists in Berlin? A look at developments there in the 1870s and 1880s sheds light on the jurisdictional wrangling over one of the essential preconditions of laboratory research in psychiatry, namely, over psychiatric cadavers.

The Politics of the Psychiatric Cadaver

The disputes in Berlin had been unleashed by the impending death of Griesinger's successor in Berlin, Carl Westphal.[177] Westphal had been Griesinger's assistant in the mid-1860s. After 1868 he headed the psychiatric and neurological wards, initially as a professor extraordinary and after 1874 as a full professor. Westphal's passing opened a strategic window of opportunity for internists. When the medical faculty was queried by the ministry of education about Westphal's incapacitation, rather then recommending a replacement, it called into question the entire arrangement that had joined the chair in psychiatry with the neurological ward. That arrangement, established for the first time in Germany with Griesinger's call to Berlin in 1865, had continued under Westphal throughout the 1870s and 1880s. But with Westphal's departure it came under direct assault from the medical faculty. The faculty was of the "unanimous opinion that the continued existence of a special clinic for nervous diseases would not benefit, but rather damage the entirety of medical education."[178] For years, they claimed, their clinics had suffered from a shortage of patients suitable to clinical instruction. Were the clinic for nervous diseases to be dismantled, then both the quality and quantity of clinical patients on their wards would improve and students would be able to complete their studies in the "*entire* field of internal medicine" much more quickly.[179] Hence, the medical faculty appealed for the neurological clinic to be dissolved and for its admission day to be transferred to the two medical clinics. With that, Griesinger's entire project of joining psychiatric and nervous disorders came under attack. What a quarter century earlier had been heralded as a milestone on psychiatry's path to an exacting medical science, was now being called into question.

The medical faculty in Berlin marshaled a number of arguments in support of its position. In essence, they all aimed at strengthening the standing of the university's two clinics for internal medicine. For one, many of the patients who were admitted to the neurological ward suffered from other diseases which, by implication, the neurological ward was not equipped adequately to handle. In addition, the fields of psychiatry and neurology had become so extensive that no single individual could reasonably be expected to master both specialties. Furthermore, at a time when demands on students were growing, a clinic for nervous diseases only contributed to the further fragmentation of their studies. Dismantling that clinic would help in concentrating the curriculum and counteracting the centrifugal forces of specialization. Most important of all, however, the medical clinics had lost large numbers of patients to the neurological ward. As a result, it had become increasingly difficult for them to cover the entire field of internal medicine. To the extent that the capacity to demonstrate the full range of diseases of the nervous system had been compromised, clinical instruction in internal medicine was inadequate.

Internists' concerns about patient volumes had been fed by the rapidly rising number of patients on Westphal's wards. Apart from demographic growth, that increase had been facilitated by a number of factors. First, Carl Westphal had petitioned for and obtained a polyclinic for neurological patients in the Charité in 1871.[180] He had argued for the polyclinic on the grounds that the costs would be minimal because the patients it admitted would be treated with electricity rather than with drugs.[181] In addition, he had appealed for the polyclinic with the express intent of expanding the number of patients on the neurological ward. He hoped that the polyclinic would both hike patient frequency on the ward and alleviate the lopsided predominance of chronic cases by admitting more curable patients. To these ends he sought and obtained permission to hold polyclinical office hours three days a week.[182] Polyclinical office hours would allow not only access to milder cases, but also facilitate admissions to the neurological and psychiatric wards.

The potential of for such office hours to increase admissions was related to the complex procedure governing patient distribution within the Charité. There, different clinicians controlled the placement of new patients on different days of the week.[183] That is, clinicians were assigned specific days on which they had first choice of patients admitted to the Charité. Upon arriving in Berlin in 1865, for example, Griesinger had entered into negotiations on this issue with the head of the clinic for internal medicine, Theodor Frerichs. The agreement that they reached saw Griesinger receiving priority over all neurological cases admitted on Saturdays.[184] Within the context of such arrangements, the advantage of polyclinical office hours lay in the fact that patients could be counseled in advance of their admission. Prospective patients who might otherwise have sought admission on any given day, could now be advised to seek admission on those specific days when Westphal had priority over the placement of neurological admissions. In this way, Westphal could use the polyclinic as a mechanism for steering admissions onto the psychiatric and neurological wards; pre-admission counseling could and did shape post-admission distribution. In the case of Westphal's polyclinic, this was done at the expense of the other two clinics for internal medicine.

Internists' worries were, secondly, exacerbated by the construction of the asylum Dalldorf on the northern outskirts of Berlin in 1880 and the subsequent closure of the city's custodial asylum (*Verpflegungsanstalt*). Dalldorf's construction prompted an administrative about-face on the part of the city. Motivated by the logistical difficulties of transporting patients to Dalldorf's distant locale, the city now needed a psychiatric hospital in the heart of Berlin. Hence, magistrates were now prepared to see the Charité serve as a forward "transit and ob-servation station" for both curable patients and for those ultimately destined for Dalldorf.[185] Having served for over fifteen years as mostly an appendage to the city's own *Verpflegungsanstalt,* after 1880 the Charité mirrored more closely Griesinger's model of an urban asylum in becoming the city's foremost psychiatric receptacle. As a result, and much to the chagrin of internists, after 1880 admissions to the psychiatric ward of the Charité rocketed.[186]

Thirdly and most importantly in the present context, even before Dalldorf opened, Westphal had been avidly working to increase the patient frequency on his ward. Esse's insistence on complete documentation had from the early 1860s prompted the city to use its own institution, rather than the Charité, as its receptacle of first resort. As a result, psychiatric admissions had fallen off rapidly.[187] Westphal complained openly and vociferously in the early 1870s about the depopulation of the psychiatric ward and delivered a battery of sta-tistics to back up his claim. He hoped to improve the situation by entering into new negotiations with the city officials in order to restore the psychiatric ward's status as a curative institution that admitted patients directly, rather than through the *Verpflegungsanstalt.* Ultimately, however, these initial efforts were for naught. Westphal was forced into retreat after city officials rebuffed his suggestions and the Charité administration responded with strong counter-arguments.[188] Finding the city unwilling to admit patients directly to the more expensive Charité and the administration equally unwilling to lower its rates, Westphal resorted to an alternative strategy.

That strategy involved having beds subsidized by the university in the form of so-called "free beds" or *Freistellen.* Westphal's strategy was given added force when in the midst of these debates, in the spring of 1874, he was offered a chair in psychiatry in Leipzig.[189] Westphal tried to exploit this offer to his ad-vantage in negotiations with the Ministry of Education in Berlin, but he was unsuccessful in extracting a firm ministerial commitment for the construction of a new clinic.[190] However, in the negotiations he demanded and ultimately received assurances that "free beds" would be introduced.[191] The great advan-tage of such subsidies was that Westphal would be able to attract and retain more patients in his wards by underbidding other forms of institutional care. State subsidies would allow his more expensive clinical wards to compete with the city's *Verpflegungsanstalt* and other private or provincial institutions.

By the same token, however, subsidized beds on the psychiatric or neuro-logical wards also competed with other clinical wards within the Charité itself, in particular with the two clinics for internal medicine. Hence, Westphal's plans were adamantly opposed by Frerichs.[192] Yet in spite of Frerichs's objec-tions and some foot-dragging by the hospital administration, Westphal achieved at least part of his aims: in early 1875 the ministry agreed to fund a total sixteen beds, eight each on the neurological and psychiatric wards.[193] The free beds were intended to serve the needs of psychiatric research and not simply clinical education. For that reason they were budgeted as expenses for "scientific purposes" and accompanied by additional funds for instruments and other research equipment.[194]

Most importantly, however, Westphal's success further exacerbated internists' concerns about their supply of cadavers. They had watched in dismay during the 1870s as the number of available cadavers fell from year to year.[195] The causes of this decline were related to the expansion of the city's own hospital system, most notably the opening of the hospitals in Friedrichhein and Moabit. These new hospitals began to compete with the Charité and syphon off many of its traditional patients. Above all the new hospital in Moabit was a thorn in the side of the medical faculty: its very proximity had done much to deprive the Charité of its "natural constituency" of patients. Not only did the new hospitals provide cheaper care, but they also focused on the treatment of less expensive so-called "internal patients," while leaving the Charité to tend to the more expensive "external patients" who it was contractually obliged to admit. Consequently, the city advised its doctors to have these choice patients admitted to city institutions rather than to the Charité.

To add to the woes of the medical faculty, ever fewer Charité patients were dying.[196] While the Charité administration greeted this decline in mortality as good news, the medical faculty was full of apprehension about the acute shortage of cadavers for research and clinical instruction. It disputed the claims of the Charité directorate and of the Ministry of Culture that the decline in deaths could be attributed to the introduction of anti-septic methods in 1872 or to fewer cases of puerperal fever and typhus.[197] Nor could improvements in the therapeutic techniques of internal medicine in any way explain the decline in deaths. On the contrary, "none of the members of the faculty involved in medical care believed that progress in internal therapy since 1872" could explain the decline in deaths. Instead, the decline in the number of cadavers was attributed to competition for patients from city hospitals. The medical faculty therefore called for negotiations with the city to alleviate the shortage of cadavers and expand the number of state subsidized hospital beds.[198]

Free beds were extremely valuable for laboratory researchers in neuropathology. They enabled psychiatrists to attract and retain patients who they deemed to be of scientific interest. They freed them from the whims of penny-pinching communities that could have their terminal patients placed in other, less expensive institutions. In effect, they served as a kind of "death row" for patients. Here, at last, was an administrative mechanism that helped academic psychiatrists retain control over patients from whom they hoped to obtain valuable neuropathological specimens.

These and other similar arrangements were common at psychiatric clinics throughout Germany. The clinics in both Würzburg and Giessen had such beds.[199] In Leipzig they were deemed an important source of corpses and designed to bind terminal patients to the hospital.[200] So eager was the director of the Leipzig clinic, Paul Flechsig, to secure a reliable source of anatomic material that he has been reputed to have pursued an outright "cadaver policy [*Politik der Leichen*]."[201] That policy combined free beds with stipulations preventing the evacuation of terminal patients so that additional autopsy material might be acquired.[202] The same policy was adopted by Otto Binswanger at the clinic in Jena. There, in the interest of obtaining more interesting pathoanatomic "material," Binswanger incurred significantly higher mortality rates in his clinic by refusing to discharge paralytic patients to the asylum in Blankenhain. Eduard Hitzig too, in his outline of the new psychiatric clinic in Halle, insisted that "it was necessary to conserve a number of cases until they have died so that students can become familiar with the anatomic nature of the given disease processes . . . .[And] a small number of beds is absolutely necessary in order to continue the [clinical] observations until the disease has run its deadly course and to confirm the anatomic basis of the [patient's] suffering."[203] In other cities, clinics regulated access to cadavers through contractual arrangements. In Munich an agreement was drawn up between the psychiatric clinic and the institute of pathology governing the procedures to be followed for all psychiatric autopsies.[204] The contract stipulated acceptable locations for the autopsies, laid out the respective jurisdictions over various body parts, and set down proper procedures of documentation.

All of these arrangements involved institutional, financial, and legal mechanisms that regulated access to cadavers and thereby formalized professional jurisdictions over the conditions of laboratory research work in psychiatry. Free beds, delayed dismissal, and formal contractual agreements were all part of a negotiated politics of the psychiatric cadaver through which academic psychiatrists attempted to secure and enhance their control over laboratory work.

The Berlin medical faculty's appeal for the dissolution of the neurological ward in the Charité left Prussian officials decidedly unimpressed. As a marginal note on the submission of the medical faculty makes clear, officials in the Ministry of Education were skeptical of the faculty's intentions. They suspected that the faculty was attempting to split off the neurological ward in order to create a third university clinic for internal medicine.[205] In the wake of the medical faculty's request, Friedrich Althoff turned to his most trusted advisor on psychiatric issues, Eduard Hitzig, and requested his expert opinion. This Hitzig provided in an extensive "Report on the question of linking academic education in psychiatry and neuropathology at Prussian Universities."[206] In a biting and at times sarcastic critique of the medical faculty's position, Hitzig strongly supported the union of psychiatric and neurological clinics at the Charité. No sooner had Hitzig submitted his report, than the medical faculty's petition was rejected.[207] Hitzig's report almost certainly prevented the Berlin medical faculty from cannibalizing not only the neurological ward, but also Wilhelm Griesinger's legacy.

The episodes involving Eduard Hitzig and Carl Westphal are instructive for what they tell us about psychiatric work in university clinics and about the professionalization of German psychiatry in the 1870s and 1880s. Both Hitzig's failure to establish an electro-therapeutic ward and Westphal's success in securing *Freistellen* for his neurological and psychiatric wards signal that ministerial and institutional support for brain research in Prussia was clearly passing from internal medicine to psychiatry. Academic psychiatrists were gaining greater access to the patients and cadavers they sought and were thereby, also securing their jurisdiction over laboratory research. The founding of the psychiatric clinic in Halle and the successful rebuff of the Berlin internists' challenge both represented strong reaffirmation and institutional solidification of Griesinger's project, combining neurology and psychiatry at Prussian universities.

At the same time, however, the experiences of Griesinger and Westphal in Berlin illustrate the very real difficulties which academic psychiatrists faced in optimizing conditions of psychiatric research. Decisions taken by internists, administrators, and civic officials all had profound effects on the clinic's economy of power and knowledge. That the Charité's psychiatric ward had first been Berlin's premiere receptacle for the mad, then after 1862 an appendage to the work house, only to again become its primary admitting hospital after 1880 illustrates how unstable, fractured, and discontinuous its economy was within larger systems of hospital administration and civic health care.[208] Similarly, the attack on Griesinger's legacy demonstrates how, within the polycratic structures of the hospital, those economies could become the objects of negotiation and contestation between rival factions.

Thus, in the Charité and elsewhere, the psychiatric clinic never attained the kind of panoptic utopia so lucidly described by Michel Foucault. Its economy was far more contingent upon neighboring institutions and professional groups. Far from being under the direct control of academic practitioners, psychiatric research was embedded in a politically negotiated institutional order and at times subject to uncontrollable third party decisions. As effective as its disciplinary mechanisms could be when brought to bear on its own populations, within larger systems of medical and psychiatric care the clinic's situation remained precarious.

CHAPTER 5

Bedside Science: Clinical Research in Heidelberg

Introduction

Of all the qualities that good psychiatric researchers necessarily possessed, none were thought more important than their visual faculties. The "opportunity to see and to observe exactly and repeatedly" was for Friedrich Nasse an essential precondition of medical training in psychiatry.[1] More important than empathy, good will, or a dispassionate demeanor was the alienist's "incisive gaze [*durchdringender Blick*] that unconsciously separated essential from inessential [symptoms] and that easily and assuredly penetrated to the core of things without the need for exhaustive research."[2] More so than for other medical specialists, it was imperative that psychiatrists "learn to see" correctly.[3] They required "instruction in observing" to sharpen their senses and to "look and listen attentively."[4] The highest laws of medical science would reveal themselves not through words or hypotheses, but through observation.

Most practicing psychiatrists in the latter half of the century, alienists as well as academics, held common inductive assumptions about the methods of their clinical research.[5] Their empiricist exhortations differed markedly from the deductive approaches of many earlier nineteenth-century psychiatrists. For men such as Dietrich Georg Kieser, still steeped in the teachings of natural philosophy, clinical observation had served wholly different aims. For Kieser clinical observation was merely an exhibition of divine natural law and a touchstone for the veracity of theoretical statements.[6] By contrast, latter nineteenth-century psychiatrists commonly believed inductive methods to be the means of arriving at, not merely verifying, scientific truth. On this point there was little to distinguish one psychiatric professional from another. In his opening clinical lecture in Berlin, Griesinger's advice to students was unabashedly empirical and could be applauded by all factions within his profession. "In the hours we will spend together don't hesitate to give yourself up to the guidance of facts. Let us investigate only that which really exists in nature; let us not always think of all sorts of applications. These will come to us if we only first learn to see correctly."[7]

In addition to learning to see correctly, it was equally important that psychiatrists see the right phenomena and especially that they see a lot of them.

For psychiatrists increasingly inclined toward positivist sentiments, quantity became a guarantor of both precision and objectivity in clinical research. Studies based on a small number of patients, or even on individual cases, were prone to inaccuracies. Reasoning along typically statistical lines, psychiatrists saw studies that drew on observations of a large pool of patients as one of the only means to escape the pitfalls of subjectivity. Tempering one's capacity to recognize nervous diseases demanded that one "see a lot."[8]

Alienists such as Laehr, Damerow, and Solbrig had long maintained that the conditions for correct and ample clinical observation were given only in the asylums. Many of their arguments advocating university clinics within asylum walls were premised on the assumption that clinical investigation could flourish only with recourse to asylum populations. The ability of alienists to observe psychiatric patients in large numbers had been the foundation of their status within the profession and their claims to perform the work of clinical research.

But, as we have seen in chapter 3, Griesinger called these assumptions into question. To recapitulate his argument as it pertained to clinical research, Griesinger believed that overcrowded asylums prevented alienists from seeing the important early phases of psychiatric disorders; alienists were instead disproportionately exposed to later, chronic stages. Overcrowding had also encouraged the application of mechanical restraints which contributed not only to the neglect of patients but also to distortions in the natural expression of patients' symptoms. Likewise, Griesinger's maxim that mental disease was brain disease helped to dislodge the claim that the asylum (as opposed to, say, the family home or the urban hospital) was the only space in which it was possible to observe uncorrupted symptoms. To the extent that mental disease was reinterpreted in terms of biological as opposed to environmental causes, the space in which mental symptoms were observed became increasingly irrelevant. Symptoms exhibited by organic diseases were less likely to vary with the patient's surroundings and could be observed anywhere, not just in the idealized environs of the rural asylum. Most importantly, if clinical research was to overcome the obstacles which its relegation to the asylums had imposed, then patient observation had to be more rigorous, systematic, and extensive. Disciplined observation became the hallmark of clinical research in university psychiatric hospitals and formed the basis of academic claims to scientific and professional legitimacy.[9] All of these arguments undermined the assumptions and empirical methods of clinical research in the asylums. Griesinger's urban asylum was an attempt to alleviate these deficiencies in clinical observation and it augured a fundamental shift in what constituted adequate conditions of clinical research.

The following chapter is an analysis of some of the institutional techniques and administrative mechanisms—in short the disciplinary economy—that academic psychiatrists deployed in order to enhance their abilities to conduct clinical research and to bolster their claims to this professional task. The chapter will consider first the waning predominance of pathological anatomy within academic psychiatry and then the resurgent interest in clinical research dating from the 1880s. Thereafter, it will assess some of the institutional characteristics of university clinics that distinguished them as centers of clinical research, including their techniques of diagnostic examination, hierarchies of observation, and surveillance wards. Finally, the case of Heidelberg's clinic in the 1890s will be used to illustrate how clinical research was influenced by extraclinical constraints. By means of analyzing the work of Germany's most prominent and influential psychiatric clinician, Emil Kraepelin, this chapter will consider how academics tried to extend clinical discipline beyond the clinic itself and to subdue the administrative environment in which they operated to the benefit of their research objectives. Kraepelin's clinic will be considered in an effort to illustrate just how intertwined research and day-to-day clinical practice were and how his seminal differentiation of the endogenous psychoses into schizophrenic and manic depressive forms emerged within the local circumstances of the Heidelberg clinic.

Neuropathology in Retreat

At the close of the century, a number of critics of neuropathology emerged within the ranks of the profession to add their voice to longer-standing alienist objections. As the fruits of anatomical research turned out to be less than originally expected, opponents from a variety of quarters began to voice their concerns more confidently. These critics believed that the somatic dominance within the profession had had a number of detrimental consequences.[10] The potential of anatomical research had been decidedly overestimated and as a result researchers had fallen victim to speculative interpretations of their laboratory results. Here the work of Theodor Meynert and Paul Flechsig stood for the over-extension of anatomical and physiological theories into the realm of what critics described as "brain mythology." The spectacular early successes of the 1860s and 1870s had not been added to in the 1880s. Research had stagnated in what had become an era of abstract theories and schematic models of brain function in which researchers appeared to take little notice of alternative theories or of contradictory evidence.[11] Such developments prompted skeptics such as Konrad Rieger in Würzburg to question altogether the usefulness of the anatomist's microscopic research.[12] Meanwhile, Paul Julius Möbius proclaimed that experiments (or, in his words, "laboratory games") had never generated any new discoveries.[13]

The enthusiasm and confidence of early laboratory psychiatrists were further dampened, because neuropathologists became entangled in their own intractable theoretical disputes in the 1890s. The same new methods of staining microscopic specimens, which had invigorated research in the early 1880s, contributed to a heated controversy among neuropathologists after 1891. The disagreements came to a head in the so-called Neuron Controversy at the annual meeting of the *Gesellschaft Deutscher Naturforscher und Ärzte* in 1893. The theoretical positions in the debate became articles of "neurological faith" and put researchers at loggerheads with one another for over two decades.[14]

The limited therapeutic applications of laboratory research work also spawned resignation and prompted many young researchers to turn their attention to hypnosis or neurology. Throughout the 1880s hypnosis became all the rage not only in the general public, but among young psychiatrists such as Sigmund Freud, Emil Kraepelin, and August Forel. A veritable flood of literature inundated the book market as authors and publishers competed for readers' interest.[15] Hypnosis seemed to provide an alternative window on the psyche that generated immediate and spectacular results (and, obviously, it did not require patients who had already died). Moreover, this wave of enthusiasm for hypnosis was compounded by the emergence of neurology as a medical specialty. From the early 1890s onward, neurologists were becoming increasingly vocal advocates of their own professional interests. In 1891 Wilhelm Erb established the *Deutsche Zeitschrift für Nervenheilkunde*—a journal which represented nothing less than a literary shot across the bow of psychiatry at the pinnacle of its neuroanatomic prestige. In the ensuing decades, neurological specialists advanced ever more assertive claims to institutional independence and to their own chairs and clinics at German universities.[16] By 1904, Erb was battling aggressively to resist what he saw as psychiatry's hegemonic hold over neurology.[17] The efforts of Erb and the contributors to his journal culminated in an open split between neurology and psychiatry in 1907 with the founding of the *Gesellschaft Deutscher Nervenärzte*. The emergence of neurology as a medical specialty in its own right could not help but compromise the neurological foundations on which Griesinger had tried to place psychiatry and aggravate a worrisome brain-drain within the profession.

Laboratory researchers also became more aware of the very real practical limits of their own neuropathological research. Detailed microscopical analysis of the brain was an extraordinarily time-consuming task that often failed to produce any information meriting the hours spent collecting it. In a paper delivered to the *Verein deutscher Irrenärzte* in 1898, Franz Nissl argued that detailed research on individual brain specimens was of scant scientific benefit.[18] Because so little was known about wide expanses of the cerebral cortex, and because of the "colossal amount of time and energy" involved in a detailed study of a single brain, extensive research on the whole of a single specimen was ill-advised. Instead, Nissl called on his colleagues to join him in restricting their investigations to a few specific locations of the cerebral cortex.

Some researchers went still further than Nissl, abandoning neuropathological research altogether in favor of alternative strategies of brain research. For example, Martin Reichardt believed that histological studies were exorbitantly time consuming and "entirely useless" when it came to distinguishing normal and pathological brain processes.[19] Instead, he embarked on gravometric investigations of brain, arguing that the study of brain weight was far less time consuming and considerably cheaper than the microscopic research.

Still other critics responded to the anatomical and physiological preponderance of the profession by placing their confidence in the precision and rigor of experimental psychology. The experimental studies and laboratories of Gustav Fechner and Wilhelm Wundt (in Leipzig) were the common source of these endeavors. These researchers came to enjoy a particularly favorable reputation among such younger psychiatrists as Emil Kraepelin, Robert Sommer, Theodor Ziehen, Konrad Rieger, and Paul Julius Möbius.[20] All were highly critical of what they considered to be a "period of anatomic calcification" in the 1870s and 1880s.[21] They looked instead to the experimental methods of psycho-physics and tried to apply them in the realm of psychiatry. These experimental psychologists framed their work in opposition to what they saw as the meager results of pathological anatomy: what remained invisible to neuropathologists in post-mortem examinations, they hoped to discover by measuring psychological reaction times or mental aptitude in living patients.[22] All of these up-and-coming, second generation clinic directors had begun to experiment with psycho-physical methods by early 1890s, and by the end of the century their work had attained considerable prominence.[23]

One of the most influential advocates not only of Wundtian experimental psychology, but also of the clinical alternatives to pathological anatomy, was Emil Kraepelin. Kraepelin was one of the few academic psychiatrists to contest the established consensus on the fusion of psychiatry and neurology that had evolved at Prussian universities.[24] In his inaugural lecture as chair of psychiatry at the Russo-German university of Dorpat in 1887, he remarked on the state of clinical science in Germany. In his opinion, the influence of Zeller's unitary psychosis had corrupted clinical research and observation well into the 1860s. As a result, clinical research had "stagnated" and it was only the work of Ludwig Snell and others that, in the early 1870s, had revived a more unbiased clinical approach.[25] Simultaneously, Kraepelin echoed the views of his mentor Wilhelm Wundt in arguing that if researchers took psychophysical-parallelist convictions seriously, they couldn't possibly endorse Griesinger's maxim that mental diseases were brain diseases. One-sided anatomical studies could advance no claim to scientific legitimacy as long as they failed to explain "psychological functions."[26] That explanation had to be supplied by clinical investigations.

These trends point to a significant and resurgent undercurrent in German psychiatry emerging in the 1890s. As Robert Gaupp observed, while the scientific psychiatry of the 1870s and 1880s was symptomatic of attempts to establish psychiatry as a medical specialty, the psychological psychiatry of the 1890s reflected how "fundamentally different" psychiatry was from the rest of medicine.[27] Gaupp's observation again casts a light on the strategic importance of pathological anatomy and physiology in the professionalization of psychiatry. Their professional function had been to advance the discipline's medicalization and to achieve its parity with other specialties within the German system of higher education. Psychological explanations of madness (be they experimental or otherwise) had been largely eclipsed within a profession seeking approbation from general medicine. Not surprisingly, therefore, early clinic directors such as Paul Flechsig in Leipzig in the 1870s and 1880s considered experimental psychology to be of very little significance to psychiatry.[28] By the 1890s, however, the very same professional status that pathology had helped to secure, now made it easier for psychiatrists to strategically distance themselves from pathological anatomy and to employ psychological models to lay claim to new professional tasks. And if, furthermore, those models were based on experimental methods, as early Wundtian psychology was, it became that much easier to substitute anatomic with psychological explanations without jeopardizing one's scientific reputation for rigor and exactitude.

Symbolic of the relative decline in the importance of anatomy and physiology within the profession was also a subtle shift in the editorial policy of the *Archiv für Psychiatrie und Nervenkrankheiten (AfPN)* as well as the emergence of a new professional journal. The *AfPN*, founded by Griesinger in the year of his death as part of his campaign to join psychiatry and neurology, was the most influential neuropsychiatric journal in Germany prior to World War One. Following Griesinger's death, Carl Westphal had become the journal's editor and, for twenty-two years, had diligently pursued Griesinger's vision. But when Westphal died in January 1890, the duties of chief editor of the *AfPN* passed to his successor in Berlin and former director of the psychiatric clinic in Strassburg, Friedrich Jolly. Although Jolly reiterated his commitment to Griesinger's legacy, he was eager to emphasize that anatomy and physiology would never be more than auxiliary sciences to psychiatry. Jolly thus sought to redress the predominance which he believed anatomy and physiology had acquired in the discipline and to reassert psychiatry's claims to primacy. For him, ultimately, the journal's work was psychiatric in character, involving "*research on the diseases of the entire nervous system and on the development of methods for their treatment.*"[29] In future, the *AfPN* would continue to lend equal attention to both psychiatric and other illnesses. But, in a subtle reinterpretation of the journal's title, Jolly deftly reduced neurology to an appendage of psychiatry by insisting that the journal was for "Psychiatrie *und* Nervenkrankheiten."[30] Thus, the bond which Griesinger had forged between psychiatry and the anatomy and physiology of the central nervous system in order to anchor his profession in scientific medicine—the same bond which had been so effective in establishing psychiatry as an academic discipline on par with other medical specialties and clinics—was reinterpreted in the early 1890s to privilege psychiatry over neurology.

This shift was also illustrated in the publication of a new journal entitled the *Monatsschrift für Psychiatrie und Neurologie*. The first issue of the journal appeared in 1897, and it was edited by Theodore Ziehen and Carl Wernicke. Both had taken a sober and skeptical view of neuro-anatomic research during the 1870s and 1880s. In particular, they sought to deflate Paul Flechsig's preeminence in German psychiatry and to deconstruct his and other "premature schematizations based on incomplete anatomical findings."[31] In their opinion the "machine" called the human brain was so complex and the contemporary understanding of it so inadequate, that clinical experience was the only reliable guide for psychiatric science. Future progress in the discipline would depend on researchers planting themselves firmly on the "ground of clinical experience" and committing themselves to "intensive clinical observation."[32]

Back to the Bedside: Clinical Research Resurgent

One of the more glaring deficits of laboratory research was its spectacular failure to deliver on promises of a system of disease classification based upon organic etiology. Over the course of the 1870s and 1880s it had become embarrassingly obvious that hopes for a complete morphological mapping of the brain, and for an exhaustive classification of mental disease on the basis of pathological anatomy, had been seriously misplaced. In other words, pathological anatomy could not fill the nosological vacuum created by the disintegration of the concept of unitary psychosis in the late 1860s.[33] One consequence of this failure was renewed concern about the lack of a reliable classification system.[34] These concerns had never been very far below the surface of professional life, but in the 1870s they acquired added urgency, especially in the face of professional disagreement over the statistical categories to be used in the census reports of the Imperial Bureau of Statistics. Compared with other branches of medicine, psychiatry's system of disease classification was fragile at best. In a lecture to the GDNÄ in 1878, one commentator likened the state of psychiatry to a country following a revolution in which people are in a state of agitation and without a guiding hand.[35] Although the speaker still held out hope for pathology to overcome this worrisome state of affairs, confidence and patience were evaporating fast. Such complaints reflected deep-seated professional concerns and have, in retrospect, prompted some historians to speak of the period as a time of "classificatory chaos."[36]

Given this state of nosological limbo and general disappointment in the results of pathological anatomy, psychiatrists began going back to the patient's bedside in search of a viable system of disease classification.[37] Having placed great credence in pathological anatomy, academics, in particular, became increasingly aware that their clinics could not be constructed solely on a natural scientific basis and that greater attention needed to be paid to clinical perspectives.[38] Some psychiatrists saw this as capitulation, researchers being left with "no other choice" than to classify mental diseases according to their "clinical manifestation".[39] But for others more skeptical of neuropathology, such as the clinician Ludwig Wille, little had been won by simply renaming "mental disorders" as "diseases of the anterior brain."[40] In fact, for neuropathology to achieve its full potential, it required first and foremost a clinically grounded nosology. Academic psychiatrists, no doubt increasingly emboldened by their growing access to psychiatric patients in university facilities, were beginning to reassess the potential of clinical research.

For their part, alienists were operating on more familiar territory when it came to clinical inquiry. In the asylums, a number of researchers had been working hard to improve their nosologies.[41] Ludwig Snell's description of monomania (*Wahnsinn*) as an additional primary form of madness alongside melancholy and mania represented one of the more widely recognized achievements of these endeavors. Snell's work was presented to the psychiatric section of the GDNÄ in 1865 and soon thereafter found rapid acceptance by Griesinger and others. Ultimately, Snell's monomania became the basis from which Kraepelin and Bleuler would delineate schizophrenia.[42] In the early 1870s, Kahlbaum's work on catatonia and Hecker's on Hebephrenia had added to Snell's work.[43]

One important statement of the methods and aims of clinical inquiry had been written by Ewald Hecker in the early 1870s. Hecker was a close colleague of Karl Kahlbaum, first in the East Prussian asylum of Allenberg and later in the Silesian town of Görlitz. There both worked as psychiatrists, Kahlbaum having purchased a private asylum and Hecker having been appointed to direct the affairs of the local public asylum. Hecker echoed Kahlbaum's long-standing dissatisfaction with the state of psychiatry and the paltry results of pathological anatomy. He too complained that the tremendous wealth of experience gathered by individual asylum directors lacked any mutually coherent and accessible form. Alienist experience had not yet been consolidated into a professional consensus on a nosology of psychiatric diseases. As a consequence, the evaluation of individual cases was inordinately difficult: "Only after years of careful observation can one arrive at some assurance that the evaluation was correct."[44] It was this inability of psychiatrists to arrive at a rapid and reliable diagnosis that continued to plague the profession. Perhaps more than anything else, psychiatry needed clearly defined nosological categories.

Hecker argued that key to establishing a clinically based consensus on psychiatric disorders was to take *disease course* into account. Under the sway of Zeller's unitary psychosis, psychiatrists had inappropriately disregarded the course of specific forms of disease in their studies. To Hecker's mind, however, the path to nosological clarity lay in the clinical work of constant and unbiased observation "of the entire course of the condition [*Affection*]."[45] Studying that course would open the way to demarcating "natural" disease categories that would certainly have to be confirmed by patho-anatomical study. However, anatomical proof was not forthcoming in the foreseeable future, due in part to the nascent state of cerebral pathology and especially to the fact that asylums rarely conducted post-mortem examinations.[46] Consequently, clinical criteria based on disease course were the only viable means of delineating disease categories. In his own work on hebephrenia and in Kahlbaum's work on catatonia, Hecker saw clinical methods that stressed disease course as having borne valuable fruit in the form of two new and clearly demarcated disease categories.[47]

Though advocating that greater attention be paid to disease course, Hecker also realized that institutional conditions hampered the investigation of the chronological development of diseases. Hecker was acutely aware that most of the patients admitted to asylums had long since passed through many of the most crucial stages of their illnesses. The patients whom he saw at his asylums in Allenberg and Görlitz had arrived "almost at the very end of the actual illness and were already, in a sense, mental cripples."[48] Significantly, in Hecker's own work on hebephrenia, it was the very early phases of the disease that were of crucial importance. Yet these were precisely the phases that he did not have the ability to examine. Therefore, in diagnosing patients as hebephrenics, Hecker had to rely on the reports of non-experts who had observed the most critical stages of a patient's condition prior to institutionalization.[49]

The case of Hecker's work and more generally the shift in psychiatric research back to the bedside was loaded with important professional implications. To the extent that one can speak, as Werner Janzarik has, of the 1870s and 1880s as an "era of Kahlbaum,"[50] and to the extent that clinical research at that time was driven by consideration of disease course, the ability to observe the early phases of that course helped to ensured professional control over clinical research. By the same token, advocating the dogma of early and rapid admission, aside from whatever therapeutic benefits that dogma may have implied, was tantamount to advancing a claim to jurisdiction over that professional labor. Taken together with Griesinger's implicit epistemological critique of alienist empiricism, the dogma of rapid and early admission provided university clinics with powerful leverage against alienist claims to clinical research.

Clinical Discipline

Of course, early admission secured only the external conditions for clinical research. The internal disciplinary regime of the institution to which patients were admitted also had to be organized in order to facilitate patient observation. It has been argued that there was no essential difference in the methodological approaches to clinical observation taken by alienists and academics. According to Gerlof Verwey, clinical observation comprised a "pedestal" on which psychiatry rested, independent of all other philosophical disagreements.[51] But even if there were common methodological or phenomenological assumptions uniting psychiatrists, their practice of clinical observation differed markedly. In short, there were great variations in terms of what psychiatrists observed and how they went about observing it. Academic psychiatrists struggled to develop more exacting forms of clinical examination than alienists had been able to muster. In particular, they sought to achieve greater depth and rigor in their observations. They drew on new kinds of instruments and new forms of clinical discipline in order to evoke the early and all but invisible prodromal symptoms of mental disease. Using these new approaches, they hoped to refine their clinical skills of diagnosis and thereby ultimately demarcate clearly defined disease entities.

DIAGNOSTIC EXAMINATIONS AND THE HIERARCHIES OF CLINICAL OBSERVATION

To examine their patients in new ways and to elicit new signs and symptoms of madness, clinicians employed a growing arsenal of instruments.[52] As they attempted to peer more deeply into the bodies of their patients, they had borrowed much in the way of medical technology from clinical medicine in order to supplement their direct observations.[53] They measured and recorded their patients' blood pressure with kymographions and their pulse with Sphygmographs.[54] Griesinger's close friend and colleague Carl Wunderlich helped introduce the thermometer into clinical research, an instrument quickly adopted by psychiatrists.[55] Psychiatrists added their own instruments for inspecting pupils and measuring patellar reflex action, cranial form, and psycho-physical reaction times.[56] As with microscopy and necroscopy, each of these instruments of clinical examination came with an economy of proper usage that researchers ignored at their scientific peril. How to set up and employ the instruments and to interpret the signs they produced were skills that demanded considerable training and practice.

One of the most striking aspects of these instruments was the great importance their usage placed on quantification and visualization in the form of graphs and charts. Numbers represented in graphical form were a persuasive means of transmitting information and of satisfying demands for precision and exactitude. So pervasive were these measuring techniques that one contemporary critic was driven to speak of the emergence of "graph psychiatry [*Kurvenpsychiatrie*]," by which he meant that portion of psychiatry that could "be expressed in numbers and curves and which had reached the highest degree of exactitude."[57]

No less quantitatively inclined were the efforts to plumb the psychological depths of patients' minds. As the nineteenth century drew to a close, one of the most promising avenues toward more precise clinical observation involved psychophysical experimentation. As noted above, Emil Kraepelin was Germany's most fervent advocate of psycho-physical approaches to clinical research. For him psychological experimentation was an answer to both the deficiencies of patho-anatomical research and the imprecision with which clinical investigations had been traditionally conducted. Psycho-physical experiments were designed to measure psychological reaction times to external stimuli, as well as various mental functions and capacities such as memory, decision making, attention span, etc.[58]

In order to understand precisely what Kraepelin hoped to achieve by using psychological experiments and what he believed to be doing differently from his alienist colleagues, it is necessary to quote him at some length. Turning again to his inaugural lecture at Dorpat in 1887, Kraepelin explained the utility of psycho-physical experiments:

> When confronting his patient and trying to establish that patient's mental condition, the alienist is armed with nothing more than the experience derived from day-to-day practice. On the basis of his acquired knowledge he may well be able to judge the diagnostic, prognostic, and therapeutic details of a case better than a laymen. But ultimately, he cannot *see* more in the patient than could a good, non-psychiatrically trained observer with a little practice and attention. If progress toward better rules of psychopathological diagnosis is possible, then we must gain access to the knowledge which remains hidden to practical, day-to-day experience [*praktischen Menschenkenntnis des täglichen Lebens*]. It appears that the investigative methods of experimental psychology hold out the most promise of at least partially filling in these gaps in our knowledge.[59]

Kraepelin's remarks are interesting for what they reveal about the concerns, aims, and hopes of clinical psychiatrists in the 1880s. For one, they make clear that the supposedly undisciplined, day-to-day experience of alienist psychiatry would no longer suffice. Kraepelin and researchers like him were in search of knowledge that was fundamentally inaccessible to alienist traditions of clinical practice. It also clarifies the diagnostic aims of clinical research. The experimental methods of psychophysics were designed to establish reliable criteria and procedures of psychiatric diagnosis.

As quantitatively exacting as these new instruments and methods were, systematic and rigorous clinical observation also depended on an institutional hierarchy of observation. While instruments and experiments might bring to light ever deeper physical and psychological signs of mental disease, more rigorous analysis of patient behavior demanded different investigative practices and disciplinary techniques. The internal organization of the clinic had to be arranged in order to provide more effective means of observation. Most important in these hierarchies were, of course, ward doctors and assistants.[60] But they were not the only ones recording patient behavior. There existed multiple and overlapping layers of observers in the clinic. Personnel in the newly constructed clinic in Halle were charged with "uninterrupted supervision and observation" of life on the wards. The head nurses were instructed to supervise the wards "day and night not only at regular hourly intervals, but especially at unexpected times."[61] Doctors in Würzburg and elsewhere received from their staff regular written morning reports summarizing the night's events.[62] Reports such as these not only documented patient behavior, it also ensconced a routine mechanism for extending the range of institutional observation beyond the hours of the doctor's actual physical presence on the wards.

These supplemental observers were part of the hierarchy of observation, tracking, and record-keeping that made more rigorous and intensified clinical research possible in the first place. Personnel and assistants were vital cogs in the wheels of clinical research. More often than not, they were charged with taking patients' temperatures, with measuring changes in their weight, with administering drugs, with writing up ward reports, and with noting changes in patients' symptoms, etc.[63] More so than microscopy, clinical research was the product social interchange on hierarchically organized and highly structured hospital wards. And since the disciplinary practice of observation was also far more labor intensive than the practice of mechanical restraint had been, it simultaneously delivered the preconditions of more exacting and penetrating clinical research. Such extensive techniques of examination, hierarchical observation, and documentation produced a wealth of clinical information on which clinicians could draw for their scientific investigations.

THE SURVEILLANCE WARD (*WACHABTEILUNG*)

At the center of such elaborate hierarchies of observation lay the surveillance wards. These were large rooms in which several patients could be closely watched and cared for in their beds. They were designed to accommodate those patients who had just been admitted to the hospital, who were suffering through acute phases of their illness, or who posed a danger to themselves or others. The first use of surveillance wards in German psychiatric institutions was a matter of some dispute. In his reform writings in the late 1860s, Griesinger had considered them to comprise the very heart of the urban asylums he called "scientific observatories."[64] In the ensuing years, Griesinger's recommendation appears to have been largely forgotten. Some alienists had apparently also called for surveillance wards, but the extent of their actual implementation is again unclear.[65] In the late 1880s, their introduction to Germany was generally attributed to Gudden's address to the annual meeting of the *Verein deutscher Irrenärzte* in 1885. However, following Gudden's death, a dispute over priority broke out in which both Albrecht Paetz and Jean Paul Scholz laid claim to having first used them in Germany.[66] By the mid-1890s, however, they were becoming commonplace, thanks in part to new Prussian building codes that required them of every large hospital.[67] By the end of the century, surveillance wards had been introduced into most German university psychiatric clinics, and they were trumpeted as the very foundation of Germany's scientific preeminence in psychiatry.[68]

One of the more elaborate and refined surveillance wards was constructed in Robert Sommer's clinic in Giessen. When that clinic opened in 1896, the entire institution was geared toward "maximal" and "subtle observation."[69] In the first year of its operation, two-thirds of all female patients and three-quarters of all male patients found themselves under "constant observation." In addition, detailed reports were made on patients' food consumption, defecation, sleep, and baths. Nor did the "principle of permanent observation" cease at the end of the day. Intensive night-time supervision of patients on the surveillance ward was maintained with the help of electrical room lighting. In fact, the electrical system was so elaborately constructed that emergency provision had even been made for short circuits so as to ensure that ward lighting could never be entirely interrupted. Attached to the surveillance wards were examination rooms where detailed lists, tables, and charts were maintained; these recorded each patient's baths, fits, and menstrual periods.[70]

Ideally, surveillance wards such as the one in Giessen were complimented by two modes of treatment: bed therapy and hydrotherapy. As its name suggests, bed therapy involved strict confinement of patients to their beds as a means of keeping them quiet and orderly. In therapeutic terms, it was designed to stabilize the circulation, reduce external stimuli, calm "agitated ganglion cells," and halt any decline of the patient's energies.[71] No less important than the physiological effects of bed therapy were its psychological consequences. Bed therapy was a conscious attempt to convince patients of their own illnesses. For nothing could so effectively reinforce their sense of being sick than lying in bed. Because psychiatrists usually considered patients' self-awareness of their illness to be the first step toward recovery, impressing upon patients that they were in a hospital, and therefore actually sick, was an important therapeutic aid. Summing up its useful effects, Clemens Neisser called bed therapy "the sovereign means for fighting states of mental excitement. Only bed therapy for all excited mental patients can lift the mental hospital to the same level and give it the same outward appearance as a hospital. And that is what the mental hospital should and wants to be! Bed therapy is the crowning achievement of the idealistic reforms of Pinel and Conolly."[72] The implementation of bed therapy was thus seen as the culmination of the policy of nonrestraint that Wilhelm Griesinger and Ludwig Meyer had spearheaded in the early 1860s. Bed therapy was the final hurdle on the road toward erasing any and all distinctions in the minds of patients and lay visitors between psychiatric and other general hospitals. After about 1890, bed therapy became increasingly common in German psychiatric hospitals.[73]

The second form of therapy associated with surveillance wards was hydrotherapy. This involved placing patients in baths for days and even weeks at a time. The baths were intended to mimic physiological processes associated with tiredness and thereby exert a calming influence.[74] Consequently, the application of hydrotherapy was deemed most useful for patients in states of agitation, especially deliriant psychotics. Skeptics worried about circulatory and dermatological dangers and warned of the potential for abuse by ward staff which could lead to neglect, scaldings, or drownings.[75] But most psychiatrists believed that the benefits in terms of improved hygiene and sedation outweighed the drawbacks. Like bed therapy, hydrotherapy was an "excellent form of hypnosis"[76] that allowed them to restrain patients without having to resort to the less palatable alternatives of isolation cells, sedatives, or straightjackets.[77] Ideally, hydrotherapy was practiced in tandem with bed-therapy, with unruly patients being moved from one to the other until the agitation had subsided. During the 1880s and 1890s, the use of hydrotherapy expanded rapidly in German psychiatric hospitals.

Advocates saw a number of advantages in the surveillance wards and their supporting therapeutic methods. For one thing, in many clinics the surveillance ward could also serve as a training ward for hospital staff.[78] There nurses and wardens could receive instruction and supervision in the proper care and treatment of patients. The ward was therefore doubly significant in terms of its disciplinary function because it extended to both patients and staff. In the words of Adolf Dannemann, it embodied the single most important characteristic of the university psychiatric clinic, namely, "the maximum supervision of the patients by the personal and of both the personnel and the patients by the doctor."[79]

The intensive observation that infused the surveillance ward also had important therapeutic and public relations benefits. Preventing patients from harming themselves, others, or the property of the institution was one of the strongest arguments deployed in its support. Surveillance wards made immediate and even preemptive therapeutic intervention easier and thereby helped to reduce rates of suicide.[80] At the same time, surveillance held out the added advantage of seeming to obviate the need for alienist practices of isolation and mechanical restraint.[81] Intense, around-the-clock observation could displace the remaining vestiges of physical restraint and help to project an image of the psychiatric ward identical to that of other hospital wards. From a public relations standpoint, therefore, surveillance wards were doubly attractive. Not only did they reduce suicide rates, but they also countered public perceptions of psychiatric hospitals as carceral institutions and projected the more salubrious image of the general hospital.

Surveillance wards also allowed university clinics to deflect criticism about their treatment of patients. Large mental hospitals usually had greater architectural flexibility in grouping and segregating patients. In fact, being able to segregate patients and place them in environments appropriate to their condition was key to the alienist practice known as "individualization." In small institutions, however, individualization was far more difficult. The smaller size of university clinics meant that patients had to be segregated in more hetero-geneous groups which, in the minds of some, was a sure recipe for institutional chaos and hence therapeutic failure. Surveillance wards, however, held out the prospect of solving this problem. Immediate intervention of ward staff to sup-press disruptive symptoms and restore the well-ordered atmosphere of a hos-pital ward would ensure that patients in university clinics suffered no ill-effects from their agitated roommates. In this way, the surveillance ward provided the opportunity to substitute intense observation for the alienist practice of archi-tectural segregation. Thus, surveillance wards took the principle of individual-ization to new heights, transforming it in good part from a task of spatial seg-regation to one of persistent examination.

The techniques outlined above (diagnostic examination, hierarchical obser-vation, patient documentation) and the clinical space in which they were chiefly deployed (surveillance ward) comprised a new disciplinary economy which was characteristic of university clinics. These techniques were well honed to the tasks of clinical research and teaching; they were the institutional preconditions by which academic psychiatrists hoped to overcome the defi-ciencies which had hobbled alienist research in the asylums. It would, how-ever, be a mistake to believe that simply introducing such techniques would suffice for the purposes of efficient clinical research. University clinics existed in far larger social and administrative environments impinging directly on their abilities to sustain research agendas. As a result, clinical discipline also involved structuring and controlling the surrounding institutional and admin-istrative environment. Creating the "scientific observatory" that Griesinger called for was one thing; but integrating clinic research agendas into the wider system of regional psychiatric administration was quite another.

Emil Kraepelin's Reorganization of the Heidelberg Clinic

I have shown above just how intertwined the interests of laboratory research at the Charité were with developments in the city of Berlin. And even in Halle, where Hitzig's clinic had been built to circumvent the strictures imposed by provincial governments, the clinic was never entirely immune from the con-straints of wider psychiatric administration. To illustrate more vividly just how clinical discipline extended beyond the bounds of the clinic itself, and to show how interwoven clinical research was with both the disciplinary prac-tices described above and the administrative environment in which clinics op-erated, an historical case study of the clinic in Heidelberg is especially instruc-tive. For it was there in the 1890s that Emil Kraepelin laid the foundations for his classification of mental disease. The clinical research leading Kraepelin to distinguish between dementia praecox and manic depressive insanity would by 1910 make him the most preeminent psychiatric clinician in Germany. At the same time, the mechanisms that Kraepelin tried to install in order to facilitate his research would deepen the gulf separating academic psychiatry from alienist practice and transform the university psychiatric clinic into a transit station designed to admit, diagnose, and discharge patients as rapidly as possible.

PSYCHIATRIC CARE IN BADEN

When Kraepelin assumed his position as professor of psychiatry and director of the clinic in Heidelberg, he found psychiatric care in the German state of Baden still laboring under the burden of the debilitating feud between the university clinics and the state asylums. For years the asylum director in Illenau, C. F. W. Roller, had succeeded in delaying the construction of a university clinic that he envisioned to be both antithetical to the very principles of alienism and a threat to his influence among state officials in the capital in Karlsruhe.[82] When the Heidelberg clinic finally was opened shortly after Roller's death in 1878, its statutes reflected his concern that the university clinic might become too powerful and autonomous within the state system of care for the insane in Baden. Although it was part of the university, and hence subject to the authority of the Ministry of Education, it had also been conceived as a health care institution of the state of Baden and so fell under the jurisdiction of the far more powerful Ministry of the Interior.[83] In other words, unlike the clinic in Halle, it was fully integrated into the state-wide system of care for the insane. The clinic had in effect a double role to play: it was at once a university run hospital in which teaching and research were high priorities and a public hospital subject to strictly regulated policies of admission, transfer, and discharge.[84] The priorities and aims associated with these dual responsibilities were very often incompatible and gave rise to acrimonious disputes that impinged on the day-to-day affairs of the institution.

The system of care for the insane in Baden divided the state into three districts, two of which were served by the university clinics in Heidelberg and Freiburg, while the third was administered by the asylum in Illenau.[85] These three institutions admitted patients directly. In addition, there was a second tier of custodial institutions (Emmendingen and Pforzheim) that were not responsible for specific geographic districts, but instead designed exclusively to relieve pressures on the frontline facilities. Emmendingen accepted transfer patients who could be engaged in productive work, while Pforzheim was responsible for long-term, chronically ill patients.[86] The smooth functioning of this system depended upon two variables: first, the institutions admitting patients directly needed to have sufficient space to accommodate them and, second, Emmendingen and Pforzheim needed the capacity to accept transfers from the three admitting institutions.

A number of factors converged to ensure that these conditions were often not met. The explosion of the patient population in the late nineteenth century placed great strains on the orderly functioning of the system and further aggravated tension between the university clinics and the asylums.[87] The difficulties posed by overcrowding were further aggravated by time-consuming bureaucratic paper-work. And when typhus broke out, asylums were sometimes forced to close, sending shockwaves reverberating throughout the entire system of care.[88] When Kraepelin arrived in Heidelberg to replace Karl Fürstner in 1891, he inherited the old tensions between university and asylum psychiatry, in a clinic that was threatened by overcrowding and that often had to reconcile conflicting academic and administrative responsibilities. Kraepelin's presence in Heidelberg did nothing to alleviate these tensions; if anything, they worsened during his tenure of service.[89]

DISPOSING CLINICAL MEANS: ON THE ARRANGEMENT OF PSYCHIATRIC FILES AND BODIES

Kraepelin began to reorganize the clinic immediately upon his arrival in Heidelberg. He wished to transform it into a more efficient research and teaching facility and, to these ends, he literally turned it on its head.[90] One of his first administrative reforms involved control over the flow of patient files to and from administrative offices. In late 1891, he complained to the Ministry of Education about the standing policy of transferring patient records between Heidelberg and Emmendingen. Kraepelin recommended that when patients were transferred, their admission files remain in the Heidelberg clinic. He argued that the files were the product of his institution's administrative labor and hence that it be Emmendingen's responsibility to approach the university clinic whenever it needed access to the files.[91] He supported his argument by stressing that the files were not only of "fundamental administrative importance," but also of "specific medical [and] scientific" interest, whereas for Emmendingen they were of "absolutely no administrative and only very subordinate medical importance."[92] The clinical necessity of quickly collecting sufficient practical documentation demanded immediate accessibility to the admission files. That accessibility could be ensured only if they remained in the clinic.

The Ministry of Education found Kraepelin's arguments compelling and moved to resolve the dispute by having copies and excerpts made of various portions of the files.[93] Crucially for Kraepelin's purposes, the ministry found that henceforth the admission file should remain in the clinic while transcripts followed patients to secondary institutions. In thus separating patients from their admission files, Kraepelin succeeded in gaining access to a much larger pool of clinical information—information that theretofore had escaped his institution. As a consequence, it became easier for him to establish and compare the course of his patient's diseases. Through the administrative reorganization of the flow of patient files, Kraepelin established an essential precondition for his practical work of collecting and comparing patient records.[94]

A year after arriving in Heidelberg, Kraepelin embarked on a second major reform initiative. In May of 1892, he disbanded the ward for semi-quiet patients and used the space to construct not only two rooms for his psychological experiments, but also a new and enlarged surveillance ward on which he introduced bed-therapy.[95] He justified this reorganization by pointing to the overcrowding in the clinic and its acute lack of laboratory rooms for scientific research. At the end of 1892, he assessed the impact of the reorganization as a complete success. He claimed to have achieved an "essential change in the entire method of treatment," which had alleviated the problem of overcrowding and reduced the number of isolated patients.[96] The architectural changes had achieved a "concentration of nursing care," so that now nearly "half of all patients were located in the large rooms of the surveillance ward under constant observation and nearly a third of them lay in bed."[97]

The construction of a surveillance ward was crucial to Kraepelin's entire conception of a university psychiatric clinic. The surveillance ward was the "focal point" of the entire institution and raised the urban asylum from "a mere repository for the insane [*Irrenniederlage*] to a *curative institution* [*Heilanstalt*]."[98] The surveillance ward was also an essential architectural and organizational component of his clinical research work. It was designed to provide intense observation of those patients who had attracted Kraepelin's scientific attention. The population of the wards included fresh admissions for whom diagnoses were still pending, patients sent by the courts for observation, and patients who were the subject of ongoing tests. The surveillance ward was the clinical space in which these patients could be scrupulously controlled, examined, monitored and documented. For Kraepelin the clinician, therefore, the surveillance ward was an important aid in establishing a reliable diagnosis and in constructing his larger classification of mental disorders.

Alongside his internal reorganization of the clinic, Kraepelin also tried to restructure the clinic's external relationship with other institutions. He did so in order to facilitate admissions and close the debilitating gap in clinical observation that spanned the early, prodromal symptoms of madness.[99] To these ends and within the means at his disposal, Kraepelin was relatively liberal in admitting patients. After he arrived in Heidelberg in 1891 the clinic experienced a marked rise in admissions.[100] Furthermore, and contrary to established practice in Baden, he advocated that patients should be allowed to initiate their own admission.[101] He also allied himself with the city magistrate in Heidelberg to urge that individuals in temporary police custody or those serving longer sentences be transferred immediately from their jail cells to the psychiatric clinic, if they exhibited symptoms of madness.[102] In addition, there is some evidence to suggest that Kraepelin sought to circumvent formal admission procedures in order to acquire cases that he felt were of particular clinical interest.[103]

Due in large part to the overcrowded system of care in Baden, Kraepelin's initiatives found little support. Asylum directors did not hesitate to point out the apparent contradiction of at once complaining about overcrowding while at the same time advocating easier admission.[104] They therefore called for a reduction of the geographic admission district of the Heidelberg clinic in order to alleviate its situation.[105] Yet Kraepelin rejected this recommendation out of hand. He believed that overcrowding was attributable not to the size of the admission district, but rather to belated admission and the uneven distribution of patients in the existing asylums. Reducing the volume of admissions would inevitably constrict the spectrum of patients available for psychiatric research and education. He insisted that his clinic could "easily handle double the number of admissions"[106] and that relief would come only from an expansion in the system of care. Ultimately, his complaints fell on deaf ears and did not result in any significant change in the statutes. However, they bear witness to the scientific importance that he placed in rapid admission and the corresponding capacity to observe early symptoms of mental illness.

Closely related to Kraepelin's attempts to make hospital admission easier were his efforts to speed up and streamline the *evacuation* of patients. From the mid-1890s, the rising number of institutionalized patients and the growing proportion of chronic patients in the clinic prompted him to complain to the state ministry about the sluggish transfer of patients to Emmendingen and Pforzheim. As early as April 1893, he wrote of the "great difficulties" in evacuating patients to Emmendingen and of his concern that the delays would cause "serious damage" to the clinic and cripple "scientific and didactic" work.[107] In June of 1896, he was again complaining to Karlsruhe that overcrowding had long since reached "entirely unacceptable levels" and that the clinic had amassed an "extraordinarily large number of unruly, violent and cumbersome" patients.[108]

Barely three weeks later Kraepelin's patience had reached the end of its tether. In a letter dated 12 July 1896, he sparked a controversy with the *Verwaltungshof* in Karlsruhe which raged for months.[109] The *Verwaltungshof* was the state administrative agency overseeing the admission and transfer of patients throughout Baden. The dispute had been touched off after the *Verwaltungshof* rejected a transfer application, insisting that Kraepelin provide cogent justification for it. The intervention of the *Verwaltungshof* was, in Kraepelin's eyes, an insult to his professional and medical integrity. In his eyes, the *Verwaltungshof* was a "*lay agency*" that could not judge the medical merits of a transfer application. Kraepelin proposed a reform in the practice of transferring patients which would employ a questionnaire to pass information on to the receiving institution. He also demanded that his clinic "immediately be given the capacity to free up space rapidly."

Kraepelin's exhortations prompted the immediate and vociferous outcry of the directorate of Illenau, the Ministry of the Interior, and the *Verwaltungshof*.[110] The *Verwaltungshof* pointed out that the Heidelberg directorate was required to supply an "obvious and exhaustive" justification of its transfer applications and that the directorate was "*very well aware*" of the problem of overcrowding in the state system.[111] The government's chief medical advisor rejected Kraepelin's criticisms and suggested that the size of the Heidelberg district be reduced in order to alleviate the overcrowding there.[112] The Ministry of the Interior agreed and accused Kraepelin of "deeming the statutes of the institution unscientific, ignoring them, and of disputing the authority of the *Verwaltungshof* as a lay agency incompetent to distribute the sick among the individual institutions. . . . Irrespective of divergent scientific opinion, the direct-orate of the clinic [i.e. Kraepelin, EJE] cannot be allowed to ignore those [statutes] at its whim; even in this instance he shall rather be able to justify its applications in accordance with the official statutes."[113]

Kraepelin found such rebuttal intolerable, and it prompted him to write an extensive memorandum concerning the transfer of mental patients out of the university clinic. He again insisted that only psychiatrists and not the *Verwaltungshof* could accurately judge transfer applications and that the current regulations were utterly useless. In order to rectify the problem, he suggested transferring patients to Illenau (i.e. to one of the other admitting institutions) or that his applications for transfer to Emmendingen and Pforzheim be given priority. He also wove therapeutic and didactic strands into his argument. For example, he insisted that if long-term patients remained in his clinic—which could not provide for their specific needs—then their health would be in acute danger. Furthermore, the accumulation of chronic cases in the clinic compromised the quality of psychiatric education and threatened to debilitate the clinic's "didactic material."[114]

Although Kraepelin was successful in heading off attempts to reduce the size of the Heidelberg admissions district, his protests did not succeed in improving conditions in his clinic. Instead the situation continued to deteriorate, prompting him to call for a wholesale "decoupling of university clinics from the state system of care for the insane."[115] Fulfilling the clinic's scientific and educational mission demanded that he should be given authority to transfer patients as he deemed necessary. It was precisely this point of contention that in 1902/3 prompted Kraepelin to leave Heidelberg and accept a position in Munich where the university clinic was less hampered by statutory constraints.[116]

DIAGNOSTIC CARDS AND THE EXTENSION OF CLINICAL DISCIPLINE

Kraepelin's concern for patient files, surveillance wards, and admissions and evacuation criteria need to be viewed in the context of his own clinical research agenda. Kraepelin showed a growing interest in the temporal course of mental diseases and in the potential that studying their longitudinal development might harbor for isolating specific illnesses and grouping them into nosological categories.[117] To this end, he had pondered a research agenda that drew on the ideas of Kahlbaum and Hecker and that stressed disease course in an attempt to replace synchronic with diachronic diagnostic criteria.[118] It was, however, not until Kraepelin was called to Heidelberg in 1891 that he began to systematically collect his clinical observations. It was only there that he found conditions he deemed suitable for rigorous clinical investigation.[119] Over the next five years—and indeed for much of the rest of his life—Kraepelin meticulously collected hundreds of patient histories. It was on the basis of these histories that he constructed the disease categories that appeared in the vanguard fifth edition of his textbook *Psychiatrie* in 1896.[120]

One of the important clinical research aids developed by Kraepelin to help chart a disease course was the so-called diagnostic card (*Zählkarte*).[121] These cards were essential tools for the construction of Kraepelin's nosology as well as a reflection of his emphasis on clinical observation and longitudinal analysis. The cards provided excerpts of the patient history and outlined the "essential characteristics of the clinical picture."[122] They were supposed to avoid technical jargon and give as objective an account of the clinical facts as possible.[123] Whenever a patient was admitted to the clinic, a new card would be prepared on which a diagnosis and course of the disease could be recorded. Even after the patient had left the clinic, the cards would continue to be updated until a final outcome could be determined. That the patient not be lost from sight upon leaving the clinic was crucial to the success of Kraepelin's research project. But one of the consequences of the project was that Kraepelin's yearly visits to the other mental institutions in Baden to check up on transferred patients further exacerbated tensions between his university clinic and the asylums.[124]

Kraepelin's diagnostic cards were, at least in name, not his own invention. They had not originated strictly as clinical research tools, but were instead derivatives of the administrative planning and policy agendas of German governments. Both state officials and alienists, whether planning new asylums, writing up reports for government officials, or simply keeping track of their own institutions, were some of the most avid tabulators of nearly every conceivable aspect of asylum life and patient disorders.[125] In their statistical inquiries, state officials in many parts of Germany had for years been using census cards, likewise known as *Zählkarten*.[126] In Kraepelin's specific case, he almost certainly filled out such census cards while working as an assistant under Franz Rinecker in Würzburg in the late 1870s. In other words, long before he developed and employed his own *Zählkarten* for purposes of clinical research, Kraepelin had been busy filling out statistical *Zählkarten* for Bavarian government records.[127]

The use of diagnostic cards and their correlation with the statistical techniques of Bavarian census takers in the 1860s and 1870s point to the expressly quantitative dimension of Kraepelin's clinical research. The construction of nosological groups, according to the criteria of a disease's course, required not only access to admission files and surveillance wards, but also to the broadest selection and largest number of patient histories possible. Only then was a satisfactory comparison, and hence a reliable grouping of individual cases, possible. Kraepelin's research agenda (not to mention the exigencies of teaching) was contingent upon an abundant supply of patients who could be tracked as they moved through the state system of psychiatric care and whose symptoms could be recorded on *Zählkarten*. From this perspective it becomes clear why Kraepelin was at once unwilling to accept any reduction of the Heidelberg admission district that might have relieved the overcrowding in his clinic and why he simultaneously encouraged a greater number of admissions.[128] The realization of his clinical research goals depended crucially on the frequency of admission and evacuation of patients.[129] While a clinic with a low patient frequency made it easier to observe a few patients over a long period of time, it simultaneously made it impossible to acquire enough patients to cover the entire spectrum of mental diseases. Conversely, a clinic with a high patient frequency made it difficult to observe the entire course of a disease, because they were so quickly moved through the clinic. Because of these institutional and systemic constraints on his research, Kraepelin felt it necessary to extend his examination of patients beyond the clinic into the asylums in order to be able to observe the entire course of a disease. He believed that the disciplinary techniques of the clinic had to be taken beyond the walls of his institution to ensure the integrity of clinical research. However, against the backdrop of his advocacy of less restrictive admissions criteria, the general crisis of overcrowding, and his own liberal policies of admission, his visits to outlying asylums met with considerable resistance.[130] As the 1890s progressed, he could rely less and less on the cooperation of his alienist colleagues.

As a consequence, analogous to the empirical gap resulting from delayed admission, there also emerged a gap in the clinical observation and documentation of the latter phases of mental disorder. As the director of a curative institution that was designed for acute cases, and in spite of all delays in transferring patients, Kraepelin found himself in danger of losing sight of the subtle mental changes in the late phases of a disease's course. Worse still, he faced considerable difficulties in verifying the terminal state of his cases; and the terminus was an essential criteria in the construction and verification of his nosological categories. Without the cooperation of asylum directors, and without knowledge of the outcome of a case, all of the earlier and time-consuming clinical observations were severely compromised, and clinical research was put in jeopardy. It is only against this backdrop of the dynamic relationship between disciplinary practices, clinical research agendas, and the state system of care in Baden that Kraepelin's clinical research acquires deeper historical significance and meaning.

THE CLINICAL UTILITY OF PROGNOSIS

When Kraepelin finally presented the auspicious results of his clinical research to the annual meeting of the *Verein deutscher Irrenärzte* in Heidelberg in

1896, he had already collected a thousand patient histories.[131] But the sharpness of the boundaries separating his nosological categories depended upon the number of cases investigated; and for him a thousand cases were far too few to arrive at final nosological clarity. As one of his colleagues noted, he "could not investigate enough cases, following their emergence, course, and outcome; he was forever preoccupied with the reworking of the thousands upon thousands of patient histories which had passed through his hands, pursuing each detail and continually grouping and regrouping what he had discovered."[132] This passionate desire to organize culminated in a nosology that ultimately revolutionized twentieth century psychiatry. But its professional implications did not stop at simply classifying patients.

Kraepelin's clinical research agenda also had important implications for the work of psychiatric diagnosis and prognosis. Alongside the development of a clinical classification of disease types, his research aimed also at securing reliable diagnostic techniques that, in turn, would open the way toward greater prognostic certainty. As Kraepelin remarked in 1896, if psychiatrists were unable to produce reliable diagnoses, then "it [became] impossible to solve the most important practical problem: reaching a prognosis. In the reliability of our prognoses lies the basis of public trust in our science, our reputation before the courts, and the ability to *teach* psychiatry."[133] Reliable prognoses would help psychiatrists to solve not just therapeutic problems, but also enhance the discipline's scientific reputation and didactic efficacy. If clinical research succeeded in developing a "teachable science of prognostics", then the discipline's authority and legitimacy would profit markedly.[134] Kraepelin had therefore attempted to integrate prognostic considerations into his disease classification. In keeping with his focus on disease course, he had placed great emphasis on terminal states as he constructed his nosology. In other words, he extrapolated backward from the outcome of patients' illnesses in order to build his disease categories.

Kraepelin's clinical research and his attempts to undergird his nosology with prognostic considerations touched on delicate professional issues. For that reason, when he presented his findings in 1896, a lively discussion ensued on the role that prognosis played in establishing categories of mental disease. Above all, it was Friedrich Jolly, then professor of psychiatry at the Charité in Berlin, who expressed doubts about drawing diagnostic conclusions on the basis of the prognosis. In Jolly's opinion, this approach to disease classification contradicted the fundamental principles of general pathology. Jolly did, however, admit to the "importance of the prognosis for the practical work of the psychiatrist."[135] Jolly thus pointed out that the emphasis that Kraepelin placed on the course of disease in his research program went hand in hand with great institutional advantages.

In these remarks, Jolly differentiated clearly between diagnostic practice and nosological research. At the same time, he also made clear just how tightly enmeshed the two were in Kraepelin's own work. In Jolly's view, Kraepelin had essentially raised the practical institutional necessity of rapidly establishing a prognosis to an instrument of disease classification. In light of Kraepelin's difficulties in evacuating patients from his clinic, Jolly's assessment seems especially notable. Indeed, in order for Kraepelin to facilitate the earliest possible transfer of patients to Emmendingen or Pforzheim, he needed to establish a prognosis as quickly as possible. Only with a prognosis in hand could he submit the application for transfer, either to Emmendingen or Pforzheim. Thus, following his arrival in Heidelberg, and from the inception of his efforts to speed up evacuation, the prognosis had been of crucial administrative importance. At the same time, that prognosis became perhaps the most fundamental criterion that Kraepelin employed in his clinical research to differentiate dementia praecox from manic depressive illness. Furthermore, the respective prognoses that Kraepelin assigned to dementia praecox (incurable) and manic depressive illness (curable) echoed the criteria of curability that governed institutionalized psychiatric care in Baden.

The importance Kraepelin placed on rapid evacuation also provides an explanation for a change in his own research methods. As part of the clinical examination and in order to refine his diagnostic techniques, he had initially required of himself and his co-workers that a diagnosis and prognosis be made within the first four weeks after admission. Then, after the patient was discharged to the asylums, his or her prognosis was to be monitored in regular and systematic examinations. In this way, it was hoped, conclusions could be drawn and corrections made in the original diagnosis. However, after 1893 and in conjunction with the renewed pressures of overcrowding, Kraepelin required that patients' prognoses be made not after four weeks, but rather immediately following their first examination in the clinic. This modification in clinical practice was designed to facilitate the rapid evacuation of patients. In the case of one patient, who was transferred to the wrong asylum, Kraepelin admitted as much to the ministry in Karlsruhe. He maintained that in his clinic it was common practice to submit applications for transfer immediately after the prognosis had been determined.[136] Thus, in the clinical practice of rapidly determining a prognosis, and immediately submitting applications for patient transfers, the priorities of Kraepelin's scientific research and the problems of an overcrowded university psychiatric clinic were inextricably intertwined.

Clinics as Diagnostic Transit Stations

By ensuring unhindered access to patient files, by constructing a surveillance ward, by following a liberal policy of admission, and by effecting the rapid transfer of chronic patients, Emil Kraepelin was attempting to reorganize the clinic in order to make it a more effective research institution. He was intensifying its internal organization and reconfiguring the protocols that governed its interaction with the outside world. The clinic was to be transformed into a funnel through which the greatest possible number of patients would be admitted, diagnosed, and then distributed to varying secondary institutions. While high rates of admission may have aggravated already crowded institutional conditions, Kraepelin welcomed additional patients to the extent that they provided him with fresh "observation material" for his research and classroom lectures.[137] Transforming the university psychiatric clinic into a transit station not only fortified claims to jurisdiction over clinical research, but more generally also put the academic psychiatrist in a position to control the work of diagnosis within the profession.

Kraepelin's view of the clinic as a diagnostic transit station through which high patient volumes could be shunted was shared by many of his colleagues. Robert Wollenberg, the director of the clinic in Tübingen, described his clinic as "nothing but a transit station [*Durchgangsstation*] from which patients were distributed to different asylums."[138] A visiting physician to the Charité in Berlin described it as a "large sifting department" in which "many of the admissions who prove to be hopelessly insane, scarcely pause on their way to the asylums at Dalldorf and Buch."[139] Similarly, Carl Fürstner conceived of his university clinic as transit station for unwanted patients.[140] In Breslau, Karl Wernicke viewed the urban asylum as a "central collection point" for all patients on public assistance, where they would be "sorted" and either released or transferred to other institutions.[141] And, finally, wherever clinics were *not* organized as transit stations, the despondency was great.[142]

The difference in frequency between urban and rural asylums was at times dramatic. For example, in the early 1890s the number of admissions to the clinic in Würzburg surpassed its total number of beds fourfold, whereas in other Bavarian asylums annual admissions reached only about half the total number of beds.[143] And in Berlin one observer remarked that as many patients were admitted to the Charité on a single day as were admitted to the asylum Nietleben near Halle in many months.[144] Pushing up patient frequencies in this way gave rise to a number of problems. A report prepared for Berlin city magistrates in 1892 elaborated on the disadvantages of funneling patients through the Charité to the asylum in Dalldorf.[145] For one, administrative work was held in limbo until the patient's final destination was clarified. In addition, the successive and rapid change of living quarters and hospital staff unduly excited patients and was considered detrimental to their care. Worse still, some patients suffering from paralysis had been admitted to the Charité in such a weak state that their subsequent transport to Dalldorf had resulted in their death.[146]

Yet beyond such consequences for patients, clinics designed as transit stations had important professional consequences insofar as they represented a redistribution of labor and with it a reconfiguration of power relations within the profession. Organizing clinics as transit stations gave academic psychiatrists the means with which to conduct clinical research and, in many cases, to exercise diagnostic control over the wider system of psychiatric administration and care. But just what did clinical research mean in this context?

Clearly, what it could not and did not mean was doctors personally spending more time examining and caring for their patients and seeing to the appropriate fit between patient and institutional architecture.[147] Instead, it meant ever more rigorous taxonomies and diagnostic techniques applied directly toward an ever smaller window on patients' lives. This in turn meant at once both the concentration of clinical research in the university clinics, as well as the consequent need to extend clinical discipline outside the institution itself and across the wider system of psychiatric care. It meant a new disciplinary regime structured less around patients' subjugation under the moral architecture of the asylum and its patriarchal director, and more around extensive and silent forms of discipline that relied on intense observation and other technologies of data collection. Normalization involved not so much fitting into the moral architecture of an idealized institutional family, than being examined, documented, and judged according to psychiatric nosologies.

Kraepelin's influential classification of psychiatric disorders was a derivative of this new economy of clinical research. However, this alone did not necessarily guarantee the enormous resonance that his nosology found among German practitioners. For its "success" was at least in part also a function of its timely appearance at a moment of nosological limbo within the profession. In the eyes of many of his contemporaries, Kraepelin's work had overcome a debilitating German "intellectual backwardness [*Sondergeisterei*]."[148] As we shall explore in greater depth in chapter 7, it appeared in the 1890s just as psychiatry was facing a wave of anti-psychiatric sentiment. Kraepelin's nosology was something around which psychiatrists could circle the professional wagons in the face of hostile public criticism. Perhaps more significantly, however, the two most important editions of Kraepelin's textbook (1896 and 1899) were published just as new regulations on medical examinations were about to be promulgated. In other words, the rapid acceptance of Kraepelin's nosology coincided with heightened demand for a teachable psychiatry with clear, concise disease categories.[149] It is to these concerns about psychiatry as a subject of academic instruction that I now turn.

CHAPTER 6

Clinical Teaching

Introduction

Certainly one of the most important professional tasks in nineteenth-century German psychiatry involved the propagation of specialized skills and knowledge. The work of psychiatric instruction was directed at both expanding the reach of professional expertise and at reproducing a professional elite. To the extent that professional legitimacy was defined in relation to specialized knowledge and practice, jurisdiction over the task of psychiatric instruction was of marked significance. Not surprisingly, therefore, teachers and their work played a pivotal role in professional development. Questions of who should teach, what should be taught, and how it should be taught were all topics of considerable portent for the discipline's professional identity and were the subject of intensive and ongoing deliberations. At stake in these debates was the division of expert labor within the profession and psychiatry's claim to constitute both an autonomous specialty within medicine and an integral and necessary component in the all-around training of every general practitioner.

Psychiatric instruction involved the dissemination of a canon of generally accepted theories and practices. Students were taught how to recognize different kinds of disease; they were instructed in what constituted proper diagnostic procedure; they were shown how to perform autopsies, microscopic examinations, and chemical tests; they learned theories of disease causation; and they were exposed to various therapeutic technologies. The dissemination of this knowledge depended upon complex and integrated arrangements of teachers, students, architectural facilities, and structured curriculums: in specially designed courses, held in architecturally segregated spaces, and using an array of didactic materials, students were supplied with knowledge deemed pertinent to their future professional practice.

Instruction was, however, not just a task of passive propagation. It was also a disciplinary operation performed on the bodies, minds, and values of students. Professional training involved the acculturation of students to specialized techniques and practices. It attempted to modify thought and behavior according to professionally accepted standards and indeed to transform or to resubjectify the very identity of the student-object. It strove toward nothing less than a resocialization and even a revaluation of the self.[1] The final products of successfully deployed pedagogic technologies were practitioners who had the capacity to exercise authority over themselves as trained professionals.

Claims to perform the work of psychiatric instruction in nineteenth-century Germany were advanced from various quarters. Alienists believed that immersion in the asylum environment was crucial for students to acquire familiarity with therapeutic techniques and indeed with the entire asylum based way of life. Neuropathologists maintained that students needed to absorb the ethos of the natural sciences or else psychiatry was in danger of degenerating into little more than a managerial and administrative science. Clinicians thought that psychiatric instruction was properly the task of internal medicine and that the foundation of the profession rested on students learning accurately to observe and interpret clinical symptoms at the bedside.

This chapter will consider the work of psychiatric instruction in Imperial Germany. What did psychiatrists believe their educational task to be? How was that task organized inside and outside the university? What constraints were placed on it? And what claims were advanced in an attempt to secure professional jurisdiction over it? Some of these questions have been addressed peripherally in previous chapters. The focus here will be on debates about psychiatry's status as part of both the academic curriculum and state licensing examinations. I will devote special attention to psychiatric instruction at the University of Jena, where Otto Binswanger lived and worked. Binswanger was one of Germany's most reputed psychiatric educators and a persistent advocate of an expanded place for psychiatry in the curriculum and examination of medical students.

Early Medical and Psychiatric Education

Medical education in Germany changed dramatically over the course of the nineteenth century.[2] Traditionally, in many German states there had existed different categories of physicians, including academically trained doctors (*medici puri*), surgeons (*Chirurgen* and *Wundärzte*), as well as midwives, barbers, and other healers. The two largest groups of medical practitioners were folk healers (*Heilpraktiker*), whose practices were rooted in local traditions, and midwives, for whom schools had been established in the eighteenth century. In Prussia and throughout Germany after 1825 this segmentation of medical training and practice was gradually reduced.[3] New state qualifying examinations erased the strict distinction between *medici puri* and surgeons. Increasingly, medical students studied surgical procedures and gynecology; surgeons, in turn, were permitted to practice internal medicine in areas where no academic physicians practiced.[4] The medical reform movement of the 1840s also pressed the cause of greater uniformity in medical education. And between 1849 and 1852 the surgical schools in Breslau, Greifswald, Münster, and Magdeburg were closed. By the early 1850s the medical profession was gradually being consolidated into a single class of academically trained general practitioners.

In the decades preceding German unification, the relationship between academic training and licensing procedures (*Approbation*) had varied widely from one German state to the next.[5] But with the constitution of the North German Confederation in 1864/66 and German unification in 1871 came more uniform standards of state licensing. The *Reichsgewerbeordnung* of June 1869 made state licensing independent of academic degrees and effectively transplanted Prussian norms to the wider confederation.[6] The structure of the examination, the *tentamen physicum,* and various other testing procedures were taken from the Prussian model and made the foundation of the new procedures. Although on paper the state examinations were standardized, examination practice continued to vary from state to state, because control over educational policy and the academic curriculum remained in the hands of the individual states and universities.[7] As a result, wide differences in university curriculums remained even after unification and influenced both the content and quality of examinations.

Accompanying these developments in medical licensing and examination were important changes in medical curriculums. After the middle of the nineteenth century, a fundamental shift took place toward hands-on training and clinical observation.[8] The course offerings of medical faculties had long stressed general education and placed primary emphasis on the acquisition of theoretical knowledge in lecture courses. The cerebral bent of instruction is witnessed in the great importance attached to the interpretation of symptoms (semiotics) and the phenomenological ordering of diseases into systematic categories (nosology). These were considered far more important than bedside instruction, to say nothing of practice in surgical techniques. Furthermore, when clinical demonstrations were held, they were generally intended to confirm and reinforce an existing theoretical canon. In 1839, the medical faculty in Berlin made its view known: the task of the medical clinic was to demonstrate "in nature" the diseases described in lecture courses.[9] Along the same lines in 1855, the professor of medicine in Jena, Dietrich Georg Kieser, believed that clinical demonstrations should illustrate "the truth of natural laws in the real life of the disease. The psychiatric clinic [was] the touchstone of the truth of theoretical psychiatry [*Psychiatrik*]."[10] Such didactic aims were characteristic of the emphasis that early nineteenth-century clinicians placed on observing nature (*Naturbeobachtung*). In this context, the task of clinical instruction placed a premium on empirical observation and did not usually extend to practical training in a sequence of examination techniques that would elicit symptoms through active intervention.[11]

However, after mid-century and in tandem with utilitarian educational reforms, medical faculties began placing greater emphasis on practical proficiency.[12] Accordingly, medical education moved away from theoretical lecture courses toward courses in the techniques of examination and diagnosis. Students were being taught not so much passively to observe the natural symptoms of disease, but to extract or elicit symptoms using a battery of standardized diagnostic skills.[13] For if no where else in the course of their careers, then, as medical students, practitioners should at least have been exposed to the techniques of rigorous and exacting clinical examination. In this respect, psychiatric clinics were conceived to be model institutions that set the standards of future conduct for young physicians.[14] Clinics were responsibile for reproducing a scientific ethos in their students, for awakening in them the "spirit of scientific aspiration," and for giving them the "key to a natural scientific understanding" of psychiatric diseases.[15]

These intentions were, however, in part counteracted by the realities of rising numbers of medical students at German universities. The 1880s saw a large influx of students into the medical faculties throughout the country. Following on the relatively gradual growth of the 1860s and early 1870s, numbers jumped precipitously after 1878 and continued to rise throughout the 1880s.[16] One of the consequences of this growth in student numbers was that the opportunities for practical clinical instruction were significantly curtailed.[17] In spite of the impressive number of new academic hospitals in the 1870s, clinical instruction often remained one-sidedly abstract and theoretical. As more and more medical students entered the universities, they received ever fewer opportunities to observe or examine patients on their own. Clinical courses at some larger German universities had upwards of four hundred or more students.[18] These circumstances helped to spur efforts to improve practical training, with debates focusing on the introduction into the medical curriculum of propaedeutic clinical courses or a practical year (*annum practicum*). From the 1870s, the *annum practicum* was an on-going topic of discussion in medical circles, and it became the focal point of reform efforts in the early 1890s.

Not withstanding these fin-de-siècle debates, practical on-the-job experience had long been the cornerstone of psychiatric training. In the second quarter of the nineteenth century, that training was almost always a nomadic, postgraduate undertaking.[19] Assuming they had the financial wherewithal to do so, young university educated physicians generally embarked on extensive travels to a handful of famous institutions. During their theory-oriented university training, they had usually received little instruction in psychiatric matters and, more often than not, had never seen a single patient suffering from mental illness. Thus, after completing their degrees and receiving their licenses to practice medicine, they now sought out practical experience in asylums in order to augment their rudimentary knowledge of mental illness. There, either as short-term visitors or as full-time assistants, they observed and participated in the daily routine of the asylum. Sometimes they were government-supported candidates who, after their travels, would help build and administer new asylums.

Upon being appointed director of the asylum in Winnenthal, for example, Ernst Albert von Zeller spent several months in training with Maximilian Jacobi in Siegburg and then traveled on to England, Scotland, and France. Ludwig Snell was dispatched on two trips by officials of the duchy of Nassau—one in 1844 to London and Paris in order to prepare him for work at the asylum in Eberbach and a second trip in 1846 to Vienna, Illenau, and Winnenthal so that he could draft plans for a new asylum in Eichberg. Such *Wanderjahre* illustrate that in the first half of the nineteenth century, professional training retained characteristics of traditional models of apprenticeship. While academic training in medicine was government regulated, specialized instruction in psychiatry was a far more informal and ad hoc affair. As late as 1878, some psychiatrists continued to complain that careers in psychiatry began only upon the appointment to the position of asylum director.[20] Thus, for most aspiring alienists, psychiatric training was on-the-job training.

In the 1860s, however, there emerged a new generation of psychiatrists whose careers had followed entirely different paths. This cohort had been trained almost exclusively within the university system. They had worked on the wards of university medical clinics and in the laboratories of newly built pathological and physiological institutes. In other words, there existed in the latter half of the nineteenth century two different career paths open to aspiring clinical directors: some came to psychiatry through the asylums (Pelman, Bumm, Jessen, Gudden); for others, such as Griesinger, Hitzig, Westphal, or Emminghaus, careers in psychiatry were pursued largely within the university. Both alternatives remained viable career paths up until the end of the nineteenth century. After 1900 career paths in psychiatry solidified and recruitment of academic psychiatrists from the ranks of alienists declined noticeably.[21]

Nothing signified psychiatry's coming of age as a medical specialty in German academics more than the establishment of full university chairs.[22] Initiatives for full chairs could come from different quarters: at times from the state and at times from university faculties. Indeed, the winding paths leading to the establishment of full academic chairs in psychiatry were as numerous as were the universities themselves. Yet one of the most characteristic paths involved a *personal union* of the positions of asylum director and university professor.[23] In this arrangement, alienists, who were generally in the employ of the interior ministries or of provincial governments, were granted university teaching posts. Depending on their academic credentials and the inclination of medical faculties, honorary doctorates or lecturing privileges (*venia legendi*) were conferred upon asylum directors. In many cases they were given positions as adjunct faculty. The ministry of the interior would usually continue to pay the director's salary and place asylum facilities at the limited disposal of the university. In turn, the ministry of education would cover the costs of research and educational materials, student transportation to the asylum, and occasionally a stipend for advanced students.

Although such cooperative arrangements had significant financial and administrative advantages for the state, medical faculties viewed them with considerable reserve. For one, because the cooperative relationship was bound to the person of the director, his departure or death inevitably voided the relationship and forced its renegotiation, usually at short notice and under unpredictable circumstances. Furthermore, the director was not employed by the university, and so his appointment as director lay beyond the medical faculty's control. Hence, medical faculties could easily find themselves confronting the fait accompli of a director's appointment, leaving them to decide only whether or not to welcome him as a new member of the faculty.[24] And worse still, if they then chose not to welcome the new director into their ranks, the ominous prospect of the state simply ignoring their corporate autonomy and appointing him to the faculty loomed large.[25] Furthermore, the difficult situation of the asylums sometimes crippled the union of clinical and alienist positions. In Halle, because of the large distance between the university and the asylum, Eduard Hitzig had to agree that he would neither become dean of the medical faculty nor receive urgent faculty circulars.[26] Problems such as these, combined with the inconveniences and impracticalities of transportation from the universities to the asylums, severely hindered the efforts to hold regular lectures and clinical courses.

Nor were personal unions between academic and alienist posts uniformly welcomed among busy alienists. The prospect of burdening alienists with academic responsibilities generated a variety of opinions which cut across the alienist/academic divide in the profession.[27] Up to the 1860s, alienists often argued that they were too busy to hold lectures or teach clinical courses. As long as the asylum was seen as the only viable locale for psychiatric training, they could point to their administrative responsibilities to undercut the advance of academic psychiatry and ensure that training would continue in the form of post-secondary apprenticeships. The administrative work of alienists was therefore one of the strongest arguments for a separation of the posts of asylum director and university professor.[28]

The force of this argument rested heavily upon the traditional familial and patriarchal ideology of the asylum, wherein university training had no place. However, the more that ideology was undermined and the preeminence of the asylum called into question, the more the alienists' administrative burdens were turned volte-face against their claim to sole jurisdiction over professional education. In other words, as soon as urban asylums became accepted as adequate receptacles for the mad, the imperative demanding the alienists' undivided attention to an institutional family became an argument excluding them from taking up full academic posts. For if, in fact, alienists had to tend first and foremost to their institutional family, then they could and indeed should not devote their time and energy to teaching medical students and staying abreast with the latest psychiatric literature. These tasks needed then to pass to academic psychiatrists. Thus, the same imperative, which earlier had fortified alienist claims to sole jurisdiction over psychiatric training, now become an acute liability and an argument against their didactic competence.

Consequently, those in favor of expanding psychiatry's academic standing were inclined to emphasize the drawbacks of the personal union model. They lamented the dire consequences arising from doctors who, as medical students, had never studied psychiatry. They attributed the generally poor state of psychiatric health care throughout Germany to the ignorance of these general practitioners. Such ignorance had given rise to consistent complaints among many psychiatrists that information on patients delivered to asylums was usually inadequate or altogether absent. Without reliable information on the patient's prior condition, therapeutic action was delayed or made more difficult.[29] In Prussia, no sooner had a system of asylums been created in the 1830s and 1840s than complaints surfaced about the quality of physicians' reports and prompted numerous ministerial interventions in the first half of the century.[30] The reports submitted by Bavarian doctors in the 1850s and 1860s were so poor that they often necessitated additional administrative paperwork and correspondence, thereby slowing admission procedures and potentially exacerbating levels of chronicity.[31] These problems, it was argued, would persist as long as university students did not study psychiatry.

Furthermore, in forensic cases, nothing less than public confidence in judicial impartiality was jeopardized by poorly trained general practitioners. By law, physicians were required to testify in court if summoned to do so. Not only the medical profession, but also the courts themselves had on several occasions been buffeted by public criticism in the wake of unreliable forensic testimony. When physicians had been called to give evidence in court cases involving mental diseases, they had often been entirely lacking in psychiatric expertise. More damaging still was the inexperience of state physicians and forensic experts, whose duties included the supervision of asylums, interdictions (*Entmündigungen*), and forensic investigations. Psychiatric ignorance among these medical professionals posed a serious threat to public trust in the judicial system.

Critics of psychiatric training in the universities agreed that such problems existed. However, they did not consider it necessary to establish chairs or clinics in order to alleviate them. Roller, for one, found the commingling of alienist and professorial duties to be wholly unacceptable.[32] In his view the clinics for internal medicine sufficed perfectly well for the purposes of psychiatric training.[33] Others believed that general practitioners had no business diagnosing psychiatric disorders. Instead, it was sufficient if doctors merely learned to recognize insanity. The work of diagnosis and treatment could be passed on to competent experts in the field and need not further burden med-

ical doctors, who were already taxed to the limit by the rapid progress of medical science. Medical faculties (especially internists) were also warily mindful
of the rapid development of the psychiatric profession. Far from unanimously
supporting additional chairs, they sometimes worried that it threatened to disrupt the balance of power within their ranks.[34]

Against the backdrop of such opposition, the arguments advanced by the
Prussian Ministry of Education for establishing the chair in psychiatry in Halle
in 1884 are particularly instructive. As noted above and in chapter 4, an intractable situation had emerged in Halle in the 1880s after the working relationship between Eduard Hitzig, who was both asylum director and professor
of psychiatry, and the provincial administration in Saxony collapsed. In this
context, the Prussian Ministry of Education had appealed for funding for
Hitzig's chair and a new psychiatric clinic.[35] Pointing to rising numbers of psychiatric patients, the ministry noted that in no other branch of medicine was
the ignorance of medical practitioners of such great import. It also emphasized
that physicians badly needed psychiatric knowledge when appearing as court
appointed witnesses. As things now stood, theoretical and practical instruction
was a joint undertaking of the university and the provincial asylum. But that
arrangement had outlived its usefulness in Halle and, by implication, elsewhere too. In its evaluation of the situation, the ministry concluded that cooperative arrangements between asylums and universities were impractical and
that they had exposed a "deep seated irreconcilability" between the goals of
the province and the university.[36] In particular, problems had arisen in appointing a director who could also serve as an academic professor. There had
been further difficulties reconciling the practical and administrative requirements of the asylum, on the one hand, and the academic qualifications demanded by the medical faculty, on the other. Furthermore, the asylum continued to lack the appropriate kind of patients for demonstration, because its
admission policy was oblivious to the needs of clinical instruction. Alongside
more subtle reminders that psychiatric clinics already existed elsewhere (in
Leipzig, Heidelberg, and Straßburg) and that university clinics served "humanitarian interests," the Ministry of Education succeeded in convincing a reluctant Ministry of Finance that the time was ripe for "organic progress" in
clinical education. The provisional clinic that resulted from these negotiations
went on to become the first "autonomous" university clinic in Prussia, with
full control over its budget and patient admissions.

The Ministry of Education's letter of 1884 is important, because it represented a shift in the policy of the Prussian government with regard to clinical
instruction in psychiatry. It moved away from a system of cooperation between the provincial asylums and the universities and thereby paved the way
for fully autonomous academic chairs and psychiatric clinics throughout Prussia.[37] And with that shift in educational policy, academic psychiatrists were
one step closer to solidifying their control over psychiatric training.

Otto Binswanger and "The Educational Tasks of the Psychiatric Clinic"

Undoubtedly one of the most well-crafted statements of the didactic tasks of the psychiatric clinic came from Otto Binswanger, director of the mental asylum and professor in Jena between 1882 and 1919.[38] Upon arriving in Jena, Binswanger undertook a reorganization of the curriculum in psychiatry. His predecessor, Friedrich Siebert, had offered only general lectures on psychiatry open to all students. Binswanger continued such lectures, but he also began clinical instruction in the winter of 1882–3.[39] Binswanger placed great importance in these courses. His assistant, Theodor Ziehen, remarked that, far more so than for other academic teachers, Binswanger made the clinical visit into "the focal point of all clinical work."[40] Binswanger's clinical courses, like those of other contemporaries, were a combination of lecture followed up by patient demonstrations. In every hour, one or two students assumed the role of *Praktikanten* and, accordingly, were charged with the examination and diagnosis of the patient.[41] Two hour courses were held twice weekly, while on Sunday morning Binswanger offered clinical visits on the wards.

When he was finally appointed full professor in 1891, Binswanger used his inaugural lecture to set down what he saw as the core pedagogic tasks of psychiatric clinics.[42] Clinical instruction in psychiatry had to train students to bring their medical knowledge to the bedside in order to disentangle the confusing panoply of a patient's symptoms and to construct transparent "pictures of the disease" [*Krankheitsbilder*]. Clinical courses would incorporate three important components: discussion of medical research and practice in both patient observation and therapeutic intervention. If successful, they would provide students with the means whereby later, in their own general practices, they could make accurate diagnostic and therapeutic decisions.

Beyond these general tasks, clinical courses also developed specific didactic responsibilities related to the character and location of mental processes. In the clinic, students unfamiliar with the symptoms and forms of madness were thrust for the first time into a "new world" that appeared entirely at odds with their understanding of medical science. Clinical instruction needed, therefore, first to reassure students that the same laws of causality governing anatomical and physiological processes also applied to psychiatric cases. Mental patients' perceptions, ideas, and acts of volition were as causally determined as other bodily processes, and defects in those processes had their seat in the anatomic structure and physiological processes of the human brain. The phenomena that students observed in psychiatric clinics were in essence no different from what they observed in other clinics. The task of the psychiatric clinic was thus to use the demonstration of psychiatric patients in order to teach students to interpret symptoms in terms of physiological psychology. Psychiatry was a supplement to instruction in physiology and, like it, was a natural science.

Clinical courses in psychiatry thus had a unique task to perform, which differed categorically from clinical instruction in other branches of medicine. According to Binswanger, other and earlier clinical courses involved little more than a collation of visible symptoms. Assessment of the patients' mental state was restricted to a simple determination on whether their state of mind was clouded or not. Clinical courses in psychiatry, however, had a far more expansive task: alongside an assessment of the physical symptoms, they involved a thorough and extensive "dissection [*Zergliederung*] of the mental processes" of a patient. Hints culled from a patient's physiognomy, posture, and movement could acquire critical diagnostic significance, especially in combination with a patients' mannerisms and verbal expressions. In addition, through extensive dialogue with the patient, the inner mental events would be explored. If successful, clinical instruction would thus expose the "inner causal relationship between all of the somatic and mental symptoms." And that success depended upon the teacher being able to "sharpen the senses of the pupil, encourage concentrated looking and listening, and ensure that the empirical facts observed [were] reworked into specific disease concepts." Only through the repeated experience of clinical observation would students come to understand the causal linkage between individual disease symptoms.[43]

Binswanger also envisioned that the technique of hypnosis could play an important role in teaching students about the relationship between soma and psyche. With the help of hypnosis that relationship could be explored as convincingly as it could be with any rigorous scientific experiment. Binswanger's hypnotist subdued his object, imposed his will upon it in the pursuit of his own investigative goals, and thereby acquired great liberty in the exploration of the mind's psychological terrain. This naturally made hypnosis a powerful research instrument. But it was a no less powerful instrument of clinical demonstration for all its ability to lay bear the significance of psychological processes in medicine. It could illustrate not just the parallels between normal and pathological states, but—in conjunction with the physical examination— could also help correlate and map psychological processes to somatic disorders. Binswanger's assessment of the importance of hypnosis for the psychiatric clinician was one—though not necessarily a typical—example of the shift away from the neuroanatomic and mechanist presuppositions of the 1870s and 1880s. In the rush to explain physiological processes in terms of chemical, physical, or mechanical models after mid-century, Binswanger maintained that the "old facts derived from observing nature" had been lost or simply ignored.[44] Clinical demonstrations employing hypnosis could help to restore a psychological dimension to psychiatry.

To bring home the importance of psychological factors, Binswanger pointed to the "modern disease concept of traumatic neurosis."[45] Also known as "railway spine" or "railway brain," the number of cases of traumatic neurosis in Germany had expanded at a breath-taking pace—an increase which Binswanger attributed to German social legislation on accident insurance. The differentiation between patients truly suffering from traumatic neurosis and those who were simulating it in hopes of receiving social welfare benefits had become one of the most hotly debated issues in German medicine in the 1880s. Binswanger lamented that medicine, in spite of all its modern instruments, had spectacularly failed to provide scientific explanations free from the patient's subjective account. He believed that this failure had prompted many physicians to view most cases of traumatic neurosis as simulation. Psychiatrists, however, knew better. For observers well trained in clinical psychiatry, the symptoms of traumatic neurosis were only too familiar. Here, then, was an important diagnosis with great social relevance and financial import. It was a diagnosis that, in Binswanger's view, only those physicians could make, who were specifically trained to recognize the subtle interaction of seemingly insignificant somatic damage and psychological disorder.

Beyond inculcating students with an awareness of the significance of psychological factors in the origins and development of mental disorder, clinical instruction had a second important task: to teach students to diagnose mental disease.[46] Here again, Binswanger drew a line between contemporary academic psychiatry and its historical predecessors. In the early nineteenth century, alienists had placed little importance in a sharp clinical delineation of different disease categories. Binswanger attributed this to a number of factors, including Zeller's *Einheitspsychose* and the anthropological moorings of alienist practice.[47] Most significantly, however, he saw it as a consequence of delayed institutionalization and of the fact that asylum patients therefore tended to exhibit monotone symptoms. Asylums had degenerated into mere receptacles for the incurably mad, so that alienists not only lacked the necessary preconditions, but they also saw no pressing need for a precise, scientific differentiation of mental diseases. But thanks to Griesinger, modern psychiatric science had finally turned the page on this era. Urban asylums had opened up the early stages of psychiatric illness to scientific investigation and thus helped preempt incurability. Above all else, therefore, the aspiring physician had an important role to play in recognizing mental diseases in their early phases, for it was general practitioners who would become psychiatric sentinels in wider society. Clinical instruction would train doctors to assess the "early stages of mental disorder" and would therefore "necessarily consist primarily in diagnostic exercises."[48]

Binswanger's inaugural lecture encapsulated the priorities of many clinical instructors in the early 1890s. In reaction to the mechanistic approaches of scientific psychiatry in the 1870s and 1880s, clinicians were reasserting the importance of psychological explanations of madness, something that their immediate predecessors had been inclined to avoid. At the same time, harvesting the fruits of laboratory and clinical research, they gave preeminence to instruction in the techniques of examination and diagnosis. Rather than disseminating intricate systems of thought or home-grown nosologies, and rather than expounding upon therapeutic approaches, students were to be trained in diagnostic techniques designed to allow them to elicit the deeper signs and symptoms of madness. Herein lay a fundamental change in the task of clinical instruction, from the simple verification of symptoms as manifestations of higher, idealized disease categories, to practice in diagnostic techniques. The goal of Binswanger and others was the production of a scientific diagnostician with psychological sensibilities, who could uncover the early symptoms of insanity in patients at large and thereby ensure more rapid institutionalization.

The Conditions and Disciplinary Practice of Clinical Demonstration

For all of their notions of what clinical instruction should achieve, psychiatrists needed more than simply ideas, if their didactic mission was to flourish. They needed a suitable and readily accessible pool of patients; they needed students listening to and recording what they taught; they needed textbooks and other materials to transport concepts and images to students and to provide them with a survey of the field; and they needed special architectural facilities that would enable them to effectively choreograph their clinical demonstrations. None of these preconditions of adequate clinical instruction were given *a priori*, and professional psychiatrists had to work long and hard to acquire them.

Over the course of the nineteenth century, what constituted appropriate *patients* for clinical demonstration changed radically from the chronic to the acute. In 1822 Friedrich Nasse had argued that chronic patients, "in whom very little remained that could be ruined,"[49] were best suited for clinical demonstration. There was no need to demonstrate curable patients, since "observation, diagnosis, prognosis, and the art of caring for the insane could be learned on incurable patients to the therapeutic benefit of the curable ones."[50] Many alienists were of the same opinion as Nasse. Damerow, for example, had also advocated using chronic patients for pedagogical purposes. Because of the sensitive nature of clinical visits, he recommended that prospective alienists spend their first year of training in custodial institutions (*Pflegeanstalten*) where they could practice their diagnostic and therapeutic skills. Damerow was confident that their "therapeutic attempts on these old patients, toward whom senior doctors were ambivalent, would benefit the asylum, if successful, and be instructive, even if they went awry."[51]

By the end of the nineteenth century, however, chronic patients were no longer really considered useful and integral components of professional training. Aside from their token representation for purposes of demonstration, directors of university psychiatric clinics came to want essentially nothing to do with chronic patients. In their opinion, it was far more important that students see the acute and fresh cases.[52] Of course, this shift had to do with the dogma of early admission and with academic research interests. But it also marked a shift in pedagogic priorities toward instruction in diagnostic examination.[53]

Most clinicians denied that patient demonstrations were harmful and instead emphasized their salubrious effects.[54] They conceded that far more caution had to be exercised in demonstrating psychiatric patients. But not all patients were unduly excited by visits; and even if they were, excitement was not necessarily harmful. And insofar as demonstrations were harmless, there was also no need to exempt any given group of patients. When officials in Heidelberg threatened to limit admission of well educated, but impecunious patients, on the grounds that they were ill-suited for purposes of demonstration, the clinic's director Karl Fürstner protested vehemently. Demonstrations were no more harmful to upper than to lower class patients. Indeed, excluding educated patients would leave the uneducated population rightly to assume that "their patients were good enough for the supposedly damaging scientific purposes of demonstration. This would cast a dark shadow across the clinic."[55]

Nevertheless, as loudly as psychiatrists might proclaim that clinical demonstration was harmless, the prospect of being used for clinical purposes put some prospective patients off and induced them to seek out alternative health care facilities. As institutionalized treatment became more common, and as the benefits of the national health system were extended into the middle classes, hospitalized patients were less obliged or inclined to endure the trials of clinical demonstration. For example academicians in Jena were very concerned that, in the wake of expanding national health care and the impending *Reichsversicherungsordnung,* they would loose their patients to facilities run by private practitioners or by medical insurance funds (*Krankenkassen*), because there patients were "not subjected to clinical demonstration."[56]

What early nineteenth-century clinicians had become accustomed to demanding from the poor, they could not necessarily demand from the well-to-do patients, who—as the century progressed—increasingly sought treatment in hospitals. While, on the one hand, the scientific aura of the university clinic certainly attracted middle-class patients, on the other hand, its pedagogical responsibilities also scared them off. The discretion in which private practitioners and alienists had long placed such paramount importance, came into conflict with the interests of scientific research and professional training. Indeed, the violation of that most valued of middle-class commodities, personal privacy, was the very precondition of clinical teaching. And the more students attended clinical courses after the 1880s, the more intrusive did didactic work threaten to become. One patient, admitted to the Charité suffering from bronchitis, was required to bare her back for hours on end while students lined up to practice their skills of auscultation and percussion.[57]

Initially, however, one of the most frustrating problems facing university psychiatrists was the lack of *students* in their classes. To judge by the complaints of many lecturers, attendance at most German universities was very poor. In spite of his best efforts, Ludwig Meyer had to concede that in the early 1870s his courses remained empty.[58] In Jena in the early 1880s, Otto Binswanger first lectured to a paultry five students and in 1884 Hubert Grashey in Würzburg counted but four students taking part in his courses.[59] Similarly, at the end of the 1880s, Carl Wernicke lamented the paucity of students enrolled in his classes in Breslau and added that the situation was little better at many other universities.[60]

Observers offered several explanations for psychiatry's inability to attract more students. Certainly the perennial problem of psychiatry's poor image in the medical profession placed constraints on its ability to recruit students. Where clinical courses were held in asylums, student attendance also depended heavily on the availability of transport and on the weather. The best efforts of universities and ministries rarely overcame these debilitating geographic and climatic hurdles. The otherwise heavy demands on students' time further compounded these problems. Pressures on the medical curriculum were a subject of constant debate among medical professionals and even led to the curriculum being expanded twice, once in 1883 to nine semesters and again in 1901 to ten. More importantly, however, courses in psychiatry were not obligatory and the subject was barely tested on state examinations. Psychiatrists complained consistently that this was the chief cause of low attendance. Without installing psychiatry firmly in the medical curriculum, student numbers would remain small.[61]

The problems of low student attendance also meant that the market for psychiatric *textbooks* remained relatively small.[62] Alienists had never had any truly compelling reason to write textbooks. While some of them had written substantial monographs, they rarely attempted to write textbooks that surveyed the entire spectrum of psychiatric knowledge. Indeed, at times alienists even exhibited a certain disdain for textbooks because of their compilatory nature, as well as their reductive simplicity and superficiality.[63] Griesinger's textbook had long been a favorite of many psychiatrists. But it had first been published decades ago in 1845 and was now rapidly showing its age in light of the advances of medical science. Thus, one of the hurdles facing academic psychiatrists in the 1870s was a lack of textbooks designed specifically for students of psychiatry.

In his opening clinical lecture in 1877, the Swiss psychiatrist Ludwig Wille complained of both the sheer lack and poor quality of available textbooks. In Wille's view "none of the existing psychiatric compendiums [gave] a truly accurate picture of contemporary psychiatry and hence [failed] to meet the standards demanded of a science."[64] Wille attributed these deficits to the transitional state in which psychiatry found itself: between an outdated psychological and phenomenological tradition and a nascent, yet still evolving neuropathological tradition. In Leipzig, Paul Flechsig was also worried that the discipline's reputation within medicine was suffering because of the poor quality of the didactic literature.[65] He was frustrated by the "very subjective character" of textbooks and by the fact that no one seemed inspired to write a comprehensive account of "all the facts." Psychiatry's reputation in other "highly developed disciplines" was crippled by the multitude of incompatible "psychiatries" published by its practitioners. And in Breslau, Karl Wernicke was similarly disconcerted by the lack of uniformity in psychiatric literature.[66] To his consternation, Wernicke found himself needing to teach students commonly accepted psychiatric principles, only to discover that such principles did not exist. What psychiatrists therefore desperately sought was a survey of the field, which at the same time integrated the findings of new research in scientific medicine. Beginning in the late 1870s, a number of new textbooks came onto the market to satisfy this demand.[67]

Clinical instruction was carried out in a number of different architectural spaces. Often courses were held on hospital wards, in make-shift lecture halls, or combinations of both. The vast majority of asylums had no facilities to accommodate academic instruction. As late as 1900 in Göttingen, lectures were held in the asylum's dining room.[68] In Erlangen, the clinic had neither an auditorium nor even wall charts, pictures, or other demonstration apparatus.[69] Even in Jena it was not until 1908 that a lecture hall for clinical demonstration was constructed; there, lecture courses had been held in regular university classrooms ill-suited for demonstration purposes.[70]

Such limitations posed few problems, as long as student numbers remained low. But at larger institutions, *lecture halls* designed specifically to accommodate clinical demonstration became indispensable architectural accoutrements to the task of professional education. Friedrich Jolly's description of the auditorium in Strassburg is revealing as much for its account of pedagogical architecture as for what it suggested about the theatrical quality of didactic work:

> Across from the central stairway is the lecture hall, flanked on both sides by a small room. The lecture hall is 6.5 meters high and receives its light through three high and broad windows along almost the entire north wall as well as through a large light in the middle of the ceiling. Seating is arranged in ascending order so that the patient being demonstrated can be seen well from every seat. Instead of a lectern, a table for performing experiments has been installed. The table holds a large, dual-purpose direct current battery, a faradizer, and all of the common auxiliary apparatus. The table is placed on rails and can be pushed to one side so that when demonstrating patients or treating them in polyclinical sessions, a large open space in front of the audience can be created. Aside from these apparatuses, alongside the blackboard in a wall-cabinet there is a Wimshurst machine which is driven by a small water-driven motor and often used in polyclinical treatment.[71]

The amphitheatric architecture, in combination with the immediately accessible electrotherapeutic apparatus, suggest the quality of theatrical performance that clinical demonstrations possessed. In many respects, they were performance rituals staged in highly functionalized architectural spaces and calculated to optimize both the exposure of patients and the impressions made on students. In support of these performances, clinics installed elaborate technological systems (ceiling lighting, electrically operated window shades, slide projectors, wall charts, etc.) that allowed for easy enhancement, projection, and manipulation of visual images.[72]

Backstage, these clinical performances were also supported by the spatial organization of the clinic. Konrad Rieger's description of the Würzburg clinic was typical of the situative preeminence accorded to the lecture hall within hospital architecture:

> The main building serves exclusively scientific and educational purposes. The lecture hall is located at the center of it all. There are two separate, entirely symmetrical buildings for each of the sexes. But they are joined to the lecture hall by covered bridges in such a way that, entirely on one level and without crossing so much as a single threshold, the beds can be conveyed without obstruction to any point on the ground floor of the entire building, especially to the podium of the lecture hall and the adjoining examination room. This conception wholly dominates the physical plant and is in itself the result of consideration given in planning to bed-therapy for those patients not entirely quiet or physically normal. If bed-therapy is to be implemented thoroughly, then it may not constantly be interrupted when patients are brought to the lecture hall or to the examination room. Thus, all of these patients are also [subject to clinical] demonstration while in bed. This eases considerably the detailed examination of the patient and saves much time.[73]

Rieger's account illustrates the tight integration of academic therapy and clinical demonstration. On the one hand, his architecture obviated any need to interrupt bed-therapy for the sake of clinical instruction. On the other hand, the same architecture extended the range of clinical demonstration to a larger proportion of the clinic's patient population. The architecture of the Würzburg clinic was indicative of attempts to overcome any conceivable obstacle (therapeutic or otherwise) to a more efficient and silently functioning demonstration of patients. It was one of the small, almost invisible technological innovations that made the clinic a more effective pedagogical theater and simultaneously conveyed its creeping panoptic culture.

Even if psychiatrists succeeded in organizing the required patients, students, textbooks, and lecture halls, clinical demonstrations themselves remained fraught with didactic pitfalls. One of the chief concerns of clinical instructors was that during a demonstration the patients would not exhibit the symptoms they were supposed to. This difficulty was especially problematic when patients were demonstrated in large lecture halls. There, more so than on the wards, a patient's characteristic symptoms might evaporate under the gaze of students. At times, merely the transport of the patients from the wards was sufficient to alter the desired symptoms.[74] One clinician was frustrated by melancholic patients who had been chosen to illustrate symptoms of anxiety: as soon as many of these patients glimpsed the students in the lecture hall, their anxiety disappeared entirely.[75] Another influential clinician warned that when manic patients were confronted with a room full of students, they often became reserved and shy and thus useless for demonstrative purposes.[76] In fact, it was often impossible to predict the success or failure of the demonstration: "maniacs often quieted down, delirious patients became lucid, and paranoic patients often feigned mental health."[77]

Although clinicians might have had difficulty eliciting from their patients the symptoms they desired, students were usually less recalcitrant and more malleable objects of didactic practice. For clinical demonstrations were also opportunities to stage and examine student performance. It was not just the psychiatric patients, but the students themselves—especially the so-called *Praktikanten*—who found themselves under observation. These students were sometimes chosen at a moment's notice and required to examine the patient and respond to professorial queries.[78] In the ensuing small daily rituals of alternating humiliation and confirmation, the students' performance was judged and normalized by the instructor before an audience of peers. Students were also admonished to maintain a serious and professional demeanor when patients were demonstrated. They were prepped to exercise the utmost restraint in their behavior and warned of the possibly damaging consequences for the patient in the event of their misconduct. If laughter arose in the course of the demonstration, it was checked by a "pantomime gesture or a '*risum teneatis amici*,' " thus inducing silence and restoring professional "dignity" to the clinical performance.[79]

State Licensing Examinations (*Approbation*)

Calls for psychiatry's stronger representation in state licensing examinations (*Approbation*) were legion throughout the latter half of the nineteenth century.[80] For the most part, however, these calls went unheeded. Prior to German unification, psychiatry comprised part of state examinations in only very few German states, including Hessen (1848), Bavaria (1858) and Hannover (1866).[81] Elsewhere little or no provision had been made for candidates to be examined in psychiatry. German unification in 1871 had raised hopes that the patchwork of medical regulations across the country could be overcome. But the harmonization of licensing procedures along Prussian lines did nothing to improve the standing of psychiatry. Nor was there much improvement in the licencing of state-employed physicians (*Physikatsprüfung*).[82] In fact, psychiatrists' hopes were soundly dashed after new imperial regulations disregarded their discipline and after numerous petitions in the 1870s were persistently ignored. Indeed, German unification had rescinded the fledgling efforts made in Hessen, Bavaria, and Hannover and thus sowed some resentment among psychiatrists in those states. As a result, it was from outside Prussia—especially from southern Germany—that efforts were later spearheaded to have psychiatry reintroduced as part of the examinations.[83]

Having seen their hopes disappointed after German unification, psychiatrists eagerly anticipated the draft version of revised examination procedures published by the Ministry of Education in 1878. Although the draft foresaw neither mandatory clinical courses nor a separate psychiatric section in the exam, an advisory board of physicians reviewing the draft recommended explicit psychiatric requirements.[84] But in spite of the board's recommendations, as well as last-minute appeals from the *Verein deutscher Irrenärzte,* the new examination procedures of 1883 all but ignored psychiatry.[85]

The Prussian government's unwillingness to support psychiatry appears to have hinged on two issues. On the one hand, the lack of facilities for practical training at all universities and the high costs of constructing new clinics spoke against psychiatry acquiring parity with surgery, gynecology, or internal medicine. On the other hand, medical faculties had intervened to oppose the stronger representation of psychiatry and other medical specialties on the examinations. In fact, commentators such as Rudolf Arndt laid the blame squarely at the feet of the academic community, which had long resisted revisions beneficial to psychiatry.[86] In Arndt's eyes, had the Prussian government taken the advice of practicing alienists rather than medical faculties, psychiatry would have long been part of the state examinations.

This failure to secure psychiatric representation in the revised regulations of 1883 unleashed a new round of professional disillusionment. Karl Fürstner, the director of the Heidelberg psychiatric clinic, had been especially active in agitating for reform and now lent his voice to the disappointed hopes of many of his colleagues. Fürstner attributed the setback solely to the considerable financial costs of constructing clinics at all German universities. Furthermore, he remarked bitingly that now students would be examined by people who had "neither the psychiatric experience nor the mental patients" required to judge the candidates' abilities.[87] Yet, complain as Fürstner might, after 1883 the debate lost much of its intensity until it was again revived at the end of the decade.[88]

In the late 1880s and early 1890s, the question of reforming licensing procedures was again taken up in medical circles. The issue assumed special prominence at the national conventions of German physicians (*Ärztetag*) in Munich and Weimar in 1890 and 1891. The *Ärztetag* was an annual meeting of the German Confederation of Doctors' Associations (*Deutscher Ärztevereinsbund*). The delegates of the confederation represented the interests of local organizations of physicians from all across the country. For several years these delegates had been watching with apprehension as the number of medical students surged upward.[89] In order to stem the flow into the medical profession, some delegates called for sharper examination procedures—including more rigorous testing in psychiatry.[90] Others objected to such recommendations and saw them as blatant attempts on the part of established physicians to ward off the competition of younger professionals entering the medical market-place.[91] Although this was vehemently denied, the exchanges made clear that expanding the examinations to include psychiatry was, in effect, an additional hurdle placed in the path of students entering the medical profession.

Delegates at the conference also debated questions of forensic competence. As long as courts could call on a general practitioner to serve as expert witnesses, doctors needed to be well versed in psychiatry. At stake was not just psychiatry's reputation, but that of the medical profession in general. As one delegate remarked, nothing was more damaging to the reputation of the medical profession than its "psychiatric ignorance in the face of judges and district attorneys."[92] This remark and the outcries of "Bravo!" which it evoked from the audience in 1890 capture the ambivalence of psychiatry's relationship to general medicine. Certainly, many could agree that no other discipline created more problems for physicians. General practitioners were well aware of the drawbacks that their association with psychiatry had for their public standing. But it was for precisely this reason that a consensus among conference participants emerged in support of psychiatrists' demands. At the close of the debates, convention delegates resolved to support the inclusion of psychiatry in the state examinations.

In this context, the debates of the *Ärztetag* were of considerable importance for the professionalization of psychiatry. They point to an area of common interest between general practitioners and psychiatrists. General practitioners had good reasons to support psychiatrists in their endeavors. They were worried about the influx of large numbers of young physicians into the medical profession and about embarrassing encounters with judges and district attorneys. In turn, psychiatrists had, in garnering the support of the general practitioners, acquired a powerful ally in attempts to overcome the resistance of medical faculties. Having psychiatry included in the licensing examinations worked to the mutual advantage of both groups.

The debates also reflected a shift away from the scientific medicine practiced in German medical faculties and psychiatry's reorientation toward general practitioners. The mechanistic and strongly somatic presuppositions of the scientific psychiatry of the 1870s and 1880s—presuppositions that had served the interests of psychiatry's medical and institutional legitimation within the university—were now becoming less important in advancing psychiatry's claim to be a medical specialty *inter pares,* and especially in bolstering its claim to jurisdiction over psychiatric instruction. Whereas in the 1870s it had been professionally advantageous to stress the discipline's affinity to the natural sciences, that affinity now undermined claims of autonomy and hence psychiatry's jurisdiction over clinical instruction. Thus, the debates of the *Ärztetag* reflected an important reorientation within the profession: academic psychiatrists were now making a claim not simply to produce natural scientists, but also to cultivate psychologically aware natural scientists along the lines described in Binswanger's "Educational Tasks of the Psychiatric Clinic."

But the professional expediency of the closer relationship between psychiatrists and general practitioners did not stop here. It extended still further to encompass the task of social prophylaxis. By raising the standards of medical training to include their discipline, psychiatrists were also extending the range of their professional knowledge and skills across a wider body of practicing physicians. While they couldn't make an expert psychiatrist out of every medical student, they could inculcate students with the basic assumptions and techniques of the discipline and thereby extend the clinic's influence outward to German society at large. Doctors well informed in psychiatric matters would be able to assess and diagnose symptoms of deviance earlier and more quickly. In other words, they would be able to serve as prophylactic agents in the larger social community. To accomplish this new task, the psycho-somatic bent of Binswanger's "physiological psychology" was aptly suited. Two petitions from the early 1890s illustrate just how academic psychiatrists drew on notions akin to Binswanger's in recasting their claims to jurisdiction over psychiatric training and simultaneously pitching the profession's socio-prophylactic utility.

The Petitions of 1892 and 1893

Psychiatrists seized on the support of the *Ärztetag* and exploited it in their further efforts to influence government policy. In the following years they crafted two petitions that argued the case for representation in state licensing examinations in far greater detail than ever before. The first petition was submitted in 1892 to the governments of several southern German states.[93] The authors of the petition hoped that through their representatives in the *Bundesrat* these states might exert pressure for the inclusion of psychiatry in the next reform of licensing regulations. The authors immediately appealed to southern German sentiments, recalling to mind how psychiatry had lost out in the wave of prussification after 1871. The petition went on to argue that psychiatry was precisely *not* a medical specialty, but rather a core discipline within general medicine and thus a necessary component in the education of every physician.[94] Interestingly, the authors of the petition cited not psychiatrists, but reports of several local physicians' associations, i.e. of general practitioners, which had been submitted to the *Ärztetag*. The petition stressed the need for doctors to consider both somatic and psychological factors when making their diagnoses. Consideration of both factors was deemed crucial to the diagnosis of the early stages of mental illness. Physicians had to be especially well attuned to these distinctions at the very outset of mental illness if they were to arrive at the proper diagnosis. Physicians could not acquire the skills necessary to make such a diagnosis, as long as psychiatry enjoyed no more prestigious place in academic life than did "Sanskrit."[95]

Nowhere was the need for subtle psychiatric diagnoses more pressing than in cases of state accident insurance. These cases, which had multiplied rapidly during the 1880s, required doctors to write up detailed patient histories. Yet physicians had never received the training they needed to meet the standards set down by state insurance regulations. "In the field [of state accident insurance] it has become clearer than elsewhere just how deficient and one-sided the training of physicians has been. Certainly, medical education as it exists today is sufficient to write up cases of gross abnormities, such as broken bones, etc. But as soon as the disorder involves the nervous system, then the current medical training received by a doctor leaves him almost incompetent to judge the case."[96] A correct medical assessment of such cases demanded intimate knowledge of the "borderline between somatic and mental abnormalities." It was thus impossible to divide body and mind up between respective specialists. Psychosomatic considerations had to comprise part of every physician's basic educational training. Significantly, in closing their remarks, the petition's authors harked back to the plenary address of Schwartz at the meeting of the GDNÄ in 1857.[97] Schwartz's address had been a general practitioner's critique of scientific medicine and—in advancing the cause of clinical training at German universities—had claimed that it was impossible to apportion "the soul to the alienist and the body to all other physicians." That the authors of the petition now cited Schwartz, heralded the waning importance of neuropathology as a strategy in professional discourse.

The second petition was drafted by the directors of university psychiatric clinics and submitted to the imperial chancellor in April of 1893.[98] Its authors hoped once and for all to argue the case for psychiatry's full inclusion in state licensing examinations. Adopting the position of the previous petition of 1892, the authors maintained that psychiatry was not a medical specialty, but rather an independent science in its own right. Most other medical specialties were viewed as appendages to internal medicine or surgery. They had been taught as part of internal medicine and, hence, they could also conveniently be tested as such. While these fields certainly had their own specialized knowledge base, there was no fundamental difference in the methods of examination. Education in psychiatry, however, was altogether different. Students of internal medicine had, as a rule, never seen psychiatric patients and had never learned how to examine them properly. Psychiatric training demanded acculturation to a fundamentally different kind of patient and familiarity with different diagnostic methods.[99] Whereas medical specialties proper differed only in terms of the "quantitative" depth of their knowledge, psychiatry was considered "qualitatively" different from internal medicine or surgery and, as such, a science in its own right; its "essence" could be grasped only if students were given ample opportunity to observe and treat psychiatric patients.

Having thus argued—in the abstract—psychiatry's status as an autonomous medical science, the petition then turned to more pragmatic questions. It maintained that recent developments in Germany had made psychiatry far more important to the "organism of the state" than had previously been recognized. The petition pointed to the great number of cases of suicide attributable to mental illness. It warned of the "horrendous murders" and the "the butchery of entire families" that had been perpetrated "in an incredibly large number of cases" by the mentally disturbed.[100] And it also drew a comparison with the cholera epidemics that had repeatedly ravaged Germany, noting that far more people fell victim to insanity than died of that scourge. In light of these facts, psychiatry needed more than ever to become a central part of every physician's training.

The petition's authors, in pointing to state accident insurance, emphasized the practical social relevance that psychiatry had assumed over the prior decade. Like the petition of 1892, they maintained that to diagnose the psychological trauma resulting from industrial or other kinds of accidents demanded the disciplined eye of well trained physicians. Moreover, keenly aware of the socio-political intentions of Bismarck's insurance program, they added a further twist to their petition: they based their arguments not only on medical merits, but also on the socially conservative political agenda of the legislation. They noted that, as a result of inadequate medical reports, legitimate insurance claims might become caught up in the courts or in a state of administrative limbo. As a result, many families might be thrust into abject poverty. Worse still, the delays in granting claims caused by the incompetence of physicians could fan the flames of social discontent. Thus, social legislation that had been designed to maintain the political status-quo and to ameliorate class divisions in Imperial Germany by binding the lower classes to state insurance programs, threatened instead to alienate those same classes, if medical expertise did not 'grease the wheels' of the programs.

One of the most striking characteristics of both petitions was the marked shift in the consensus from just two decades before. During the 1870s and 1880s the reputation of psychiatry as a medical specialty had depended in large measure on its ability to embed a specific organ, the brain, in anatomy and physiology. But in order for it to be included in state licensing examinations, psychiatrists now had an interest in arguing the case for their distinctiveness within medicine. If psychiatry was merely an extension of anatomy and physiology, then it was more difficult to endorse its autonomous inclusion in the examinations. If, however—as academicians now argued—it differed "qualitatively" from other medical disciplines by providing students with unique skills to diagnose the subtle distinctions between psyche and soma, then their claims to didactic jurisdiction could be markedly enhanced vis-à-vis internal medicine. At the same time, however, arguing the case for "qualitative difference" now necessarily left them open to criticism that they were reverting

to the cerebral speculations of the past. Since the 1840s, psychiatry had defined itself as a profession largely in sharp somatic opposition to the "speculation" and "psychology" of romantic psychiatry. That it now found it professionally advantageous to return to psychosomatic arguments, also raised the
specter of past errors and challenged the historical identity of the discipline.

Psychiatrists could respond to such criticisms in at least two ways. First,
the experimental psychology practiced by Kraepelin became a budding field
of psychiatric research.[101] If psychiatrists chose to "go psychological" when
they argued for their discipline's inclusion in state licensing examinations,
then they might at least do so in the guise of an exacting, Wundtian experimental psychology of the kind Kraepelin was attempting to introduce into his
discipline. The context of the psychological turn around 1890, as well as attempts to see psychiatry included in licensing adopted into the medical examination, thus help *in part* to explain why Kraepelin's research was greeted
with such interest and mimicked by many of his contemporaries.[102] Second,
psychiatrists could and did redouble their attacks on laymen, quacks, and especially clerics, in order to reaffirm their standing as medical professionals
and scientists. In the early 1890s, psychiatry came under direct assault from
the public and from conservative religious and political leaders such as Adolf
Stoecker and Heinrich Treitschke. These attacks sprang from a series of spectacular court cases and revelations involving the maltreatment of psychiatric
patients in mental hospitals. Both petitions had noted the rising crescendo of
anti-psychiatric sentiment; both had tried to exploit public criticism to push
their demands for more intensive psychiatric training. These public criticisms
and psychiatrists' robust responses to them will be considered in detail in
chapter 7 below.

The Binswanger-Schultze Dispute

The petitions of 1892 and 1893 did not go unnoticed among academic colleagues. In fact, they prompted a further dispute, which from 1893 to 1896,
overlapped with the ongoing debate about state licensing reform. The dispute
pitted Otto Binswanger against the professor of gynecology at the university of
Jena, Bernhard Schultze.[103] The gist of their disagreement over psychiatry's full
adoption into state examinations concerned the question of priorities in the
dissemination of knowledge to future medical practitioners. Schultze argued
that, over the course of the nineteenth century, state examinations had obliged
students to cover an ever widening collection of medical specialties. Areas such
as gynecology, physiology, pathological anatomy, ophthalmology and most
recently in 1883, public hygiene, had acquired special representation in the examinations. At the same time, however, Schultze believed that the medical curriculum had not expanded apace. As a result, the addition of each new specialty had been at the relative expense of other fields. Schultze believed that

widening the examinations required a simultaneous extension of the general medical curriculum.[104] If such an extension was not forthcoming, however, then revisions in the existing curriculum had to be weighed against the resulting detriment to other disciplines. In view of these growing pressures within the medical curriculum, revisions became a question of renegotiating the priorities over what was taught in the scarce number of semesters available.

In Schultz's mind, psychiatry was a rather low priority in relation to other branches of medicine. Compared with the larger number of surgical or gynecological cases, medical practitioners would be far less likely to need psychiatric expertise in their day-to-day practice. Beyond that it was not even the task of general practitioners to treat those few psychiatric patients whom they did encounter. At most, general practitioners would have to ensure simply that mental patients were brought to an asylum. While the ability to establish a diagnosis might be of some small benefit, ultimately such decisions lay with alienists and could only be established reliably after institutionalization and close observation on asylum wards. If, due to the extreme difficulty in diagnosing psychiatric disorders, alienists alone were competent to perform such tasks, then there was little use in having all medical students tested in psychiatry.

Nor was it necessary that general practitioners possess in-depth psychiatric knowledge in order for them to fulfill their forensic responsibilities. Schultze was under no illusions as the to great importance of forensic questions for both the individual and for the state. No one could expect a general practitioner, who at best had spent a semester or two practicing in a psychiatric clinic, to be able to meet the high standards expected of forensic specialists. However, precisely because forensic cases were so important they needed to be placed in the hands not of general practitioners, but of state physicians and other full-fledged experts. For these specialists, Schultze advocated rigorous post-graduate psychiatric training.

Otto Binswanger was quick to counter Schultze's assertions. Binswanger agreed that it was not and could not be the task of clinical instruction to provide medical students with specialized training in psychiatry. But he did insist that students be far better versed in psychiatry than Schultze thought necessary. They not only needed to diagnose their patients, but also to assess the "social and forensic significance" of psychiatric cases in order to preempt suicide and criminal behavior. Beyond this carceral argument, however, Binswanger also resorted to a classic statement of the dogma of rapid admission. Because of the slow admission procedures to state asylums, it was paramount for general practitioners to have extensive psychiatric knowledge of the early stages of psychiatric disorders in order to prevent acute cases from developing into chronic ones, which would then waste away as "mental ruins" in the asylums. If the initial treatment outside the asylum were in the hands of a psychiatrically competent general practitioner, not only could the patient be saved, but the community and the state would be relieved of the sad responsibility of forever caring for this "invalid member of the social organism."

Binswanger also differed with Schultze on the question of forensic cases. While Binswanger too called for improved post-graduate training for state physicians, he did not agree that highly trained experts absolved medical faculties of their responsibility to provide students with basic forensic knowledge in psychiatry. As much as it may have been desirable to have forensic experts involved in every case, the large volume of cases made it impossible to limit all forensic work strictly to state employed physicians. Inevitably, every general practitioner would have to be relied upon to make basic judgements about defendants' individual responsibility (*Zurechnungsfähigkeit*) and competence to dispose of their own affairs (*Dispositionsfähigkeit*). And by the same token, legislation on accident and invalid insurance had resulted in a "massive influx of cases of so-called traumatic neurosis" that demanded psychiatric expertise. Finally, Binswanger believed that preliminary observation of forensic cases was essential in order to obtain a full clinical picture. Forensic work done early and well would save the courts countless hours of work at later stages of the legal process.

A final argument of Binswanger's harked back to debates of the 1850s and 1860s between alienists and neuropathologists. Like the petition of 1892, Binswanger took aim at the neuropathological predominance of the past two decades and stressed the need of all physicians to pay greater attention to the psychological condition of their patients. The practicing physician no longer adhered to the "patho-anatomical viewpoint" which had come to dominate medicine of late. Instead, the "progressive deepening and expansion of the medical sciences" demanded better preparatory training in "psychology as well as psychiatry." Thus, for Binswanger in the early 1890s, psychiatry grounded its medical legitimacy not strictly in neuropathology, but also in its access to the recesses of the human psyche and its influence on the health of the individual. Academic psychiatrists were now recouping the psychological tradition they had earlier shunned in order to gain the approbation of scientific medicine. And in doing so they were staking their claim to perform the work of clinical instruction and ultimately social prophylaxis. With the promulgation of revised regulations on state licensing in 1901, including clinical course requirements in psychiatry and a separate examination section tested by psychiatric specialists, those claims acquired legal sanction.

Fabricating Psychiatric Sentinels

The new licensing regulations acted as a catalyst to academic psychiatry. Although clinics had long been considered a prerequisite for the adoption of psychiatry into licensing examinations, in 1901 there were still universities with-

out an independent clinic. At these universities, however, the regulations reinforced calls for new psychiatric hospitals.[105] The new regulations also raised
significantly the number of students attending psychiatric courses. The shortage of students, which had often plagued the discipline prior to 1900, disappeared as a topic of discussion in professional circles. With more students
came also more lecture fees and, of course, a stronger bargaining position vis-
à-vis state education ministries for all manner of wants and needs, from additional assistants to laboratory equipment.

But the new regulations were not greeted with unrestrained joy. They were
also a source of apprehension and concern. At least initially, the new regulations cast an embarrassing light on the continuing divergence of psychiatric
terminologies, theories, styles of teaching, and therapeutic approaches. After
hailing the regulations as a great achievement, Robert Gaupp complained that
psychiatrists were now expected to teach a widely accepted canon of psychiatric knowledge and practice, even though they still couldn't "even understand
one another."[106] If students would now be expected to diagnose and treat psychiatric disorders, then they had the right to expect that, regardless of where
they had studied, they would receive standardized training and that their expertise would be applicable throughout the empire.

Others, however, such as the professor of psychiatry in Marburg, Franz
Tuczek, were more optimistic. Tuczek had no doubt that, after a long and arduous journey, psychiatry had finally become an "empirical descriptive, and
experimental discipline of the natural sciences."[107] In the wake of advances in
anatomy and physiology, psychiatry's task now lay in establishing causal linkage between psychological and cerebro-physiological processes. He believed
that experimental psychology held the key to establishing these linkages and
that, as such, psychiatric science recognized that mental illness afflicted the entire personality of the patient. Psychiatrists therefore had something important
to offer all students preparing for general practice. Because it took account of
both somatic and psychological symptoms and placed special emphasis on the
distinct traits of the individual patient in a way that other branches of clinical
medicine did not, psychiatry was in a unique position to help "educate medical
thought and action.[108]

Psychiatry's inclusion in licencing examinations was highly significant, but
it was not the only realm into which psychiatric education was expanding. The
Prussian Ministry of Education had also begun organizing a far-reaching program of post-graduate courses in 1897. The courses became part of a major
expansion of post-graduate and continuing education spearheaded by the *Zen-
tralkomitee für das ärztliche Fortbildungswesen* and designed chiefly for government health officials and county physicians.[109] Continuing education
courses were offered at several psychiatric hospitals, including the clinics in
Berlin and Munich, the asylum in Illenau and at the new academies for practical medicine in Cologne (1904) and Düsseldorf (1907).

These courses complemented other professional efforts to organize and disseminate psychiatric knowledge and to exert greater influence over civil servants and neighboring disciplines.[110] For example, Emil Kraepelin believed that the state should force jurists to take courses in psychiatry, and he actually offered such courses in Heidelberg and Munich.[111] Furthermore, a Prussian ordinance of 1902, urging courts to hear the expertise of district physicians in psychiatric cases, prompted the VdI to endorse continuing education courses for alienists and to establish a commission on postgraduate education.[112] In 1910 voices could be heard calling for railroad doctors to be trained in psychiatry, and in 1912 a proposal to the medical faculty in Würzburg recommended that an "Institute for Case Reporting" be established in order to improve the quality of professional expertise in foro.[113]

These strategies reiterate the socio-medical and political significance of the new didactic economy within the profession. Psychiatrists argued that *every* medical student should be trained and tested in psychiatry in order to be able to recognize mental illness outside the asylum and to do so at the earliest possible moment. With that, they were staking a professional claim to diagnose and take therapeutic action on *ever less* marginal forms of mental deviancy across *ever wider* expanses of Imperial German society. In other words, the new didactic economy entailed a simultaneous lowering and broadening of the threshold of sensitivity toward mental deviance. Universities did not so much need to train students to be experts in diagnosing every form of insanity, as they needed to train future general practitioners to act as psychiatric sentinels at large, able to diagnose the initial, prodromal stages of mental deviance. All of the instruments of this didactic economy, including lecture halls, textbooks, examinations, etc. were thus important means of projecting clinical technologies outward into broader society and buttressing claims to speak to important ills on the very fringes of insanity.

Another medium through which professionals tried to project their own clinical practices across German society was the psychiatric polyclinic. And it is to the polyclinic that this study now turns.

Social Prophylaxis:
Psychiatric Polyclinics

Introduction

Some historical accounts have argued that, following Wilhelm Griesinger's death, most university psychiatrists no longer recognized that they had explicitly social responsibilities and that they increasingly closed themselves off from broader society.[1] It has been suggested that because of their obsession with neuropsychiatry and systematic psychopathology, university clinics were no longer in a position to respond effectively to the social challenges facing German society. No doubt, psychiatry faced a number of new social challenges as the century drew to a close. National health and accident insurance legislation in the mid 1880s had inundated psychiatrists with new responsibilities: as expert witnesses for insurance companies, the state railway administration, and other corporate organizations. The rising levels of alcohol consumption and bourgeois concerns about it in the 1880s filled their institutions with inebriated "patients." And numerous other fin-de-siècle concerns about nervousness, mental exhaustion, syphilis, crime, and degeneration posed daunting challenges for psychiatrists.[2]

But far from ignoring these challenges, psychiatrists responded to them by redefining their work in more explicitly socio-prophylactic terms. They were not only aware of, but also moving their discipline—nolens volens—in the direction of greater responsiveness and openness toward social issues. Psychiatry's social expansion in the 1890s was noted by a number of contemporary observers. The professor of psychiatry in Marburg, Franz Tuczek, described his patients as "social beings" and "mental illness" as a "sociological concept."[3] Robert Gaupp, the young new director of the psychiatric clinic in Tübingen, remarked that psychiatry was far more than simply a medical specialty, because it extended outward to touch on the larger socio-political questions of the age.[4] At the clinic in Giessen, a young psychiatrist named Adolf Dannemann believed that psychiatry was "as much if not more a social than a medical science."[5] And looking back from the vantage point of 1913, the cerebral pathologist Alois Alzheimer noted the "increase in the social importance of psychiatry" over the last twenty-five years.[6] As these quotations suggest, far from closing down and becoming lost in the details of laboratory or clinical research, academic psychiatry was repositioning itself to address social questions and simultaneously extending its jurisdictional reach in subtle, new, though perhaps less visible ways. Psychiatry was making itself simultaneously more accessible to the general public and expanding its jurisdiction across a widening expanse of personal and social ills.[7]

This chapter investigates the social expansion of academic psychiatry in the years leading up to World War One. It will look first at a new generation of psychiatrists emerging in the 1890s for whom theories of heredity and degeneration carried powerful persuasive force. It will then treat the energetic antipsychiatry movement in the 1890s that sharply scrutinized the work of these professionals. After considering some of the varied psychiatric responses to its critics, the chapter will then turn to psychiatric polyclinics (i.e. outpatient facilities) established at most universities in the 1890s and early 1900s. In the face of sustained public criticism, the polyclinic served to demonstrate the social utility of the profession and to dismantle barriers of mistrust and prejudice separating mental hospitals from society at large. If, as many psychiatrists assumed, the profession's poor image rested on public prejudices, then the polyclinic was an important medium for putting those misconceptions right. More so than in any other clinical space, it was the place where professionals interacted with the general public. In the decades preceding World War One, it represented an important portal through which psychiatric expertise could reach patients and relatives without the need to resort to formal institutionalization.[8] As such, psychiatric polyclinics were an important professional strategy deployed especially by academic psychiatrists to overcome and indeed further dissolve the boundaries separating their institutions from German society.

A New Generation of Psychiatrists

A new generation of psychiatrists was coming up through the professional ranks in the 1880s and 1890s.[9] They had been born following the revolution of 1848 and entered university after German unification in 1870/71. They had been raised in the heady years of German national prowess, but were also tempered by the economic contraction of the late 1870s. They had come of age in an era of heightened social consciousness, but also of grave middle-class concern about the growing strength of social democracy. They were also the first generation to have been exposed to Darwinian concepts as part of their academic training. The mix of social ferment and Darwinian theories of heredity proved fertile ground for the development of the ideas of social Darwinism, degeneration, and cultural pessimism that became so prevalent among the educated middle classes in Wilhelmine society in the years prior to World War One. By 1890 the influence of these younger psychiatrists was making itself strongly felt within the profession, and by 1905 it had become predominant.

Among the most important topics to occupy the attention of this new generation were Darwinism and the etiological implications of hereditarian theories for psychiatric disorders.[10] These debates were inevitably characterized by a standard model of disease etiology that posited a dual cause in the emergence of psychiatric disorders. Most psychiatrists tended to believe that when a congenital disposition (*Anlage*) combined with the pressures of the environment, they "caused" many (especially endogenous) forms of mental illness. When environmental factors acted on a congenital disposition in the "struggle for survival [*Kampf ums Dasein*]," they were viewed as the operative components in the pathogenesis of many psychiatric disorders. Such assumptions were very widespread in German psychiatric circles after about 1890. In ubiquitous statements, psychiatrists expressed their great concerns about the dangers that "congenital psychopathic defects" (*psychopathische Minderwertigkeit*) posed for the social life of the nation. Coupling these concerns with theories of degeneration, they worried about supposedly irreparable damage done to patients and extrapolated their assumptions to the larger social and national body. The prevalence of such ideas was so great that Klaus Dörner has quite correctly argued that Griesinger's legacy was now compounded by a further maxim: mental illness was not only a brain disease but now too a hereditary disease (or *Erbkrankheit*).[11]

Some historians have associated the growth of hereditary theories with widespread therapeutic pessimism in psychiatry at the turn of the century.[12] It is, however, more accurate to say that degeneration theory shifted therapeutic work (and optimism) into the spheres of prophylaxis and socio-biological education and reform. For if congenital defects could not be cured, then they might still be prevented from arising in the first place or at least rendered "harmless" once they had arisen. This conviction opened up space for a new kind of social psychiatry in which prophylaxis and public enlightenment came to be seen as the only viable forms of therapeutic action that could redress the specter of congenital defects.[13] This had profound implications for psychiatric practice. For example, in the context of hereditary theories, institutionalization took on new meaning as a prophylactic undertaking, since it prevented sexual reproduction and thus served to counter the forces of hereditary degeneration.[14] In other words, to be institutionalized meant to become the object of the profession's expanding prophylactic work and of a psychiatric therapy administered to the larger social body. In this sense, the flip side of hereditary theories can be understood as a new kind of social psychiatry writ large as public psycho-hygiene.[15]

One important indicator of the arrival of these ideas was this new generation's ascent to full academic chairs after 1900. A quick glance at the frequency with which chairs in psychiatry changed hands in Germany reveals a sea change after the turn of the century. Between 1900 and 1906 a wave of departures spread across large expanses of the academic corpus and ended in the departure of many of Germany's most senior psychiatrists.[16] The first quiver was registered in early February 1900 when German psychiatry's elder statesman and longest serving Ordinarius, Ludwig Meyer, died in Göttingen. Shortly thereafter, with the death of Rudolf Arndt and the retirement of Peter Willers Jessen, positions at Greifswald and Kiel opened up. In 1902 the members of the medical faculty in Freiburg found themselves seeking a replacement for their colleague Hermann Emminghaus. And then, in the two years from 1903 to 1904, five of the country's most distinguished and influential psychiatrists departed the academic stage: two of them, Carl Pelman in Bonn and Eduard Hitzig in Halle, were close confidants of the ubiquitous Prussian government counsel Friedrich Althoff; another, Friedrich Jolly at the Charité in Berlin, had held the most prestigious psychiatric post in the land; a fourth, Anton Bumm, was the director of the psychiatric clinic in Munich, the capital of Germany's second largest state, Bavaria, and had been charged with the design and construction of what in the first decade of the twentieth century would be hailed as Germany's most modern psychiatric clinic; and the fifth, Franz Meschede, had administered psychiatric affairs at the university of Königsberg for over a quarter of a century. Together with the deaths of Carl Wernicke in Halle and Karl Fürstner in Straßburg, these psychiatrists had held their posts on average for nearly twenty years, and so their departures generated an enormous vacuum into which a whole new generation of psychiatrists was drawn. In retrospect, therefore, Ludwig's departure in 1900 can be interpreted as a symbolic changing of the guard, an exodus of an entire generation of psychiatrists, who were all born in the second quarter of the nineteenth century, had usually received their psychiatric training in the asylums, and had laid the foundations of psychiatry as an academic discipline. With their departure came a new generation of psychiatrists, who began to redefine professional work in more explicitly socioprophylactic terms.

Professionals in the Public Eye: Anti-psychiatry in the 1890s

Psychiatrists of this generation worked in the face of considerable public scrutiny and suspicion. Indeed, one of the formative events touching on the professional careers of this generation of psychiatrists was the emergence of a nascent anti-psychiatry movement in the 1890s.[17] A number of factors contributed to the emergence of this movement and fed public skepticism about psychiatric work. In general terms, the anti-psychiatry debates were fueled by greater public sensitivity to social and (especially after the 1893 cholera epidemic in Hamburg) medical concerns, as well as the rising expectations of a more self-conscious civic middle-class that was able to formulate and advance its own demands.[18] However, one of the more specific catalysts in this historical process was a change in German poor laws coupled with attempts on the part of Protestant agencies to expand their influence over welfare services and to exploit the opportunities created by the new law. To understand the issues involved in the anti-psychiatry debates, we must therefore turn briefly to the poor laws and the interests of church-sponsored psychiatric hospitals.

POOR LAWS AND PROTESTANT WELFARE AGENCIES

The anti-psychiatry movement had been sparked in good part by a change to the Poor Law of 1871 (*Unterstützungs-Wohnsitz-Gesetz*).[19] When it was originally promulgated, that law had made local communities financially responsible for the care of the poor when they fell ill. Provinces, however, were saddled with far less financial responsibility for psychiatric care; they could, if they deemed it necessary, provide financial support, but were not required by law to do so. In the years after German unification, owing chiefly to the forces of rapid industrialization and domestic migration to urban centers, communities were confronted with staggering financial obligations for the support of their poor and sick citizens. Officials in many communities and provinces sought to save money by putting off the construction of expensive new mental institutions and instead contracted private entrepreneurs and/or subsidized religious institutions. In this way they hoped to relieve the financial pressures on their budgets and alleviate institutional overcrowding. In other words, these institutions were put in charge of indigent patients for whom local officials and provinces were otherwise legally responsible. As a result, private and religious asylums experienced rapid growth in the 1870s and 1880s. In the Rhineland, for example, by the early 1890s nearly 800 patients were being cared for by the state outside its own institutions.[20]

In 1891, the Poor Law as it applied to Prussia was revised to alleviate the financial burdens on local communities. The Prussian provinces were made responsible for ensuring adequate institutional care of the insane. What according to the law of 1871 had not been legally binding on the provinces, now became their responsibility.[21] The revision of the law raised the specter of using provincial funding not for the construction of new state-run institutions, but for the cheaper alternative of subsidized asylums operated by Protestant organizations, especially those of the *Innere Mission*.[22] The law also posed a particular danger to urban asylums. The transfer of financial responsibility from communities to the provincial assemblies threatened to make it more difficult to negotiate the construction of urban asylums in smaller, less affluent cities.[23] Thus, although the anti-psychiatry debates of the 1890s quickly expanded to encompass many other issues, one of the most important questions that had provoked the disputes was how provinces would respond to the new poor laws. Would they construct expensive new asylums? Or would they subsidize and out-source psychiatric care to private and church-run institutions?

This question was especially urgent for psychiatrists, because Protestant welfare agencies were actively working to expand their influence over hospital and welfare services.[24] The post-unification economic crisis and the accompanying social tensions had pushed social questions to the forefront of public consciousness and reinvigorated Protestant engagement in the field of social assistance.[25] The *Innere Mission* had become more actively involved in caring for the urban poor; also, Adolf Stoecker's new Christian-Social Party, founded in 1878, had enlivened Protestant interest in social questions. Furthermore, in the 1880s national health legislation had opened up a wide field of activity for both Protestant and Catholic health care services. The energies of these welfare efforts strengthened in the early 1890s after the coronation of Wilhelm II, the repeal of the anti-Socialist laws, and the resurgence of Catholic welfare agencies following the *Kulturkampf*. In 1891, a collection of highly influential Protestant social reformers had rallied under the banner of a new organization, the Lutheran Social Congress, hoping to put Protestant ethics to work in the alleviation of social ills. A kind of "pastoral socialism" gripped a small but influential group of activists within the church who sought to reach out to the poor and the disaffected working classes.[26]

This Protestant reform movement also extended to the field of psychiatry. In 1889, Friedrich Bodelschwingh, one of the driving forces behind the work of the *Innere Mission,* founded the Association of Lutheran Asylum Clergy (*Verband Deutscher evangelischer Irrenseelsorger*). The association's first annual conference was held that same year in Bielefeld, the home of Bodelschwingh's own hospital for epileptics. The declared aim of the association was to improve religious services in the asylums and to coordinate Protestant efforts in response to expanding Catholic welfare services in the Rhineland. The initiators of the association had circulated a questionnaire to clergy working in asylums prior to their first meeting and used the responses to criticize the constraints placed on asylum clergy and to bolster their calls for more Protestant asylums.[27] Particularly contentious about the work of the association was that it sought to establish more asylums not just for incurable patients, but also to extend the range of Protestant influence to include hospitals for curable patients. In the words of one skeptical participant, the conferences were convened not with the intent of discussing the practical problems of asylum clergy, but rather with the intent of creating a "new religious psychiatry."[28]

One of the most contentious issues in the anti-psychiatry debates became the question of nursing staff (*Wärterfrage*) and, in particular, whether it should be recruited from religious orders.[29] Secular hospital staff had been a source of constant concern among psychiatrists. They were nearly unanimous in lamenting its poor training and want of moral fortitude. Some viewed the nursing staff as little more than "ill-suited, irresponsible, and degenerate elements."[30] The *Wärterfrage* was especially acute in university clinics, where the staff tended to be less well paid than in asylums. As a consequence, clinics lost many of their nurses to other asylums and suffered very high rates of turnover in the 1890s.[31] The turnover rate was further aggravated by their urban location, which made it easier for staff to find more lucrative employment elsewhere. Given the difficulties faced in securing a reliable source of staff labor, religious orders promised to bring a degree of stability to psychiatric nursing and reduce patient abuse. At the same time, however, directors worried about their influence on the quality of care and the internal organization of the hospital. Psychiatrists were quick to point out abuses that had occurred under the auspices of Protestant nurses. In the heated polemics of the early 1890s, they suggested that Protestant nurses might hold patients morally responsible for their illnesses, try to convert them, or even resort to exorcism. Without the guidance of psychiatric science, and especially a doctor at the head of every mental hospital, they believed that Christian care would inevitably lead to patient abuse.

THE KREUZZEITUNG ARTICLE

In the context of all these and other developments,[32] an article appeared on 9 July 1892 in the conservative Prussian *Kreuzzeitung* that sent shockwaves reverberating through the psychiatric community.[33] Although the article was unsigned, it was at least inspired if not actually written by Adolf Stoecker.[34] The article pointed to a series of recent scandals in which asylums had been accused of illegally interning psychiatric patients. In light of many recent abuses, Stoecker maintained that new laws needed to be implemented to protect the "civil rights" of innocent citizens. Those rights were too important to be left to the discretion of lawyers and medical experts. Instead, cases of interdiction and institutionalization needed to be placed in the hands of a "commission of independent men" that enjoyed the trust of their fellow citizens. The article also called for sharper controls on asylums, especially private enterprises.

This attack on psychiatry was of no small political importance. The *Kreuzzeitung* was the political organ of a small but highly influential group of Lutheran conservatives on the far right wing of the German political spectrum. The common goal of the paper's supporters was the resurrection of a Christian-conservative state in the face of growing liberal and socialist influence. In a battle for the soul of the German Conservative Party in the 1880s, these supporters waged unrelenting battles against the National Liberals and against Bismarck's right-of-center *(Kartell)* government. Hoping to mobilize lower and lower-middle-class voters, they strove to transform the conservative party into an active, socially oriented, and broad-based political organization.[35] They envisioned a grass-roots political party energized by a missionary Christian zeal: they would battle the corrupting influence of modern society, revitalize the estates and corporate organizations, lead the people back to Christianity and reverse the nation's dizzying descent into moral decadence.

For the greater glory of the Hohenzollern monarchy, they dreamed of dismantling secular capitalism and siphoning off the rapidly growing support for social democracy. In accordance with this Christian-social project, the *Kreuzzeitung* had supported the social programs of Bismarck and, later, Wilhelm II. Yet its advocates never succeeded in attracting the broad-based support they yearned for. Furthermore, although staunchly monarchist, the virulently theocratic, anti-capitalist, and anti-Semitic convictions of the group evoked the opposition and wrath of both Bismarck and Wilhelm II. In the early 1890s the *Kreuzzeitung* and one of its most avid supporters, Adolf Stoecker, were instrumental in regrouping the conservative party and became a spearhead of conservative opposition to the ruling Caprivi government.[36] Thus, the *Kreuzzeitung* article clearly had political aims which went beyond the narrower scope of criticizing psychiatric care in Wilhelmine Germany. It was one of many attempts to mobilizes public opinion with the intent of destabilizing the Caprivi government. It sought to tap into public concern about unlawful incarceration and exploit it for the political ends of the Christian conservative opposition.

While the impact of the *Kreuzzeitung* article on the national political scene is difficult to assess, it had far more tangible effects in the narrower confines of psychiatric discourse. Naturally, psychiatrists interpreted the article in the context of expanding church interest in the field of psychiatric care. The more Stoecker and his associates succeeded in undermining the public trust in psychiatric institutions, the better stood the chances of Bodelschwingh to advance his own agenda.[37] The prospect of having provincial governments invest heavily in Protestant hospitals represented a serious competitive challenge to state-employed psychiatrists. They looked on in dismay as ever more private institutions sprang up in reaction to increased provincial demand for psychiatric services.[38] In their eyes, the fact that the provinces were subsidizing asylums run by the church represented not only a throwback to the religious cast of institutions in the early nineteenth century and the *traitment morale,* but also a direct challenge to the scientific principles that they had worked so hard to instill in their profession.

The official psychiatric reaction to these developments came at the annual meeting of the *Verein Deutscher Irrenärzte* in Frankfurt in 1893. There, Fritz Siemens and August Zinn delivered scathing attacks against Bodelschwingh, Stoecker, and the Association of Lutheran Asylum Clergy.[39] They both painted harrowing pictures of the influence of religious orders on psychiatric care and exposed the links between Stoecker's appeals for better asylum supervision and the interests of Protestant hospitals. Siemens and Zinn were especially annoyed with the more or less explicit assumption that religious orders might, on the basis of their long experience of caring for incurable patients, now begin building asylums for curable ones as well. In conjunction with the *Innere Mission,* the Association was aiming to "to take from doctors the reigns of authority over mental asylums and place them back in the hands of the church."[40] Faced with such challenges to their professional authority, participants at the meeting unanimously approved a catalogue of resolutions condemning hospitals run by religious orders and calling for legislation to ensure that all psychiatric facilities be run by medically trained experts.

Although the resolutions passed by the *Verein* went unheard in state ministries, an inflammatory debate ensued and consumed its combatants over the next several years.[41] Psychiatrists and clergy traded volleys about exorcism or seventeenth-century witch hunts, on the one hand, and cold scientific materialism, on the other. Psychiatrists branded so-called "pastoral psychiatry" for interpreting psychiatric disease as the product of demonic forces and individual sin; Bodelschwingh and his associates disputed any claims of psychiatrists to a monopoly over the care for the insane, even pointing to psychiatry's own failure to produce a reliable system of classification for psychiatric disorders.

Alongside attacks from the leaders of the *Innere Mission,* numerous critical accounts of the conditions of patients held in psychiatric institutions began to appear in print. During what one psychiatrist described as an "era of mistrust,"[42] first-hand accounts of scandalous abuses spread out across the front pages of the national press. Jurists responded with draft legislation and a panoply of recommendations for reform. Most prominent among these recommendations were the so-called *Göttinger Sätze*[43] which were drafted by a group of conservative jurists advocating reforms in the procedures of interdiction. Also, a number of reports emanated from a spectacular trial in the early 1890s that involved Carl Pelman, head of the psychiatric asylum in Bonn.[44] These early accounts formed the basis of what in the latter half of the 1890s grew into a full fledged reform movement, calling for laic oversight of the asylum system and imperial legislation on psychiatric institutions. Although driven by different assumptions and goals, this movement ultimately extended across the entire political spectrum. Initially it had broken out into wider public discourse following the right-wing attacks of Stoecker in 1892 and 1893. After 1895, however, anti-psychiatric sentiments spread to left-of-center liberal and social democratic parliamentarians and the movement began to consolidate itself around a number publications and associations.[45] As a result, the psychiatric profession came under intense pressure concerning procedures of interdiction, admission, and discharge. By the first decade of the twentieth century, psychiatrists found themselves confronting an increasingly well organized and vocal opposition that drew its support from former patients and relatives across a wide spectrum of the political landscape.

THE MELLAGE TRIAL AND PRUSSIAN REFORMS OF 1895

What ultimately helped deliver psychiatrists from their embattled station in the 1890s was, ironically, a further scandal and ensuing litigation.[46] In a nutshell, the so-called "Mellage trial" of 1895 involved abuses visited upon a Scottish patient while in an asylum run by a Catholic religious order near the town of Aachen. The abuses had been uncovered by a local restauranteur (Mellage) and reported to officials. After state inspectors found no wrongdoing, Mellage proceeded to publish his story of patient abuse in the national press. As a result, the religious order promptly began libel proceedings against Mellage and his supporters. But the proceedings only further exposed the abuses in the asylum, thereby discrediting church-run asylums and revealing the wholesale failure of state inspectors to execute their duties.

Once the courts had exonerated Mellage, smug psychiatrists were quick to exploit the embarrassment it had brought upon religious orders and the state. They saw the trial as the logical consequence of the provincial policy of relying on religious orders to care for the insane. The trial opened the way for psychiatrists to take aim at provincial care for the insane, branding it a "quagmire" far beneath the standards of other "civilized states."[47] The Mellage trial, in the graphic words of one psychiatrist, had lanced a boil and "emitted an a enormous mass of putrid, stinking pus."[48] Others complained loudly to Prussian officials that the resolutions of Frankfurt in 1893 had been "systematically ignored" and that government policy had succumbed to "formal bureaucratic procedures . . . administered without the help of experts."[49] The consequences of these failures were the shocking abuses exposed by the trial.

In order to defuse the rising crescendo of criticism, the Prussian government was spurred into action. Once the trial ended, the issue of reform was brought before the Prussian House of Representatives. Within four months the government had implemented substantial reforms involving the state's inspection policy and regulations governing admission and discharge from psychiatric hospitals.[50] The regulations set standards for asylum directors, including at least two years experience in a large asylum or university clinic. Provincial officials were instructed to dismiss doctors whose qualifications were unsatisfactory. The new rules also set down stricter criteria for inspection committees. Finally, the regulations set up guidelines on proper documentation of all institutionalized patients. Similar reforms were put into effect in Bavaria, Württemberg, and Baden.[51]

But these regulations did not mollify psychiatry's critics. For years to come, the Mellage trial helped to spur calls for national legislation on mental hospitals.[52] In fact, the defense attorney in the Mellage case went on to voice his demands for legislation on the floor of the *Reichstag*. Again prodded into action, in April 1897 the government queried the German states about the need for imperial legislation. The initiative found only tepid support outside Prussia and was opposed by the powerful interests of the German Lawyers Association and the Association of State Medical Officers.[53] As a result, in 1902 the German government finally announced that legislation would not be forthcoming, effectively putting psychiatric reform on the "back burner" of national politics.[54]

The response of psychiatrists to the administrative reforms of 1895 and to the looming prospects of national legislation were decidedly ambiguous.[55] Some psychiatrists welcomed the regulations of 1895 as the fulfillment of long-standing needs. But most were extremely wary of any increased state supervision. They especially feared that their professional interests would be sacrificed to the exigencies of the political process—that *Sachlichkeit* would succumb to *Parteilichkeit* in any attempt to regulate their profession at the national level. Consequently, they preferred to rely on administrative regulations rather than on formal legislation, convinced that their ability to persuade ministerial officials of the need for policy reform was far greater than their ability to steer favorable national legislation through the rough waters of party politics.[56]

For all the satisfaction psychiatrists may have found in seeing church-run institutions accused of mishandling their patients, the anti-psychiatry movement and the reform initiatives that followed in its wake were also profoundly disconcerting. While public scandals such as the Mellage trial may have blunted the advance of religious asylums, they also resulted in regulations that impinged on the profession of psychiatry as a whole and did little to relieve the pressures facing their embattled discipline. The anti-psychiatry movement heightened public scrutiny of psychiatric hospitals, zeroing in on the legal and administrative threshold of the institution as defined by policies of admission and discharge. Public scrutiny also penetrated more deeply into the psychiatric hospitals. As one academic clinician complained, newspaper accounts of the scandals made their way back into psychiatric hospitals where they compromised the authority of psychiatrists within their own institutions and endangered any hard-won trust doctors may have established with their patients and staff.[57] In short, the scandals brought with them intensified public scrutiny at all levels of psychiatric work. They placed psychiatrists under the critical purview of state inspectors, of public watchdogs, journalists, and politicians, and even of their own institutionalized patients. This intensified scrutiny shaped the work of psychiatrists and mobilized them into action in defense of their professional reputations. In the ensuing years, they worked hard to overhaul the pejorative image of their profession and began building a public relations infrastructure to answer their critics' charges.[58] An important part of these endeavors included efforts to redefine their work in terms of social prophylaxis.

Revamping the Profession's Image

It has been argued that in the 1890s psychiatrists responded either aggressively or with a wall of silence to attacks "from below," while at the same time remaining loyal to the state "above."[59] This was often true, especially if one focuses on the polemical literature of the 1890s. However, by polarizing the analysis in terms of the state versus society, this assessment also oversimplifies the dilemmas faced by professional psychiatrists. Psychiatric responses were much more complex and ambivalent than this interpretation suggests. Psychiatrists had a genuine interest in improving their reputation and they were well aware that they desperately needed to win "the support of public opinion" for their work to bear fruit.[60] They were simultaneously reluctant to make themselves pliable instruments of the state's public security interests. They certainly looked to the state to enforce professional standards of practice, but they did so in the expectation that the state would accede to their professional expertise.[61] If the anti-psychiatry movement taught psychiatrists anything, it was the acute danger they faced if their hospitals became instruments of state repression and incarceration. Psychiatrists, such as Otto Binswanger, therefore demanded "the freest and most unimpeded admission to mental hospitals. Patients and relatives should not have to endure the time-consuming and embarrassing intervention of state officials, who convey a police-like quality" to the entire admissions process.[62] When psychiatrists looked to the state for more thoroughgoing regulations, they did so with mixed feelings: they at once worried that those regulations would disregard their own interests and at the same time hoped that they would provide a solid legal footing on which they could justify their actions in the face of the accusations of their critics and detractors. Therefore, in gauging the responses of psychiatrists to the anti-psychiatry movement, it is useful to look more closely at the explicitly professional motives that guided their efforts to correct public misconceptions and project a positive image of their discipline.[63]

One of the most visible manifestations of these efforts was a change in nomenclature. Psychiatrists moved to change both the names of the institutions in which they worked, and their own professional title. In light of the damaging scandals of the 1890s, many sought to jettison such pejorative labels as *Irre, Irrenanstalt,* or *Irrenarzt* and replace them with terms more amenable to the public ear, such as *Gehirnheilanstalt, Nervenheilstätte, psychiatrische Klinik.*[64] Most prominently, the *Verein deutscher Irrenärzte* adopted the new name *Deutscher Verein für Psychiatrie* at its annual meeting in Jena in 1903. In Heidelberg the official name *Irrenklinik* was dropped.[65] In 1902 the asylum in Jena was renamed from *Irren-Heil- und Pflegeanstalt* to *Psychiatrische und Nervenklinik.*[66] In Würzburg, Konrad Rieger too saw great public relations advantages in avoiding the name "*Irrenabteilung*" or "*Irrenklinik,*" preferring instead "*psychiatrische Klinik*" or better still "*Nervenklinik.*"[67] Furthermore, the builders of new clinics, such as those in Giessen (1896), Kiel (1901), and Munich (1904) distanced themselves from the stigmatized term *Irren* by designating them psychiatric and/or neurological clinics.

Efforts to improve the profession's image also extended to the more efficient dissemination of information. A more rapid and coordinated response to the charges of psychiatry's opponents was key to nipping criticism in the bud. One of the intentions of a new journal first issued in 1899 by Johann Bresler was to do precisely that. The weekly, which after 1902 appeared under the title *Psychiatrisch-neurologische Wochenschrift* (*PNW*), was an eclectic and hybrid undertaking that juggled the professional interests of both psychiatrists and neurologists and delivered to its readers a potpourri of issues pertaining to day-to-day professional practice. Hoping to act as a central clearing house for the profession, it had been born of the arduous battles of the 1890s with the anti-psychiatry protest movement. Bresler hoped that the journal would provide a common medium through which psychiatry could respond to its critics, deflect public criticism of the profession, and quickly defuse potential scandals.[68]

Bresler's initiative remained the work of a single individual. But gradually psychiatrists began laying more formal groundwork for their own public-relations apparatus.[69] As early as 1893, Carl Pelman, professor of psychiatry in Bonn, had called for a central body to protect psychiatrists from unwarranted criticism.[70] On the initiative of Emil Kraepelin, the VdI established a "Commission for the Preservation of Professional Interests" in 1907.[71] Proposals were also advanced to set up a news bureau to disseminate information to the press.[72] In 1912, a commission brought together psychiatrists and representatives of the *Reichsverband der deutschen Presse* in order "to verify objectively all reports of admissions and treatment" which had given rise to public criticism.[73]

Academic psychiatrists were particularly adept at turning the anti-psychiatry sentiment of the period to their own advantage. Far more so than their alienist colleagues, they were in a position to capitalize on the crisis of the profession's public image. For one, the atmosphere of scandals contributed to a greater willingness on the part of relatives to see their family members committed to university clinics rather than an asylum. As a result, clinic directors registered tangible increases in their admissions statistics.[74]

Some academics even relished the heightened scrutiny under which psychiatrists found themselves. Carl Fürstner, the director of the clinic in Straßburg, tried to seize the anti-psychiatry mood of the 1890s as an opportunity to continue educating the public about mental illness. He hoped to exploit the scandals by exposing prejudice and bias in published accounts. Never, he believed, had the public's interest in psychiatry been so great. Hence, ironically, the aura of scandal and heightened public sensibility enveloping the discipline might just be the key to improving the profession's reputation.[75] Among many other things, Fürstner recommended that relatives be allowed to visit patients not just in special visiting rooms, but also on the wards of the hospital as well. He believed that this would help dispel false impressions about the care of patients in psychiatric institutions. Interestingly enough, Fürstner's suggestion was made with very clear disciplinary goals in mind. Allowing relatives onto the wards would not only enlighten them, but also check their criticism. The continual presence of other patients and visitors on the wards imposed "a certain reserve" upon relatives so that they could be controlled in an "inconspicuous manner."[76]

The crisis of professional image also represented one of the strongest arguments for psychiatry's inclusion in state licensing examinations. Doctors who lacked psychiatric training heightened the dangers of unlawful incarceration and ensured the persistence of negative public stereotypes. Carl Fürstner believed that the main cause of the anti-psychiatric mood in the country could be attributed to general practitioners who had failed to serve as intermediaries between the specialists and the public.[77] Because general practitioners had received no academic instruction in psychiatry, they were incapable of correcting public misconceptions about the discipline. Konrad Rieger also rushed to bolster the profession's position on professional education. According to him, "in order to quiet the public" about unlawful incarcerations, better psychiatric training was needed of all doctors.[78] Some even argued that if more doctors were training in psychiatry, then disciplinary oversight of nursing care on the wards would be easier, thus solving the *Wärterfrage* and further ameliorating public criticism.[79] Hence, after 1892 public scandal fueled the debate in Prussia and elsewhere about psychiatry's inclusion in medical licensing examinations.[80]

Psychiatric Polyclinics

Among the many different means of dismantling the barriers of mistrust separating mental hospitals from society at large, perhaps none was more important for academic psychiatry than out-patient or polyclinics. Medical polyclinics had existed at many German universities since the early 19th century and had been designed chiefly as academic courses with didactic aims in mind.[81] Over the course of the century, however, they became more closely associated with poor relief. In fact, according to one account, the "natural environment" of the polyclinic was the delivery of medical services to the poor in university towns.[82] Often polyclinics were operated on the basis of contractual arrangements between universities and local welfare agencies as supplementary dispensaries of medical services otherwise provided by poor relief. In exchange for these medical services, polyclinical visitors became the objects of clinical research, instruction, and ultimately socio-prophylactic intervention.

One of the first psychiatric polyclinics to be established was at the Charité in Berlin, where in 1872 Carl Westphal opened a *Poliklinik für Nervenkranke* and linked it to the neurological ward.[83] It was modeled after the polyclinics of the pediatric and ophthalmological wards and was used by Westphal to investigate borderline conditions.[84] Other early polyclinics existed in Halle and Strassburg. According to Hitzig, the clinic in Halle had a polyclinic from its inception. It was a provisional facility in 1885, and after the new clinic was constructed in 1891, the polyclinic occupied three rooms of the new building.[85] In

Strassburg, polyclinical facilities had been introduced in the years following the clinic's construction in 1886.[86] Elsewhere, in 1879 Carl Fürstner established an "*Ambulatorium*" for epileptics in Heidelberg, which consisted of twice weekly office hours in which the relatives of epileptics could receive medical advice.[87] During the 1890s, psychiatric polyclinics were also established at the universities in Breslau and Königsberg. Most polyclinics, however, were not constructed until the late 1890s and early 1900s.[88]

Sometimes polyclinics were spatially segregated from the rest of the clinic. In Leipzig, for example, an annex to the clinic was constructed in 1906 to house the rooms of the polyclinic, together with a new lecture hall and rooms for photographic exposures. This spatial segregation lent poignant expression to the tight architectural and institutional mesh connecting outpatient care, pedagogical demonstration, and photographic fixation. The annex had also been placed at the fringe of the clinic, not only to prevent its bustling activity from disturbing other patients in the hospital, but also to make it "directly accessible to the outside [world]."[89]

The potential of polyclinics to expand the pool of patients seen by clinicians was enormous. In Berlin in 1909 the polyclinic employed 12 physicians who together treated 6000 patients a year.[90] That same year in Breslau, admissions to the polyclinic were more than two-and-a-half times that of the psychiatric ward itself.[91] In Jena in 1895, over forty percent of all admissions to the clinic came through the polyclinic.[92] Thus, polyclinics gave psychiatrists unprecedented access to large patient volumes and even drew criticism for their routinizing effect on medical diagnosis. But given the threats that rival provincial, civic, and confessional institutions posed in the delivery of psychiatric services, polyclinics were relatively inexpensive means of responding to these challenges by expanding the reach and social utility of clinical means.

Psychiatric polyclinics employed a number of different therapeutic instruments.[93] Reports on polyclinical facilities speak of "hot air therapy," "vibration therapy," and massage as some of the more exotic forms of treatment. Suggestion (including but not restricted to hypnosis) was also an important form of treatment in polyclinical settings. By far the most common form of treatment, however, was electrotherapy. Electricity was used primarily as a form of pain-relief, especially for head aches and neuralgic complaints. An elaborate literature on different kinds of electricity and their proper application evolved over the course of the 1870s and 1880s while psychiatrists gradually developed and refined their therapeutic techniques.[94] Above and beyond the basic physical laws of electricity, polyclinical practitioners had to learn the correct points of application, the type of electricity, and the appropriate frequency and voltage with which to apply electricity. Their work demanded an exact topographic correlation between the mode of application and the nervous disorder to be treated. They thereby transformed the bodies of their patients into three-dimensional electrotherapeutic spaces—spaces governed by the theoretical assumptions and therapeutic techniques of electrotherapy.

Polyclinical physicians also employed more traditional forms of medical advice. They counseled their patients in all manner of daily affairs from physical fitness to mental hygiene. Similarly, prescription medicines and dietary instruction were among the most common forms of therapeutic advice. In treating nervousness, simple hygienic directions on the conduct of the patient's daily routine was an important aspect of the polyclinic's mission. How long to sleep, when to rise, what and when to eat, whether to consume alcohol and how much—these were all questions critical to the therapeutic restructuring of patients' lives. Typical of this type of out-patient advice were the recommendations made by Eduard Hitzig to the influential Prussian official Friedrich Althoff, who had been suffering with "symptoms of nervousness." After reassuring Althoff that his symptoms were not organically based, but merely functional, Hitzig advised: "The most important thing is *regularity!* Within limits, it's not so important whether you begin work an hour earlier or later, as long as these times are never deviated from. The same is true for meals. In particular I recommend satisfying one's hunger not all at once in one meal. Instead, breakfast and lunch should be substantial—a few eggs or a portion of meat. [. . . Dinner can] be more frugal."[95] Hitzig then went on to recommend that "under no circumstances" should Althoff engage in serious paper work after dinner. Instead he should do some light reading. In the morning, or while working, cigars were ill-advised; they should be limited to three per day. A bottle of good wine was perfectly acceptable. In short, Hitzig was advising his famous patient to lead a disciplined and regular lifestyle, much as doctors had throughout the nineteenth century. Yet now he was doing so with the persuasive force not so much of Hitzig's character, as of an entire branch of medical science with its own elaborate institutions and disease concepts.

The Professional Utility of Polyclinics

Throughout the 1890s and early 1900s psychiatrists marshaled a number of arguments in justification of psychiatric polyclinics. A few concrete examples can illustrate just what they believed the professional function of the polyclinic was. One of the most concise statements of the polyclinic's professional utility came from the director of the clinic in Strassburg, Carl Fürstner. According to Fürstner, the benefits of the polyclinic included getting

> the public in the habit of seeking professional advice even for apparently innocuous mental anomalies. In this way prophylaxis can be improved: proper treatment can prevent psychoses from arising and the patient and his family can be protected from unpleasant consequences. . . . In easily accessible polyclinics we can provide medication, advice and instruction. We can also advise on re-

moving the patient as soon as possible from his harmful environment and placing him in an institution before his chances for recovery dissipate. The polyclinic also allows for out-patient treatment of many diseases closely related to the psychoses, such as epilepsy, hysteria, and hypochondria. These are forms of mental illness which are more familiar to the psychiatrist than to the internist. They are also forms which are especially valuable for the purposes of psychiatric education. Finally, the polyclinic has yet another advantage. The polyclinic can be visited in a casual way [*ungeniert*] by those former patients who still need the supervision and advice of a physician. Furthermore, the polyclinic [is a place] of constant interaction between doctors and the lay public. It is therefore especially well suited to dispel the prejudices which . . . to this day dominate public opinion about mental disease and related issues.[96]

Fürstner was not alone in propagating these views. Many of the same claims were expressed by colleagues at other German universities as well. One particularly notable example is the case of Giessen. There, polyclinical rooms had existed in the psychiatric clinic from its inception in 1896. To acquire those facilities, the clinic's director had to overcome the staunch objections of the medical faculty.[97] Once the clinic did open, doctors working in the polyclinic had a number of diagnostic tools at their disposal, including instruments for performing blood tests, for testing sense perception, ophthalmological and craniometric instruments, means for measuring reflexes and producing three-dimensional representations of knee reflexes.

Beyond the opportunities provided by its "wealth of material" in "prodromal and initial stages," the polyclinic in Giessen also had more far-reaching public relations and prophylactic aims. In the words of Adolf Dannemann, a doctor in the clinic and the chronicler of the hospital's construction:

The polyclinic fulfills an important task in relation to the wider public. The public, after overcoming a certain resistance to the term *Irrenanstalt,* soon realizes the great advantage which the direct advice of specialists can offer. There are many 'nervous' conditions which, although they accompany mental symptoms or are otherwise related to psychiatry, don't signal actual mental disease. This large group of patients who suffer from neurasthenia and hypochondria receive useful advice based on psychiatric principles. Once the polyclinic . . . has become known in the community, the psychiatrist will be able to establish contact with the public. This contact will allow him to fulfill many of the tasks of his discipline as a social science.

Dannemann went on to emphasize the usefulness of the polyclinic in providing former psychiatric patients with follow-up advice and support. He believed that Griesinger himself had had just such post-institutional care in mind when he designed his urban asylum. Dannemann thus envisioned the polyclinic as escaping the odium attached to other psychiatric hospitals and functioning as a point of dissemination of psychiatric advice. If the advantages of the polyclinic were duly exploited, then "[public] perceptions of the nature and purpose of mental hospitals would at last be brought up to date." This, in turn, would ease public access to the clinic and thus facilitate its socio-prophylactic task. In other words, the most important aim of the polyclinic was to prevent the "social damage resulting from ignorance about the early symptoms of insanity and to enhance public understanding of psychiatric things."[98]

Potentially, this meant an enormous expansion of the social responsibilities of the psychiatric clinic. Coupled with a polyclinic, the psychiatric clinic would no longer be an institution of last resort harboring the indigent sick, but rather a general psychiatric hospital serving as an integral component within the community health care system. In the past, psychiatric institutions had been receptacles for individuals who had been socially marginalized and who had demonstrated that they could not live on their own outside the asylum. Now, however, psychiatric institutions would admit "all patients who might benefit from psychiatric help."[99] As Dannemann and others envisioned them, polyclinics—replete with their armature of diagnostic and therapeutic technologies—had an integral part to play in the profession's reorientation toward greater socio-prophylactic tasks.

Würzburg was a further example of attempts to cast the polyclinic as an instrument of socially oriented psychiatry. There the polyclinic had been established in 1903 as a private institute. Its chief advocate, Wilhelm Weygandt, had argued for the polyclinic on a number of the grounds.[100] It would, for one, service numerous disease categories such as the early stages of psychosis, functional neuroses, and mentally abnormal children. In providing treatment for these patient groups, it would also fill an important gap in medical education, namely, in the demonstration of fresh, nervous cases. It would become possible, Weygandt argued, to exploit these "borderline" conditions, since the polyclinic would allow for a "greater concentration of the scattered patient material." After Weygandt left Würzburg in 1908, his successor Martin Reichardt attempted to have the polyclinic incorporated into the university as an independent institute.[101] Reichardt justified this request by arguing that he intended to establish what he called an "Institute for Social Medicine" or, alternately, an "Institute for Case Reporting [*Begutachtung*]." This reorganization was designed to satisfy two important didactic aims. First, it was to teach the fundamentals of writing up good case reports on accident victims sent to the clinic for observation by insurance agencies. And second, he hoped to turn the polyclinic into an institute that would specialize in teaching students to recognize and treat nervous diseases. Reichardt couched his request in terms of "social medicine," emphasizing the great prophylactic importance of better medical training in the social causes of disease. He also stressed that medical students needed to acquire a better "psychological understanding" of their craft in order for them to fight the "national disease [*Volkskrankheit*]" of nervousness.[102]

A final example of the emergence of psychiatric polyclinics in Germany is the case of Göttingen. There the polyclinic was established in 1901 at the urging of the newly appointed professor of psychiatry August Cramer.[103] The polyclinic had been created ostensibly to counteract the deficiencies of the local asylum, where a lack of acute cases had crippled psychiatric instruction.[104] According to Cramer, the polyclinic was of great importance, because it would allow students to see not just "artifacts of the asylum" but also the "lighter, nervous and mental disorders" which they were likely to encounter in their daily practice.[105] Students needed to see these types of patients so that they could "intervene preemptively" in the interests not only of the patient, but of the national economy and the body politic. Cramer also insisted that the polyclinic carry the name "Nerven-Klinik," so that it would be sought out by "psychiatric patients who usually prefer to be considered nervous rather than insane."[106] Cramer discerned the fruits of such public relations efforts in the fact that the polyclinic appeared to enjoy public confidence: during the year 1903/4 it treated more than six hundred patients in over four thousand appointments.[107]

What made the polyclinic in Göttingen exceptional was its integration into a web of other institutions of psychiatric care in the province of Hannover. The polyclinic was essentially an easily accessible ante-chamber to an array of other institutions, including the nearby large provincial asylum, a far smaller university psychiatric clinic, and a sanatorium for nervous patients in Rasemühle. The sanatorium, in particular, was a construction unique for its time. According to its statutes, it was accessible only through the polyclinic. It was specifically designed for those lower-class patients who were suffering from nervous disorders, but who were not considered mentally ill. It provided patients an affordable opportunity to "relax" and "escape the daily monotony and misery" of their lives. Significantly, it was built to "avoid all characteristics of an asylum" and was instead modeled after a family hotel or *pension.* The sanatorium even went so far as to abolish the gendered segregation of the institution in order to allow for "unconstricted relations between the sexes."[108]

In an address to the provincial parliament of Hannover in 1903, Cramer outlined his views on the prophylactic aims of the sanatorium in Rasemühle.[109] There he appealed to the concerns of listeners, warning them of the dangers that mental illness posed to the "cultural and monetary values of the state." Psychiatric disease was just as pressing a public health issue, Cramer declared, as other afflictions such as tuberculosis, alcoholism, and sexually transmitted disease. Indeed, mental hygiene was intimately associated with the fight against alcohol and syphilis, since these "enemies of humanity" could directly spawn both nervous exhaustion and mental disease.[110]

The linkage of the polyclinic and the sanatorium reflected the central prophylactic intent of the entire system of psychiatric care in Göttingen. As director of the polyclinic, the sanatorium, the provincial asylum, and the psychiatric clinic, Cramer oversaw an elaborate and highly integrated system for the delivery of psychiatric services.[111] Each of the institutions complemented and buttressed the others in support of a common prophylactic goal. In these efforts Cramer was in step with other attempts by psychiatrists to create more specialized institutions to match the various groups of patients they were treating and to mesh them administratively with their own clinics.[112]

In assessing these three polyclinics in Giessen, Würzburg, and Göttingen, it becomes clear that they offered a number of professional advantages to academic psychiatry. First and foremost, polyclinics were superb advertisements for the psychiatric clinic, as well as strategic responses to the charges of the anti-psychiatrists. They embodied precisely the image of openness and accessibility that psychiatrists wished to project in light of public skepticism. In the public eye, polyclinics could help to redefine the image of psychiatric work from more carceral tasks to expert advice, state-of-the-art therapy, public hygiene, and even bio-social engineering. They therefore held the potential to extricate clinical psychiatrists from their dire association with public security issues. Polyclinics also undercut the competition of private institutions for nervous patients and thus held out the prospect of significant financial gain.[113] Moreover, polyclinics were a rich source of precisely the kind of patients whom academic psychiatrists most valued in terms of teaching and research. For such patients exhibited the milder, boarderline symptoms that young physicians were far more likely to encounter in their daily practice and that could help hone faculties of observation and diagnosis in society at large. It is therefore hardly surprising that psychiatrists took great pains to emphasize that polyclinics were intended for individuals who were explicitly *not* mentally ill in any medical or legal sense.

This had extremely important ramifications not only because it encouraged individuals to visit the polyclinic, but also because it allowed the polyclinic to circumvent rigorous state regulations on mental hospitals. State regulations governing admission to psychiatric hospitals were not enforced in polyclinics.[114] This gave them an important intermediate function, providing services to an outpatient community and simultaneously acting as a gateway toward easier admission into the psychiatric clinic proper. Not surprisingly, therefore, a large portion of patients in psychiatric clinics initially entered through polyclinical facilities, sometimes bypassing more formal admission criteria to the larger clinic itself.[115] Polyclinics thus further established academic psychiatrists as arbiters of normality in so far as they enhanced academic jurisdiction over decisions of who was "fit" to be institutionalized and how patients were distributed within the system of care. It was in polyclinics that the borderline states inaccessible even to the regular university psychiatric clinic could be brought within the pale of psychiatric science and be diagnosed, treated, and if necessary steered to more specialized facilities for further treatment.

Finally, polyclinics also directly addressed pressing issues of mental hygiene and social prophylaxis. They helped psychiatrists to redefine their professional work, to capture and exploit new professional tasks, and to enhance their own social utility in the eyes of a critical public. The work of prophylaxis had always been implicit in the dogma of early and rapid admission. But in the 1890s the anti-psychiatry movement, the "social question," and theories of heredity and degeneration all infused prophylactic endeavors with a greater sense of urgency. The polyclinic addressed these concerns and in the process helped to facilitate the redeployment and extension of the clinical work of academic psychiatrists outward into German society.

Social Prophylaxis and Borderline States

Academic psychiatrists at the turn of the century were keenly interested in a number of issues concerning public hygiene and borderline states. They faced a wide range of social problems and sought to intervene to prevent or alleviate many of them. To greater or lesser degrees, they considered it their professional responsibility to apply their expertise toward the solution of these problems. While a full account of these endeavors will not be provided here, a cursory glance can serve to point out some of the many fields to which psychiatrists turned their attention.

One such area of pressing social concern was the problem of overburdened school children. One of the first psychiatrists to enter the imperial German debates was Ludwig Snell, who warned his professional colleagues of the dangers of excessive schoolwork. In a lecture to the GDNÄ in 1873, Snell had spoken of the classroom's potential for causing "nervous and mental disorder," "digestion problems," and other "anomalies in life of the brain and nerves."[116] Snell attributed these problems to the "mechanical scheduling of the [pupil's] entire day." He hoped to remedy this situation in a variety of ways, including more physical education and a more "psychologically appropriate" mode of instruction which fostered an "organic relationship" between different course subject matter. In addition, less emphasis needed to be placed on language and far more on observation—in other words, on the pupil's "eye." Snell's remarks were a precursor to more extensive discussion on the question of overburdened children in the early 1880s.[117] In 1883 Carl Westphal and Rudolf Virchow even treated the question in a report for the Scientific Commission for Medical Affairs.[118] The issue had been given added urgency by rising rates of suicide among school children; in the late 1890s, it became the subject of numerous papers at GDNÄ meetings. [119]

National insurance legislation had also pushed the "social treatment" of patients to the forefront of medical attention.[120] The programs of sickness, accident, and retirement insurance that were implemented over the course of the 1880s and then expanded in the ensuing decades all formed part of an integrative strategy designed by Otto von Bismarck to bind the loyalties of the lower classes to the state and thereby undermine the growing strength of social democracy.[121] In the wake of the insurance laws, university clinics were increasingly called upon by various agencies to prepare expert opinions on applications for accident benefits.[122] Many of these cases were diagnosed as suffering from "traumatic neurosis" in the aftermath of industrial accidents. One of the chief concerns was the abuse of the insurance system by workers feigning insanity in hopes of collecting benefit checks. Psychiatrists developed labels to describe the symptoms of such patients, including "retirement hysteria" or "accident hysteria." The diagnosis of these accident cases was of particular concern to psychiatrists because of the danger of being duped by patients simulating mental illness.[123] If psychiatrists could not distinguish between individuals who were truly suffering mental distress and those who were simply feigning madness, then the reputation of their discipline was in jeopardy. Hence, psychiatrists needed more refined techniques not just to diagnose the core forms of madness, but also the subtle variations of nervous disorders on the borderline between mental health and illness.

Alcoholism had also been the subject of repeated debates and petitions in psychiatric circles during the late nineteenth century.[124] On several occasions, professional associations found cause to deal with the problem.[125] In a petition to the ministries of culture and the interior in 1877, the *Verein deutscher Irrenärzte* called for state intervention in the fight against alcoholism—a problem that had taken on the proportions of a national emergency. They recommended that asylums for alcoholics should be established and that the state recognize that alcoholics were the victims of their own "pathological state-of-mind."[126] However, in anticipation of opposition from jurists, the *Verein* refrained from recommending changes in existing laws. Instead, their petition only appealed to state officials to carry out statistical surveys in hospitals, mental asylums, and poor houses in order to ascertain the extent of the problem. By the end of the 1880s, alcoholism had become a persistent professional problem. Concern about alcoholism went hand-in-hand with a rapid rise in the number of cases of alcohol induced delirium from the mid-1880s. On the Charité's psychiatric ward, and at other metropolitan clinics, such cases could comprise nearly forty percent of admissions.[127]

In addressing these social problems, psychiatrists attempted to diversify their institutions and colonize the borderline between sanity and insanity.[128] As World War One drew nearer, they were calling for a plethora of subsidiary institutions to accommodate different segments of the population of borderline patients. Carl Fürstner recommended that corporate associations (*Berufsgenossenschaften*) build sanatoriums for their workers and that patients be admitted to them through the university clinics.[129] In Bonn the polyclinic was attached to a facility for treating alcoholics.[130] Similarly, after moving to Munich in 1904, Emil Kraepelin tried to have special asylums constructed for alcoholics in order to allow him to transfer these patients out of his clinic.[131] Robert Sommer was an eager advocate of so-called Quiet Halls or *Ruhehallen*, which he displayed at the hygiene exposition in Dresden in 1911. Sommer's *Ruhehallen* were intended to provide nervous urban visitors temporary respite from the frantic pace of city life.[132] Special asylums designed to treat nervous patients (*Nervenheilanstalten*) emerged in the 1890s and mushroomed in number.[133] Of especially great interest were asylums for lower-class nervous patients (*Volksheilstätten für minderbemittelte Nervenkranke*) like that constructed at Rasemühle near Göttingen. Great interest in such institutions evolved during the 1890s, due in part to the writings of Theodor Benda and Paul Julius Möbius.[134] Their therapeutic agenda was premised on the assumption that work (including gardening, animal husbandry, forestry, etc.) was the most effective means of treating nervous disorders in the lower classes. All of these proposed institutions were symptomatic of the growing psychiatric interest in borderline states and prophylactic strategies.

If there was one single common denominator that united the new generation that had been called to chairs in the first decade of the twentieth century, it was their acute interest in these borderline conditions. In opening the new clinic in Munich in 1904, Emil Kraepelin pointed the way by reminding his colleagues that they still had "broad border regions to conquer."[135] And in 1906, Adolf Bickel informed students of medicine that psychiatry's chief concern was borderline states and prophylaxis.[136] In 1910, August Cramer remarked that the progress made in research into borderline conditions was in large part attributable to the work of university clinics.[137] This view was echoed by others for whom university clinics had "made possible the expansion of psychiatric research and knowledge into a new field, into the large field of borderline mental states in the broadest sense of the word."[138] Certainly, interest in borderline or prodromal states between mental health and disease was not new, especially among advocates of early institutionalization.[139] But it grew from the 1880s alongside theories of degeneration that brought a sense of urgency to locating prodromal symptoms and delineating nebulous boundary zones.[140] In colonizing this intermediate space, the long-standing interest of psychiatrists in recognizing the subtle early signs of madness merged with an interest in isolating physical characteristics of hereditary degeneracy. Here psychiatrists could appeal to higher social, cultural, and national purposes in order to justify the expansion of their professional jurisdiction over mental and social deviance.[141]

At this confluence of prodromal and hereditary "symptoms," the janus-faced nature of prophylactic work became especially apparent and acute. On the one hand, prophylaxis meant the prevention of mental illness; it meant taking steps to ensure that insanity did not arise, and as such it was part of efforts to provide medical health care services to the community. On the other hand, prophylaxis also meant protecting the community from the potential dangers of psychiatric patients before that danger had necessarily manifested itself. It meant identifying and securing those individuals who had not yet, but who potentially could pose a threat to the body politic. In other words, psychiatric prophylaxis claimed to go further in protecting two important social values: public health and public security. The first of these social values depended on psychiatrists establishing public trust, whereas the second involved them exerting more direct social control. We have already seen above how the polyclinic was a strategy to improve public trust in the profession and thereby to enhance the prophylactic efficacy of academic psychiatry. But how did the polyclinic and the study of borderline states also serve the interests of public security?

To answer this question, we must turn in conclusion to forensic debates about criminal accountability at the turn of the century. Paragraph 51 of the German criminal code stipulated the limits of criminal accountability in cases of mental illness: "A criminal act is not present if, at the time the crime was committed, the perpetrator was in a state of unconsciousness or if he suffered a morbid disorder of the intellect which precluded him from exercising his free will." The criminal code was an expression of the idealistic tenets of the German legal tradition. It posited the free will of the individual as a precondition of accountability and thus of punishment. Individuals lacking free will could not be held accountable for their deeds. Accordingly, the only distinction recognized by the law was that between mental health and mental illness. Individuals could either be held accountable or not. There was no other alternative, and in cases of doubtful accountability judges were prone to decide in favor of unaccountability according to the convention: *in dubio pro reo.*

However, those tenets were severely challenged by psychiatrists in the last half of the nineteenth century.[142] Influenced by Cesare Lombroso's positivist school of criminology,[143] many psychiatrists refuted the idealist assumptions of the legal code and argued vehemently that the legal definition of accountability contradicted the findings of psychiatric science.[144] Not only was the assumption of human free will contrary to the determinist principles of science, but the law's provisions did not do justice to the multifarious intermediate mental states existing between individuals in full possession of their mental faculties and those who could not be held accountable for their actions. They maintained that studies of degeneration had revealed how important borderline symptoms were in any judgment of accountability. In particular, the law could not account for the so-called "mentally deficient [*geistig Minderwertige*]."[145] Psychiatrists therefore lobbied for greater flexibility in the criminal code, advocating the introduction of the concept of reduced accountability [*verminderte Zurechnungsfähigkeit*] in order to accommodate individuals who, although not, strictly speaking, mentally ill were nevertheless mentally impaired.[146]

The debate between psychiatrists and jurists on these questions were prolific and came to a head at the meeting of the German Association of Lawyers in Innsbruck in 1904.[147] There August Cramer and Emil Kraepelin argued for the incorporation of more flexible legal statutes to account for borderline condition of the "mentally deficient."[148] In his address on the "Penal Treatment of

Mentally Deficient Individuals," August Cramer drew a clear distinction between "mentally deficient," which he defined as a medical condition amenable
to scientific investigation, and "reduced accountability," a legal term that he
considered foreign to medical science. Cramer took pains to stress that unlike
reduced accountability, mental deficiency was a term that could be clearly defined and demarcated. Mental deficiency was a borderline condition midway
between health and mental illness. It differed from mental health in that individuals showed "several symptoms" of mental illness, but, taken together,
these clinical symptoms did not indicate any explicit mental disease. Demonstrating mental deficiency required one to show first that an individual is not
mentally healthy and then second that he or she was not mentally ill in any scientific or legal sense. In this way "the boundaries on both sides could be fixed
and the borderline state established."[149] Cramer emphasized that his definition
was a clinical one, based upon empirical observation and that both jurists and
physicians needed to study these cases. In addition, he attributed the progress
in arriving at these clinical truths to the work done in psychiatric polyclinics.
"I believe it to be an important sign of progress that at one university after another polyclinics for mental and nervous diseases have been built. As a result,
knowledge about borderline states will expand in ever widening circles to ever
more experts. Only on the basis of purely clinical cases can we draw conclusions about the forensic treatment of the mentally deficient."[150]

By substituting the term mental deficiency for reduced accountability, psychiatrists effectively sought to usurp jurisdiction over legal judgments of accountability. At the debates in Innsbruck in 1904, conservative jurists were un-
derstandably worried that the adoption of the term mental deficiency would
lead to a "psychiatrization of criminal law."[151] Nevertheless, a resolution was
adopted reformulating paragraph 51 of the criminal code to conform more
closely with the views of psychiatrists and to provide for treatment in special
asylums for "mentally deficient" individuals. The adoption of the resolution in
Innsbruck all but assured its subsequent adoption into law.[152]

Cramer and other psychiatrists could place such great emphasis on borderline conditions in the their arguments because they had the ability to study
them in patients visiting their polyclinics.[153] This ability helped them to back
up professional claims to enhance public health and security. As instruments
of social prophylaxis, polyclinics represented an interface at which the disciplinary technologies of the clinic became enmeshed with larger forces of social
control and normalization in society. In other words, polyclinics not only supplied advice on mental hygiene to the public at large, but also enhanced the
abilities of professionals to speak with authority about issues that seemed to
lie at and even beyond the margins of madness. They helped psychiatrists lay
claim to jurisdiction over these margins and to colonize them with the disciplinary technologies of clinical psychiatry.

Conclusion: Clinical Psychiatry and the Politics of Professional Practice

This study has been about the psychiatric profession in Germany in the half century prior to World War One. It has placed a particular kind of psychiatric institution—the university psychiatric clinic—at the center of its analysis and investigated the division of expert labor within the profession. In doing so, it has considered both the kinds of work that psychiatrists performed and the jurisdictional disputes that arose in relation to those kinds of work. It has argued that the university psychiatric clinic represented a new economy of power and knowledge within the profession and that academic psychiatrists constructed that new economy in the process of attempting to secure jurisdiction over specific professional tasks.

The university psychiatric clinic came to be a functionally well ordered architectural space in which various professional tasks were segregated. The clinic provided the facilities and equipment for laboratory research. Its wards were organized to accommodate the demands of clinical investigation. The clinic included a lecture hall for the instruction of students in the "science" of psychiatry. And it had a polyclinic to advance the cause of prophylactic intervention. Allowing for inevitable variations over time and place, the tasks to which academic psychiatrists laid claim were ensconced in specific institutional spaces within the psychiatric clinic. This functional segmentation of space distinguished university psychiatric clinics from other earlier receptacles for the mad and made them distinctly "modern" institutions. These different spaces, the professional tasks performed in them, and the debates that enveloped clinical work have provided this study with its organizational structure.

This study has been premised on an understanding of university psychiatric clinics as disciplinary institutions. That is to say, they were facilities in which complex institutional regimes governed and conditioned the conduct of their populations. It was as such that they became the locales in which psychiatric knowledge was generated and tested, disseminated to students, and applied toward socio-medical problems. They represented new scientific, didactic, and prophylactic environments, designed to make the execution of these tasks more efficient and hence improve the overall efficacy of psychiatric labor. In this sense, they were elaborate economies of power and knowledge: they comprised extensive repertoires of arguments, strategies, administrative structures, financial instruments, and material tools, all of which were designed to facilitate effective research and teaching, as well as to maximize the social utility of psychiatric means.

But these disciplinary economies were neither omnipotent nor autonomous. Throughout this study I have emphasized that they were embedded in a politics of professional practice, and as such highly contested and the objects of recurrent negotiation at various scientific, institutional, and socio-political levels. For example, as centers of laboratory research, clinics certainly instilled norms of scientific behavior that expressed the great value that psychiatrists had come to place in various techniques of post-mortem observation. Furthermore, it was precisely these techniques that made it possible to extract meaningful images in the first place and that shaped the way in which madness was interpreted. At the same time, however, laboratory work was contingent upon what I have called the politics of the psychiatric cadaver. In Berlin and elsewhere throughout Germany, reliable access to and jurisdiction over the material conditions of that work (cadavers, microscopes, etc.) was hotly contested and ultimately subject to negotiation and compromise. In other words, the disciplinary economy of the laboratory—although by no means ineffective—remained unstable, fractured, and discontinuous.

The same can be said for university clinics as centers of clinical research. In juxtaposition to the experiential investigations of alienists, university psychiatrists defined their clinical labor much more in terms of intensive observation and documentation. Clinical research now meant applying standardized techniques of examination; it meant fabricating strategies of uninterrupted observation; and it meant exploiting the clinical information derived from these methods in the construction of psychiatric nosologies. The surveillance ward helped to bring and hold puzzling cases within the gaze of the doctors and ultimately to incorporate them into the fold of psychiatric nosology. But optimizing the disciplinary strategies of clinical research always involved discursive contests over professional work. As the case of Heidelberg illustrates, clinical research depended upon the statutory arrangements within a wider system psychiatric administration (criteria of admission and evacuation) and upon the vagaries of extending clinical technologies beyond the walls of the institution itself (anamnestic and prognostic reports). It involved the reconfiguration of the protocols governing the clinic's relations with other institutions and state authorities. In this respect, the disciplinary economy of clinical research remained contingent upon the political vicissitudes arising from competing administrative and intra-professional jurisdictions.

In addition to being centers of research, university psychiatric clinics were also responsible for professional training. Clinics were instruments of professional reproduction, charged with disseminating specialized knowledge and ensuring that students acquired the normed skills necessary to diagnose mental illness. Moreover, the clinic's didactic labor was not limited to training psychiatric experts. With psychiatry's adoption into state licensing exams, that work was also performed on prospective general practitioners. As teaching hospitals, psychiatric clinics were primed to extend and multiply many times over the conceptual paradigms and diagnostic technologies practiced within their walls. This extension of clinical discipline implied at once both an enormous widening, but also a lowering of more rigorous clinical standards. But, again, before medical students could become sentinels of madness in wider society, the conditions of possibility for their training as nascent professionals (textbooks, lecture halls, curriculums, etc.) had to be negotiated with professional rivals, state ministeries, or other local interest groups. The didactic economy of the psychiatric clinic was thus embedded in a politics of professional practice that could confound or modulate efforts to extend disciplinary strategies into the daily conduct and social spaces of doctors practicing throughout the country.

The potential reach of university psychiatric clinics was also enhanced by the prophylactic aims of the polyclinic. Polyclinics facilitated the dissemination of expert advice into the community and in the process also brought new groups of patients within the purview of academic clinicians. They drew on the subtle techniques of suggestion and authoritative advice in order to assess and normalize borderline personality disorders. They could serve at once to regulate the behavior of individuals living outside the institution and to colonize the space separating mental health from illness. "Polyclinical discipline" was clinical discipline at its minimalist best. However, the deployment and incitement of polyclinical practices across non-institutionalized populations hinged on that perennially fragile commodity of public trust. In fact, as illustrated by the challenges facing the profession from religious institutions and the anti-psychiatry movement in the 1890s, public mistrust and skepticism participated in the fashioning of these very practices. That is to say, it was partly in response to pejorative images of psychiatry that its practitioners were recasting their labor in more prophylactic and socially amenable forms. This reconfiguration of the discipline—indeed, its renegotiation in relation to society—is a vivid illustration of just how intimately bound up psychiatry's polyclinical work was with the visions of psychiatry that danced in the public mind's eye.

Finally, I close this monograph on an historiographic note. One of the most enduring themes in the history of German psychiatry has concerned the extent of the profession's carceral functions and its proximity to the state. Social historians have often viewed psychiatric institutions as essentially instruments of state repression, making little distinction between the state and the psychiatric profession.[1] However, this study suggests that assumptions about the social control and medicalization of patients "from above" have long been over-stated.[2] In their focus on the state and their top-down concepts of power, these interpretations have tended to ignore or discount the disciplinary effects of psychiatric practices themselves. There were plenty of reasons for psychiatric professionals to have an interest in seeing people institutionalized without needing to rely so heavily on the motivations of the state to explain the expansion of institutionalized populations. And there were equally many reasons for psychiatrists to want to escape from their reputation as tools of state repression. Regardless of whether state control over non-institutionalized populations was increasing or not, psychiatrists too were doing everything in their power to make their institutions more accessible and diversified, at times even contrary to the state's insistence on tighter regulatory controls over admission.

The professional development of psychiatry, at least as far as university clinics were concerned, seems to have been directed less toward heavy-handed incarceration, than toward more subtle preemptive and prophylactic measures. In fact, in addressing the social questions of their day, academic psychiatrists were in tune with a more general trend toward providing social services ("*sociale Fürsorge*")[3] and prophylaxis. From the 1880s, German social policy witnessed a "paradigm-change from repression to prophylaxis," from institutionalized care (*geschlossene Fürsorge*) to non-institutional, community care open to all citizens (*offene Fürsorge*).[4] Psychiatry was as much a part of these developments as was the rest of German medicine. Although far-reaching recommendations for community based care remained peripheral within the discipline,[5] psychiatrists were nevertheless actively responding to the social questions of their day and polyclinics were visible institutional expressions of these efforts.

It is important to stress that while psychiatrists identified with the security interests of the state and at times acted as the "long arm of the law," disciplinary consequences also followed from their *own* professional work. For example, the professional imperatives implicit in the dogma of early and rapid admission prompted psychiatrists to encourage unregulated admission to psychiatric institutions and so to undercut legal safeguards against unlawful incarceration in the interest of research, teaching, and therapeutic efficiency. Similar tendencies can also be seen in psychiatrists' resistance to national legislation on psychiatric care and in their efforts to see the criminal code changed to reflect the findings of psychiatric science. The last example, in particular, demonstrates the encroachment of psychiatric practices into the realm of judicial process. At stake in the ensuing jurisdictional disputes over borderline mental states was the range of the rule of law and its potential displacement by an extra-legal disciplinary space.

Understanding professionalization in terms of jurisdictional contests and in conjunction with economies of power and knowledge therefore touches on important questions about the strength of liberal values and the relationship between the law and psychiatry in Imperial Germany. The anti-psychiatry movement is a case in point. To the extent that public sentiments were fueled by concern about unlawful detention, those concerns can be read as barometers of liberal and democratic values. In the 1890s, bourgeois critics of psychiatry feared that their highly prized civic rights would be compromised by institutionalization in overcrowded asylums for the poor. They feared their own subsequent "civic death [*bürgerlicher Tod*]"[6] as respectable middle class citizens if they were ever interned in a psychiatric hospital. Their concerns were directed not so much at the state, as at the supposedly unfettered influence of psychiatrists. Therefore, the rising crescendo of public criticism can be taken as a sign of heightened sensitivity for liberal and democratic values.

But public concern was janus-faced. It focused not just on illegal *in*carceration, but also premature *de*carceration of patients presumed to be dangerous deviants. If the middle classes were concerned about "their own" going into psychiatric institutions, they were equally, if not more concerned about "their other" coming out of them. Psychiatrists were only too aware of this double standard, and it even prompted one academic psychiatrist to exalt his work as the very protection of the rule of law and patients' individual rights.[7] Indeed the profession's own ambiguities illustrate the more general uncertainties of liberalism in Wilhelmine Germany, at once hoping to cure the growing social ills besetting the nation and at the same time fighting to preserve its practitioners' own tenuous social position. Hence, while the anti-psychiatry movement of the 1890s can be read as a sign of resurgent liberal values, it was no less a signal of the encroachment by psychiatric professionals on civic rights and the rule of law.[8]

One might therefore plausibly ask just how extensive and effective were these disciplinary strictures in Wilhelmine Germany? While this study has focused narrowly on psychiatric clinics and cannot gauge the wider impact of the clinic's disciplinary economy in German society, it has sought to demonstrate that psychiatrists had at least mobilized much of the cultural machinery needed to expand the profession's influence across civil society. Furthermore, it has stressed that the mobilization of this machinery evolved to a considerable degree from psychiatrists' own work and professional concerns. In other words, clinical discipline was not reducible to state power.[9] But if we are to understand power relationships in Wilhelmine society, then it will be important to recognize that the practices of professional work were themselves inherently political and that they represent not simply the extension of state power, but its nascent transformation into new "rationalities and technologies of power."[10] It is therefore the politics of professional practice as it relates to various actors, including but not limited to psychiatrists, that deserves further historical attention and that has been the object of this study's sustained examination.

Notes

Chapter 1

1. Heinrich Laehr, *Fortschritt?—Rückschritt!,* vol. 1 (Berlin: Oehmigke, 1868), 26.

2. Emil Kraepelin, *Die königliche Psychiatrische Klinik in München* (Leipzig: Barth, 1905), 31-2.

3. Gustav Kolb ranked them at the pinnacle of all psychiatric institutions in public consciousness. G[ustav] Kolb, ed., *Sammel-Atlas für den Bau von Irrenanstalten,* pt. A (Halle: Marhold, 1907), 75.

4. Compare also Karl Jaspers, *Allgemeine Psychopathologie* (Berlin: Springer, 1913), 326–33 and Gerolf Verwey, *Psychiatry in an Anthropological and Biomedical Context,* Studies in the History of Modern Science, eds. Robert Cohen, Erwin Hiebert, Everett Mendelsohn, vol. 15 (Dordrecht: Reidel, 1985).

5. Werner Janzarik, "Die klinische Psychopathologie zwischen Greisinger und Kraepelin im Querschnitt des Jahres 1878," in *Psychologie als Grundlagenwissenschaft,* vol. 8 of *Klinische Psychologie und Psychopathologie,* ed. Helmut Remschmidt (Stuttgart: Enke, 1979), 52.

6. August Cramer, "Die preußischen Universitätskliniken für psychisch und Nervenkrankheiten," *Klinisches Jahrbuch* 24 (1910): 185.

7. The concepts of power and discipline employed in this study are in large measure indebted to the work of Michel Foucault, *Discipline and Punish,* trans. Alan Sheridan (New York: Random House, 1977), especially his chapter on "The Means of Correct Training," 170–94.

8. See for example Gunter Herzog, *Krankheitsurteile* (Rehburg-Loccum: Psychiatrie-Verlag, 1984), 82–147, 167–71, 217–38.

9. Foucault, *Discipline and Punish,* 194.

10. See Jan Goldstein, "Foucault among the Sociologists," *History and Theory* 23 (1984): 170–92.

11. Carl Westphal, *Psychiatrie und psychiatrischer Unterricht* (Berlin: Hirschwald, 1880), 20-1.

12. C[arl] Moeli, *Zur Erinnerung an Carl Westphal* (Berlin: Hirschwald, 1890), 12.

13. See J. B. Friedreich, *Systematische Literatur der ärztlichen und gerichtlichen Psychologie* (Berlin: Ensslin, 1833; reprint, Amsterdam: E. J. Bonset, 1968).

14. Paul Flechsig, *Die Irrenklinik der Universität Leipzig und ihre Wirksamkeit in den Jahren 1882–1886* (Leipzig: Veit & Comp., 1888), 58.

15. Dörner, *Bürger und Irre,* 2d ed. (Frankfurt/M: EVA, 1984), 13.

16. Dörner, *Bürger und Irre;* Dirk Blasius, *'Einfache Seelenstörungen'* (Frankfurt/M: Fischer, 1994); Doris Kaufmann, *Aufklärung, Bürgerliche Selbsterfahrung und die 'Erfindung' der Psychiatrie in Deutschland, 1770–1850,* Veröffentlichungen des Max-Planck-Institutes für Geschichte, vol. 122 (Göttingen: V&R, 1995); Hans-Georg Güse and Norbert Schmacke, *Psychiatrie zwischen bürgerlicher Revolution und Faschismus,* vol. 1 (Kronberg: Athenäum, 1976); and Achim Thom, "Erscheinungsformen und Widersprüche des Weges der Psychiatrie zu einer medizinischen Disziplin im 19. Jahrhundert," in *Zur Geschichte der Psychiatrie im 19. Jahrhundert,* ed. Achim Thom (Berlin: VEB Verlag Volk und Gesundheit, 1984), 11–32.

17. Harry Oosterhuis, *Stepchildren of Nature* (Chicago: University of Chicago Press, 2000); Udo Benzenhöfer, *Psychiatrie und Anthropologie in der ersten Hälfte des 19. Jahrhunderts* (Hürt-

genwald: Guido Pressler, 1993); Michael Hagner, *Homo cerebralis* (Berlin: Berlin Verlag, 1997); Volker Roelcke, *Krankheit und Kulturkritik* (Frankfurt/M: Campus, 1999).

18. Schmiedebach, *Psychiatrie und Psychologie im Widerstreit,* Abhandlungen zur Geschichte der Medizin und der Naturwissenschaften, ed. Rolf Winau and Heinz Müller-Dietz, vol. 51 (Husum: Matthiesen, 1986); Thomas-Peter Schindler, "Psychiatrie im Wilhelminischen Deutschland" (Med. diss., Free University Berlin, 1990); Joachim Radkau, *Das Zeitalter der Nervosität* (Munich: Hanser, 1998). See also the more general surveys of Werner Leibbrand and Annemarie Wettley, *Der Wahnsinn* (Munich: Karl Albers, 1961); Bernhard Pauleikopf, *Das Menschenbild im Wandel der Zeit,* 2 vols. (Hürtgenwald: Guido Pressler, 1987); and Joachim Bodamer, "Zur Entstehung der Psychiatrie als Wissenschaft im 19. Jahrhundert," *Fortschritte der Neurologie, Psychiatrie und ihrer Grenzgebiete* 21 (1953): 511–35.

19. See Ann Goldberg, *Sex, Religion, and the Making of Modern Madness* (New York: Oxford University Press, 1999) and Frank Ortmann, "Die Entstehung der Psychiatrie in Jena" (Med. diss., University of Jena, 1983). Some older studies have also looked beyond individual institutions in search of larger typologies of hospital architecture. See Dieter Jetter, *Grundzüge der Geschichte des Irrenhauses* (Darmstadt: WBG, 1981).

20. On the professions in Germany, see Geoffrey Cocks and Konrad Jarausch, *German Professions, 1800–1950* (New York: Oxford University Press, 1990); Charles McClelland, *The German Experience of Professionalization* (Cambridge: Cambridge University Press, 1991); Konrad Jarausch, *The Unfree Professions* (New York: Oxford University Press, 1990). See also Geoffrey Cocks, *Psychotherapy in the Third Reich* (Oxford: Oxford University Press, 1985); Kenneth Ledford, *From General Estate to Special Interest* (Cambridge: Cambridge University Press, 1995); Jeffrey Allan Johnson *The Kaiser's Chemists* (Chapel Hill: University of North Carolina Press, 1990); Kees Gispen, *New Profession, Old Order* (Cambridge: Cambridge University Press, 1989) and Ulfried Geuter, *Die Professionalisierung der deutschen Psychologie im Nationalsozialismus* (Frankfurt/M: Suhrkamp, 1988). On the German medical profession see Claudia Huerkamp, *Der Aufstieg der Ärzte im 19. Jahrhundert,* Kritische Studien zur Geschichtswissenschaft, eds. Helmut Berding, Jürgen Kocka and Hans-Ulrich Wehler, vol. 68 (Göttingen: V&R, 1985); Ute Frevert, *Krankheit als politisches Problem 1770–1880* (Göttingen: V&R, 1986); Annette Drees, *Die Ärzte auf dem Weg zu Prestige und Wohlstand,* Studien zur Geschichte des Alltags, eds. Hans J. Teuteberg and Peter Borscheid, vol. 9 (Münster: Coppenrath, 1988); and Arleen Tuchman, *Science, Medicine, and the State in Germany* (Oxford: Oxford University Press, 1993).

21. See Nikolas Rose, *Inventing Our Selves,* Cambridge Studies in the History of Psychology, ed. Mitchell G. Ash and William R. Woodward (Cambridge: Cambridge University Press, 1998), 12.

22. In this I am following Nikolas Rose, who understands psychiatry in terms of transformation rather than extension of state power. Rose views psychiatry as "a domain that is 'disciplined'" in relation to certain practices and problems of government, is dependent for its epistemology on certain institutional forms and regimes of judgement in relation to human conduct, and as that 'know-how' which makes certain 'power effects' possible." Rose, 18.

23. On the concept of assemblages and self-governance alluded to here see ibid., 22–40.

24. Andrew Abbott, *The System of Professions* (Chicago: University of Chicago Press, 1988), 59.

25. Compare also the distinction between "cultural authority" and "social authority" in Paul Starr, *The Social Transformation of American Medicine* (New York: Basic Books, 1982), 13.

26. Haraway's term is "simian orientalism," by which she means in reference to Western primatology "the construction of the self from the raw material of the other, the appropriation of nature in the production of culture." Donna Haraway, *Primate Visions* (London: Verso, 1992), 11. See also Kaufmann, *Aufklärung.* For an example from the period see Heinrich Laehr, *Über Irrsein und Irrenanstalten* (Halle: Pfeffer, 1852), vii–viii.

27. In a similar vein, see Kathryn M. Olesko, "Commentary: On Institutes, Investigations, and Scientific Training," in *The Investigative Enterprise,* eds. William Coleman and Frederic L. Holmes (Berkeley: University of California Press, 1988), 299, 324.

28. See Klaus Dörner, "Wir verstehen die Geschichte der Moderne nur mit den Behinderten vollständig," *Leviathan* 22 (1994): 367–90.

29. Public relations work represents a further important task of academic psychiatrists, but which is difficult to nail down in an institutional context. Here it can best be considered as a derivative of clinical teaching in the sense of *Aufklärungsarbeit*. Of course, there were any number of other academic and administrative duties which psychiatrists performed, but these were not tasks specific to them or otherwise constitutive of their professional identity.

30. See for example the general tone of Carl Wernicke, "Zweck und Ziel der Psychiatrischen Kliniken," *Klinisches Jahrbuch* 1 (1889): 218–23.

31. Two significant and ultimately influential therapeutic reforms in Germany—psychoanalysis and community care—were decidedly not products of academic psychiatry. Nor was the colony system actively endorsed by academics.

32. When it suited their particular interests, clinicians even admitted as much. See the Directorate of the Psychiatric Clinic Heidelberg to MdJKU, 6 May 1897, Nr. 1045, PKUH VIII/4.

33. The greater rigor in German usage is in part a consequence of the resolutions of the German physicians' association, which restricted the use of the term clinic or polyclinic to institutions engaged in teaching. However, administrative courts in Germany had long refused to rule that the use of the term *Klinik* be limited strictly to teaching institutions. See *Aerztliches Vereinsblatt* 17 (1890): 467.

34. See *[Brockhaus'] Allgemeine deutsche Enzyklopädie für die gebildeten Stände: Conversations-Lexikon*, 1852 ed. and 1894 ed., s.v. "Klinik."

35. This definition corresponds roughly to what Eduard Hitzig termed psychiatric clinics "in the stricter sense." Eduard Hitzig, *Bericht über die Wirksamkeit der Universitäts psychiatrischen und Nervenklinik zu Halle* (Halle: Gebauer-Schwetschke'sche Buchdruckerei, 1887), 6. Obviously, no technical definition can ever fully grasp the historical diversity of psychiatric institutions.

Chapter 2

1. Blasius, *Friedrich Wilhelm IV, 1795–1861* (Göttingen: V&R, 1992), 215–6. On the political situation in Prussia in 1857 and 1858, see Günther Grünthal, "Das Ende der Ära Manteuffel," *Jahrbuch für die Geschichte Mittel- und Ostdeutschlands* 39 (1990): 179–219.

2. On the impact of railroads, see Hans-Ulrich Wehler, *Deutsche Gesellschaftsgeschichte*, vol. 2 (Munich: Beck, 1987), 614–31.

3. Wolfram Siemann, *Gesellschaft im Aufbruch* (Frankfurt/M: Suhrkamp, 1990).

4. Heinrich Damerow, "Ein Blick über die Lage von Irrenanstaltsfragen der Gegenwart," *AZP* 19 (1862): 174–5.

5. There are no comprehensive studies of the social composition of cohorts of psychiatric professionals. See Eric J. Engstrom, "The Birth of Clinical Psychiatry" (Ph.D. Dissertation, University of North Carolina at Chapel Hill, 1997), 28, note 6. See also Heinrich Laehr and Max Lewald, *Die Heil- und Pflege-Anstalten für Psychisch-Kranke des deutschen Sprachgebietes* (Berlin: Georg Reimer, 1899), 335. On the social composition of physicians in general, see Huerkamp, *Der Aufstieg der Ärzte*, 61–78.

6. Review of Wilhelm Griesinger's *Die Pathologie und Therapie*, in *CblDGPgP* 9 (1862): 146; Carl Friedrich Flemming, "Über einige der nächsten Aufgaben der Psychiatrie," *AZP* 21, supplement (1864): 50.

7. On early psychiatric institutions, see Dieter Jetter, *Zur Typologie des Irrenhauses in Frankreich und Deutschland (1780–1840)* (Wiesbaden: Steiner, 1971), 119–173 and id., *Grundzüge*.

8. With the notable exception of Ernst Albrecht Zeller, most alienists at mid-century, including Jacobi, Flemming, Damerow, and Roller were advocates of such mental hospitals. See C. F. W. Roller, *Die Irrenanstalt nach allen ihren Beziehungen* (Karlsruhe: Müller'sche Buchhandlung, 1831) and Heinrich Damerow, *Über die relative Verbindung der Irren-Heil- und Pflege-Anstalten* (Leipzig: Otto Wigand, 1840).

9. Laehr, *Über Irrsein und Irrenanstalten*, 229, 233; id., *Die Heil- und Pflege-Anstalten*, 334–5.

10. See "Neue Bahnen für das preussische Irrenwesen," *ZblNP* 41 (1891): 152. On the different jurisdictional constellations, see [Moritz] Jastrowitz, "Über die Staatsaufsicht über die Irren-anstalten," *AZP* 34 (1878): 713–24.

11. Such a schism was not specific to psychiatry; in fact, it was characteristic of medical affairs in general in Prussia from the 1820s onward. See Ragnhild Münch, *Gesundheitswesen im 18. und 19. Jahrhundert* (Berlin: Akademie Verlag, 1995), 66–7.

12. Rural isolation was a "fundamental necessity of [the asylum's] vitality" according to C. F. W. Roller, *Psychiatrische Zeitfragen* (Berlin: Georg Reimer, 1874), 32.

13. Maximilian Jacobi, *Über die Anlegung und Einrichtung von Irren-Heilanstalten* (Berlin: Reimer, 1834), 5. See likewise Laehr, *Über Irrsein und Irrenanstalten,* 108–14.

14. Leupoldt, 30, 47. According to Leupoldt, the daily routine of the asylum was supposed to become "second nature" to the insane. Ibid., 47.

15. Laehr, *Über Irrsein und Irrenanstalten,* 121.

16. See Rudolf Lemke, "150jähriges Jubiläum der Nervenklinik an der Friedrich-Schiller-Universität Jena," *Wissenschaftliche Zeitschrift der Friedrich-Schiller-Universität Jena, Mathe-matisch-Naturwissenschaftliche Reihe* 4 (1954–5): 367 and "An die Leser," *If* 1 (1859): 2–3. On the same phenomenon elsewhere, see David Rothman, *The Discovery of the Asylum* (Boston: Little and Brown, 1971); Anne Digby, *Madness, Morality, and Medicine* (Cambridge: Cambridge University Press, 1985), chapters 2 and 3; and Ellen Dwyer, *Homes for the Mad* (New Brunswick: Rutgers University Press, 1987), 57.

17. See Carl Friedrich Flemming, *Die Irren-Heil-Anstalt Sachsenberg bei Schwerin im Groß-herzogtum Mecklenberg* (Schwerin: Kürschner, 1833), 13.

18. Bopp, "Antrag," *Jahrbuch der gesammten Staatsarzneikunde* 3 (1837): 555.

19. C. F. W. Roller, *Grundsätze für Errichtung neuer Irrenanstalten* (Karlsruhe: Müller'schen Buchhandlung, 1838), 91.

20. See Dietrich Georg Kieser, *Elemente der Psychiatrik* (Breslau: Weber, 1855), 279–81 and 286.

21. Alfred E. Hoche, *Jahresringe* (Munich: Lehmann, 1934), 120.

22. Thus August Solbrig speaking at the GDNÄ meeting in Dresden in 1868, *AZP* 25, supple-ment (1868): 88. In an obituary, Solbrig was praised as one of the "most efficient and assiduous leaders of the patriarchal system." Eugen Lachner, "Nekrolog: Solbrig," *CblDGPgP* 18 (1872): 190.

23. Roller as cited by Michael Kutzer, "Die Irrenheilanstalt in der ersten Hälfte des 19. Jahrhunderts," in *Vom Umgang mit Irren,* eds. Johann Glatzel, Steffan Haas and Heinz Schott (Regensburg: S. Roderer, 1990), 71. The term "regime" is taken from contemporary discourse. See, for example, Carl Friedrich Flemming, *Pathologie und Therapie der Psychosen* (Berlin: Hirsch-wald, 1859), 285.

24. Carl Wilhelm Ideler, "Über psychiatrische Klinik," *Medicinische Zeitung* 2 (1833): 99. See also Walter Artelt, "Die Gründung und die ersten Jahrzehnte der Berliner Medizinische Fakultät," *Ciba-Zeitschrift* 7 (1956): 2575.

25. Cited in Lemke, 367. See also Ortmann, 109–11 and Anton Müller, *Die Irrenanstalt* (Würzburg: Stahel, 1824), 39.

26. On the term "domestication," see Andrew Scull, "The Domestication of Madness," *Medical History* 27 (1983): 233–48.

27. Maximilian Jacobi, "Irrenanstalten," in *Encyclopädisches Wörterbuch der medicinischen Wissenschaften,* eds. D. W. H. Busch et al. (Berlin: Veit et Comp., 1839), 173; Laehr, *Über Irrsein und Irrenanstalten,* 117; Damerow, *Über die relative Verbindung,* 107; J. C. A. Heinroth, "Ein Wort über Irren-Anstalten," afterword to *Über die Verrücktheit,* by M. Georget, trans. Johann Christian August Heinroth (Leipzig: Weidmann, 1821), 413; Roller, *Grundsätze, 75.*

28. Damerow, "Ein Blick," 148 and id., *Über die relative Verbindung,* 107.

29. Flemming, *Pathologie und Therapie,* 286. See also Emil Löwenhardt, "Über den Zeit-punkt der Übersiedlung von Geistes- und Gemüthskranken in Irrenanstalten," *If* 1 (1859): 23–7.

30. Compare Müller, *Die Irrenanstalt,* 60–67 and Engstrom, "The Birth," 29–34.

31. Heinrich Laehr, "Rundschau in Preussen," *AZP* 22 (1865): 327 and his *Über Irrsinn und Irrenanstalten,* 118.

32. Heinrich Neumann, "Zum Non-Restraint," *AZP* 28 (1872): 679. But see also his *Gedanken über die Zukunft der schlesischen Irrenanstalten* (Wohlau: Leuckart, 1848), 24–6.

33. Cited in Elisabeth Eberstadt, "K[arl] A[ugust] von Solbrigs Liebe zu den Irren," in *Um die Menschenrechte der Geisteskranken,* ed. Werner Leibbrand (Nürnberg: Die Egge, 1946), 43.

34. Damerow, *Über die relative Verbindung,* 229.

35. See Jacobi, "Irrenanstalten," 77–9.

36. Cf. Wilhelm Griesinger, *Die Pathologie und Therapie der psychischen Krankheiten* (Stuttgart: Krabbe, 1861; 3d edition reprint, Amsterdam: Bonset, 1964), 472 and Kahlbaum, "Die klinisch-diagnostischen Gesichtspunkte der Psychopathologie," *Sammlung Klinischer Vorträge* 126 (1877): 1128.

37. Damerow, "Ein Blick," 150.

38. Thom, "Erscheinungsformen," 11.

39. For accounts of German psychiatry in the early nineteenth century and the disputes between *Psychiker* and *Somatiker* see Otto Marx, "German Romantic Psychiatry," *HP* 1 (1990): 351–81 and *HP* 2 (1991): 1–25; Pauleikhoff, 187–91; Dörner, *Bürger und Irre,* 244–79; Leibbrand and Wettley, *Der Wahnsinn,* 465–508; Goldberg, *Sex.*

40. See Kaspar Max Brosius, "'Der Umschwung in der Psychiatrie'," *If* 10 (1868): 33 and the views of Solbrig cited in Eberstadt, 46.

41. A bellwether in this respect were the contributions to Jacobi's and Nasse's *Zeitschrift für die Beurtheilung und Heilung der krankhaften Seelenzustände,* 1 (1838).

42. Brosius, "Wieder ein Wort über die Vorurtheile über die Irren-Anstalten," *If* 2 (1860): 11.

43. Cited in Lachner, 190.

44. "Association der Irrenärzte," *If* 4 (1862): 72.

45. Laehr, "Rundschau in Preussen," 326. See, for example, the disputes in Erlangen and Bonn: Academic Senate of the University of Erlangen to SMIKSA, 19 December 1847 and Medical Faculty to Academic Senate, 8 November 1847, BHStA, MK 11488; Medical Faculty Circular, 16 January 1848, UAB, MF 1102.

46. See Carl August Wunderlich, *Geschichte der Medizin* (Stuttgart: Ebner & Seubert, 1859), 345 and Obersteiner, "Grundzüge einer Geschichte des Vereins für Psychiatrie und Neurologie in Wien in den ersten fünfzig Jahren seines Bestehens (1868–1918)," *Jahrbücher für Psychiatrie* 39 (1919): 2. Such opposition was characteristic of much wider resistance to specialization in academic medicine. See Huerkamp, *Der Aufstieg der Ärzte,* 104; Hans-Heinz Eulner, *Die Entwicklung der medizinischen Spezialfächer an den Universitäten des deutschen Sprachgebietes,* Studien zur Medizingeschichte des neunzehnten Jahrhunderts, eds. W. Artelt and W. Rüegg, vol. 4 (Stuttgart: Enke, 1970), 26–7; and Awraham Zloczower, *Career Opportunities and the Growth of Scientific Discovery in 19th Century Germany* (New York: Arno Press, 1981), 28.

47. For those provisions see §§ 66–70 of the *Prüfungsordnung* in Bickel, *Wie studiert man Medizin?* (Stuttgart: Wilhelm Violet, 1906), 114–5.

48. See, for example, Paul Börner, "Die Zukunft der wissenschaftlichen Hygiene in Deutschland," *Preußische Jahrbücher* 56 (1885): 234–66.

49. Bonhoeffer, *Die Geschichte der Psychiatrie in der Charité im 19. Jahrhundert* (Berlin: Springer, 1940), 1. Similarly, Eulner, *Die Entwicklung,* 261.

50. For a concise critique of psychiatry's "blind imitation" of medicine and its costs, see Dörner, "Psychiatrie und Gesellschaftstheorien," in *Psychiatrie der Gegenwart: Forschung und Praxis,* Grundlinien und Methoden der Psychiatrie, ed. K. P. Kisker et al., vol. 1, 2d ed. (Berlin: Springer, 1979), 780–1.

51. At the forefront of this critique were the contributors to the *Correspondenzblatt der deutschen Gesellschaft für Psychiatrie und gerichtliche Psychologie.* On the *Correspondenzblatt,* see below.

52. Heinrich Neumann, *Der Arzt und die Blödsinnigkeits-Erklärung* (Breslau: Gosohorsky, 1847), iii–iv.

53. Carl Friedrich Flemming, "Was heisst Fortschritt in der Psychiatrie und welches ist sein Weg," *AZP* 16 (1859): 177.

54. Flemming, "Über einige der nächsten Aufgaben der Psychiatrie," 50.

55. Brosius, " 'Der Umschwung,' " 24.

56. "Bericht über die Versammlung in Landau und Speyer vom 11. bis 20. September 1861," *AZP* 18 (1861): 793.

57. Wilhelm Griesinger, "Vorwort," *AfPN* 1 (1868): iii.

58. Westphal, *Psychiatrie und psychiatrischer Unterricht,* 23. Similarly, Laehr, "Rundschau in Preussen," 325; also see his "Gegen einen Vorwurf Virchows," *AZP* 27 (1871): 751–3, and Ideler as cited in Adolf Dannemann, *Die psychiatrische Klinik zu Giessen* (Berlin: S. Karger, 1899), 23.

59. Eberstadt, 38. See also Carl Friedrich Flemming, "Über Notwendigkeit, Nutzen und Benutzung der Irren-Heilanstalten," *ZBHkS* 1 (1838): 705.

60. Adolf Albrecht Erlenmeyer, "Rechenschaftsbericht über die ersten 5 Jahre der Gesellschaft," *CblDGPgP* 5 (1858): 145. Cf. also P[eter Willers] Jessen and W[illers] Jessen, "Vorlagen für die vierte Versammlung deutscher Psychiater," *AZP* 20, Supplement 2 (1863): 1–33.

61. Roller, *Psychiatrische Zeitfragen,* xi.

62. Neumann, *Lehrbuch der Psychiatrie* (Erlangen: Enke, 1859), 167: "Es giebt nur eine Art der Seelenstörung. Wir nennen sie das Irresein." On Neumann, see Mario Lanczik, "Heinrich Neumann und seine Lehre von der Einheitspsychose," *Fundamenta Psychiatrica* (1989): 49–54; Pauleikhoff, 257–78; Heinz Henseler, "Die 'Analytische Methode' des Psychiaters Heinrich Wilhelm Neumann" (Med. diss., University of Munich, 1959).

63. Heinrich Damerow, for example, insisted that training in the asylums should be praxis oriented and should *not* include systematic lectures. Damerow, *Über die relative Verbindung,* 208.

64. Kahlbaum, *Die Gruppierung der psychischen Krankheiten und die Einteilung der Seelenstörungen* (Danzig: A. W. Kafemann, 1863), 5, 4. Kahlbaum saw his own work as a "necessary step in the further development of scientific psychiatry." Ibid., 132.

65. Ibid., 61.

66. Eduard Hess, "Zum fünfzigjährigen Bestehen der Kahlbaum'schen Nervenheilanstalt zu Görlitz," *ZblNP* 28 (1905): 770.

67. Kahlbaum, "Die klinisch-diagnostischen Gesichtspunkte," 1133.

68. Kahlbaum, *Die Gruppierung,* 177.

69. Rudolf Arndt, *Die Psychiatrie und das medicinische Staats-Examen* (Berlin: Reimer, 1880), 4. Laehr considered the courts' mistrust of psychiatric experts to be one of the most pressing problems of the 1860s. Laehr, "Rundschau in Preussen," 324.

70. Kahlbaum, *Die Gruppierung,* 55–6.

71. Jessen and Jessen, 3. In their recommendations the Jessens were responding to (and substantially revising) a list of 19 so-called 'Carlsruher Thesen,' which Carl Flemming had put forward in 1858. See "Die psychiatrische Sektion der Naturforscherversammlung in Carlsruhe im September 1858," *AZP* 16 (1859): 178–81.

72. Jessen and Jessen, 11.

73. Ibid., 16.

74. Flemming, "Über einige der nächsten Aufgaben der Psychiatrie," 51.

75. Damerow, "Ein Blick," 187.

76. Laehr, "Rundschau in Preussen," 314.

77. See Ernst Köhler, *Arme und Irre* (Berlin: Wagenbach, 1977).

78. Damerow, "Ein Blick," 152, 151. See especially 186–9.

79. Laehr, "Rundschau in Preussen," 324.

80. Damerow, *Über die relative Verbindung,* 260–1.

81. Damerow, "Einleitung," *AZP* 1 (1844): xlv and "Einladung an die Irrenanstalts-Directoren zur Benutzung gemeinschaftlicher Schemata zu den tabellarischen Übersichten," *AZP* 1 (1844): 430–40.

82. See Damerow, "Die Zeitschrift," *AZP* 3 (1846): 18 and also the appendix to Laehr, *Über Irrsein und Irrenanstalten;* also see his "Die Irrenanstalten Deutschlands," *AZP* 22, no. 5 and 6 (1865) and the various editions of Laehr, *Die Heil und Pflegeanstalten für Psychisch-Kranke des*

deutschen Sprachgebietes (1875, 1882, 1891, 1899, 1907, 1912). Laehr was also instrumental in establishing an association for the exchange of asylum reports that helped scattered and irregularly published hospital literature reach a wider audience of alienists.

83. See J. L. A. Koch, *Zur Statistik der Geisteskrankheiten in Württemberg und der Geisteskrankheiten überhaupt* (Stuttgart: Kohlhammer, 1878), 1–23; Roller, *Psychiatrische Zeitfragen,* 113–130; and for Prussia Albert Guttstadt, "Die Geisteskranken in den Irrenanstalten," *Zeitschrift des königlich preussischen statistischen Bureau* 14 (1874): 201–248h. See also Engstrom, "The Birth," 68, note 156.

84. Guttstadt, "Die Geisteskranken," 203.

85. See "Bericht über die Sitzung des Vereins der deutschen Irrenärzte zu Leipzig am 13. August 1872," *AZP* 29 (1873): 466. See, for example, the proposal of the *Medizinisch-Psychologische Gesellschaft* in *AfPN* 2 (1870): 506–13, and the report of Wilhelm Sander, *Über Zählblättchen und ihre Benutzung bei statistischen Erhebungen der Irren* (Berlin: Sittenfeld, 1871) as well his exchange with Laehr in *AfPN* 3 (1872): 502.

86. See Guttstadt, "Die Geisteskranken," especially 248–248d. Alienists later complained that the Prussian government had ignored their recommendations and imposed its own statistical categories. See *AZP* 38 (1882): 721.

87. Cf. Guttstadt, "Die Geisteskranken," 218, 237; and Georg Buschan, review of "Läßt sich eine Zunahme der Geisteskranken feststellen?" by L[udwig] W[ilhelm] Weber, *ZgNP* 3 (1911): 109–110.

88. Gerhard Baader, "Stadtentwicklung und psychiatrische Anstalten," in *'Gelêrter der arzenîe, ouch apotêker': Beiträge zur Wissenschaftsgeschichte,* ed. Gundolf Keil, Würzburger Medizinhistorische Forschungen, vol. 24 (Pattensen: Wellm, 1982), 239–53.

89. Blasius, *Einfache Seelenstörungen,* 80.

90. Ursula Gast, "Sozialpsychiatrische Traditionen zwischen Kaiserreich und Nationalsozialismus," *Psychiatrischer Praxis* 16 (1989): 78–85.

91. See Directorate of the Psychiatric Clinic Heidelberg to MdJKU, 24 April 1883, Nr. 468, GLA 235 3565 or Eduard Hitzig to Curator of the University of Halle, 13 September 1883, GStA PK, IHA, Rep. 76Va, MgUMA, Sect. 8, Tit. X, Nr. 17, Bd. I, Bl. 136–44.

92. See Guttstadt, "Die Geisteskranken," 225. In Baden county hospitals were exploited. See Roller, *Psychiatrische Zeitfragen,* 39–51 and the Decree of the Ministry of the Interior, 20 May 1884, GLA 235-3565, Nr. 8944.

93. On these views, see Neumann, *Gedanken,* 18–9; Damerow, "Ein Blick," 187–9; Heinrich Laehr, "Privatanstalten im Dienst der öffentlichen," *AZP* 34 (1878): 102–6; Max Huppert, "Über die beste Art der öffentlichen Irrenfürsorge in Deutschland," *Schmidt's Jahrbücher* 144 (1869): 322–8; Heinrich Laehr, "Die Bildung von Vereine Behufs Verbesserung der öffentlichen Fürsorge für Irre," *AZP* 30 (1874): 50–2; also Roller, *Psychiatrische Zeitfragen,* 39–51.

94. For this reason, family care is conspicuous by its absence in the above register of solutions. See Brosius, "Wieder ein Wort," 15–6.

95. I am employing the term dogma here not so much to cast doubt on the therapeutic effectiveness of early intervention, as to convey the breadth of its acceptance and the depth of conviction with which alienists advocated it. For a succinct statement of the dogma, see Jacobi, *Über die Anlegung,* 309, footnote. See also Heinroth, "Ein Wort," 417. Similar views were expressed by English alienists. See Andrew Scull, Charlotte MacKenzie and Nicholas Hervey, *Masters of Bedlam* (Princeton: Princeton University Press, 1996), 95, 171, 192.

96. In many areas, such as Baden, Saxony, Bavaria, Württemberg, and Westphalia, the state echoed these alienist concerns, sometimes also providing financial incentives for early admission. Cf. Engstrom, "The Birth," 74–5 and Thomas Küster, ed., *Quellen zur Geschichte der Anstaltspsychiatrie in Westfalen.* Forschungen zur Regionalgeschichte, ed. Karl Teppe, vol. 26 (Paderborn: Schöningh, 1998), 168–70, 206–7.

97. See for example the claim of P[eter Willers] Jessen, "Über die in Beziehung auf Geistes- und Gemüthskranke herrschende Vorurtheile," in *Amtlicher Bericht,* ed. G. A. Michaelis and H. F. Scherk (Kiel: Akademische Buchhandlung, 1847), 56–61. Interestingly, clinicians would later argue that it was not the negative, but rather the positive image of university clinics that con-

tributed to overcrowding. In 1891, for example, Eduard Hitzig claimed that psychiatry's very success in cultivating the public's trust had contributed to families' greater willingness to place their relatives in psychiatric institutions. As a result, the psychiatric profession had finally succeeded in tapping the natural reservoir of madness which was now surging forth and taxing institutional capacities to their limits. Eduard Hitzig, "Rede gehalten zur Einweihung der Psychiatrischen und Nervenklinik zu Halle a.S.," *Klinisches Jahrbuch* 3 (1891): 123–4; similarly, A[lois] Alzheimer, "25 Jahre Psychiatrie," *AfPN* 52 (1913): 855–6.

98. August Solbrig, *Verbrechen und Wahnsinn* (Munich: Cotta, 1867) 4, 5.

99. Peter Hamann, "Peter Willers Jessens ehemaliges Asyl Hornheim in Kiel," *Historia Hospitalium* 12 (1977–8): 89.

100. Peter Willers Jessen, *Das Asyl Hornheim, die Behörden und das Publicum* (Kiel: Homann, 1862), iv.

101. See the administrative orders of 7 May 1859, 20 June 1859, and 25 April 1862 in Hermann Eulenberg, *Das Medicinalwesen in Preussen*, 3d ed. (Berlin: Hirschwald, 1874), 44–6. On similar issues in England see Daniel Hack Tuke, *Chapters in the History of the Insane in the British Isles* (London: Kegan, Paul, Trench & Co., 1882), 190–6, 522–7; Trevor Turner, " 'Not Worth Powder and Shot,' " in *150 Years of British Psychiatry, 1841–1991*, eds. Hugh Freeman and German Berrios (London: Athlone Press, 1991), 3; Scull, *Masters*, 6.

102. Admission to Prussian asylums (both public and private) after 1825 could legally be ordered only by the local courts or the police and was contingent upon a state physician's (*Physikus*) report. See the circular of the MInn and MgUMA of 16 February 1839, cited in Heinrich Unger, *Die Irrengesetzgebung in Preussen* (Berlin: Siemenroth & Troschel, 1898), 19.

103. Damerow, "Ein Blick," 160. See also Neumann, *Gedanken*, 19.

104. See the ministerial order of 25 April 1862 in Unger, 19–20.

105. On early nineteenth century psychiatric journals, see Heinrich Damerow, "P[ro] M[emoria] An Deutschlands Irrenärzte, "*Medicinische Zeitung* 10 (1841): 33–42; Gundolf Keil, "Deutsche psychiatrische Zeitschriften des 19. Jahrhunderts," in *Psychiatrie auf dem Wege zur Wissenschaft*, ed. Gerhardt Nissen and Gundolf Keil (Stuttgart: Thieme, 1985); Robert Linke, "Psychiatrische und Neurologische Zeitschriften im 19. Jahrhundert" (Med. diss., University of Düsseldorf, 1979). Cf. also Friedreich, 1–5 and Walter Brunn, *Das deutsche Medizinische Zeitschriftenwesen seit der Mitte des 19. Jahrhunderts* (Berlin: Idra, 1925), 26–9.

106. *Jahresbericht über die Leistungen und Fortschritte auf dem Gebiete der Neurologie und Psychiatrie* 1 (1897): iii. So rapid was the growth of psychiatric knowledge that journals were forced to devote increasing amounts of their space to reviews of contemporary publications, including the *Centralblatt für Nervenheilkunde, Psychiatrie und gerichtliche Psychopathologie* (1878ff), *Jahresbericht über die Leistungen und Fortschritte auf dem Gebiet der Neurologie und Psychiatrie* (1898ff), and the review section of the *Zeitschrift für die gesamte Neurologie und Psychiatrie* (1910ff).

107. Damerow first outlined the project in his "P[ro] M[emoria]," 33–42. On the *AZP*'s early history, see also Winfried Berghof, "Heinrich Damerow (1798–1866): Ein bedeutender Vertreter der deutschen Psychiatrie des 19. Jahrhunderts" (Med. diss., University of Leipzig, 1990), 96–124 and Bodamer.

108. The Prussian state purchased 50 subscriptions to the journal and granted Damerow access to ministerial archives. Damerow, "Die Zeitschrift," 2. A further ten subscriptions went to the Grand Duchy of Baden. See *AZP* 5 (1848): 112.

109. Damerow, "Einleitung," *AZP* 1 (1844): v.

110. Damerow, "Die Zeitschrift," 7.

111. Laehr, "Vorwort," *AZP* 15 (1858): 1.

112. See the lamentations of Jastrowitz, "Über die Staatsaufsicht," 717–21.

113. Dörner, *Bürger und Irre*, 19, 280. Cf. Helmut Plessner, *Die verspätete Nation:* (Stuttgart: Kohlhammer, 1959).

114. Ackerknecht described the *AZP*'s editors less regressively as representatives of a "transitional generation" of philosophical anthropologists. Erwin H. Ackerknecht, *Kurze Geschichte der Psychiatrie*, 2d ed. (Stuttgart: Enke, 1967), 62.

115. Damerow, "Einleitung," i–ii. From its inception the title page of the *AZP* read "published by Germany's alienists." At first the alienists published the journal "in association with forensic doctors and criminalists," symbolic of their early close affiliation with *Staatsarzneikunde*. But after Laehr became chief editor in 1857 that association was abandoned.

116. Damerow, "Die Zeitschrift," 11–12.

117. Laehr, "Vorwort," 2, 3.

118. See for example Roller, *Psychiatrische Zeitfragen*.

119. Damerow, "Einleitung," iii. For a subtle interpretation of that debate, see Verwey, 1–36. See also Benzenhöfer, *Psychiatrie und Anthropologie*.

120. The distinction between theory and practice was also fought out linguistically with *Psychiatrik* denoting the art or science of healing and *Psychiatrie* the actual practice. See Dietrich Georg Kieser, "Psychiatrie oder Psychiaterie?" *AZP* 5 (1848): 136–8.

121. Damerow, "Einleitung," iii–iv.

122. Ibid., vi, xlviii. This emphasis on practice has also been noted by Otto Marx, "Wilhelm Griesinger and the History of Psychiatry," *Bulletin of the History of Medicine* 46 (1972): 534.

123. On difficulties mobilizing alienist participation see Damerow, "Die Zeitschrift," 13–17.

124. Flemming, "Was heisst Fortschritt," 177.

125. Laehr, "Vorwort," 2.

126. For longer articles, an *Archiv der deutschen Gesellschaft für Psychiatrie und gerichtliche Psychologie* was published alongside the *Correspondenzblatt* between 1858 and 1872.

127. "An die Leser," *CblDGPgP* 3 (1856): 1, 147.

128. "An die Leser," *CblDGPgP* 1 (1854): 1.

129. Until 1863, the journal's full title was *Der Irrenfreund: Eine Volksschrift über Irre und Irrenanstalten, sowie zur Pflege der geistigen Gesundheit*; thereafter, *Der Irrenfreund: Eine psychiatrische Monats-Schrift* and from 1875 with the explicit appendix "for general practitioners."

130. A list of contributors can be found in *If* 16 (1874): iii–iv.

131. "An die Leser," *If* 1 (1859): 2.

132. See Brandau, "Wie sind Geisteskranke in ihren häuslichen Verhältnissen zu behandeln," *If* 3 (1861): 38.

133. Cf. Kaspar Max Brosius, "Über die Vorutheile gegen Irre und Irrenanstalten," *If* 1 (1859): 105–10 and his "Wieder ein Wort."

134. For a cursory survey of early psychiatric societies, see Carola Herold, "Untersuchungen zur Organisations-Geschichte der Psychiatrie in Deutschland" (Med. diss., University of Marburg, 1972).

135. On German liberalism, see Konrad Jarausch and Larry E. Jones, eds., *In Search of a Liberal Germany* (New York: Berg, 1990); Dieter Langewiesche, *Liberalismus in Deutschland* (Frankfurt/M: Suhrkamp, 1988); and James Sheehan, *German Liberalism in the 19th Century* (Chicago: University of Chicago Press, 1978).

136. See the lamentations of Heinrich Laehr, "Bericht über die Versammlungen deutscher Irrenärzte zu Frankfurt a.M. und Giessen im Jahre 1864," *AZP* 21, supplement (1864): iii.

137. *AZP* 27 (1871): ii.

138. "Psychiatrischer Verein der Rheinprovinz," *AZP* 24 (1867): 539.

139. On the GDNÄ, see Frank R. Pfetsch, *Zur Entwicklung der Wissenschaftspolitik in Deutschland, 1750–1914* (Berlin: Duncker & Humblot, 1974), 252–313.

140. Cf. *AZP* 4 (1847): 1–18. On the different sections of the GDNÄ, see Hermann Lampe, *Die Entwicklung und Differenzierung von Fachabteilungen auf den Versammlungen von 1828 bis 1913*, Schriftenreihe zur Geschichte der Versammlungen deutscher Naturforscher und Ärzte, ed. Hans Querner, vol. 2 (Hildesheim: Gerstenberg, 1975), 277–80.

141. Paul-Otto Schmidt, *Asylierung oder familiale Versorgung*, Abhandlungen zur Geschichte der Medizin und der Naturwissenschaften, vol. 44 (Husum: Matthiesen, 1982), 73–4.

142. See the report of Jessen in "Bericht über die Versammlung in Landau und Speyer," 799–804.

143. Ibid., 802.

144. For Pfetsch, 309, "the GDNÄ understood itself from the outset as a 'purely' scientific organization which closed itself off from utilitarian interests, 'Praxis,' and political activity."

145. Oscar Schwartz, "Über die Stellung der Seelenheilkunde (Psychiatrie) zur Naturforschung und insbesondere zur praktischen Medicin," in *Amtlicher Bericht,* ed. J. Noeggerath and H. F. Kilian (Bonn: Carl Georgi, 1859), 66, 67, 69. Schwartz went on to complain about the poor psychiatric training of physicians and to call for clinical courses in psychiatry at all universities.

146. Significantly, this first plenary address to the GDNÄ on a psychiatric topic since Jessen had spoken in 1847 was not published in the *AZP.*

147. See Moritz Smoler, "Die Section für Psychiatrie und Staatsarzneikunde in Stettin," *CblDGPgP* 10 (1863): 298–9.

148. Of the 339 members in 1858, 223 were forensic experts (*Gerichtsärzte*), only 73 or less than a quarter were alienists, and 43 were practicing physicians. See *CblDGPgP* 5 (1858): 146–7. For more details on the society, see Engstrom, "The Birth," 94–5.

149. Thus Erlenmeyer in his address to the DGPgP in 1856, *CblDGPgP* 3 (1856): 146.

150. Critics of this view claimed that treatment outside the asylum would lead to a detrimental "popularization" and "despiritualization [*Entgeistung*]" of the professional art. Members of the society countered these charges by sponsoring a prize essay: "How are the beginnings of insanity to be treated?" "An die Leser," *CblDGPgP* 5 (1858): 1.

151. Herold, 36.

152. See Erlenmeyer's address to the DGPgP in 1856, *CblDGPgP* 3 (1856): 146.

153. "Erklärung," *AZP* 11 (1854): 358–9.

154. See "Bericht über die Versammlung in Landau und Speyer," 799.

155. For more details on the early history and composition of the *Verein,* see Engstrom, "The Birth," 96–8; Schindler; and Carl Pelman, "Zur Geschichte des Deutschen Vereins für Psychiatrie," *MMW* 53 (1906): 760–1.

156. Roller, *Psychiatrische Zeitfragen,* 68.

157. See Gabriele Feger, "Die Geschichte des 'Psychiatrischen Vereins zu Berlin,' 1889–1920" (Med. diss., Free University Berlin, 1983).

158. See Bernhard van Gülick, "Die Geschichte des 'Psychiatrischen Vereins der Rheinprovinz' 1867–1930" (Med. diss., Free University of Berlin, 1992) and *AZP* 24 (1867): 539ff.

159. Schmiedebach, *Psychiatrie und Psychologie.*

160. See, for example, Jacobi, "Irrenanstalten," 179. University officials also argued this point. See Bopp, 547.

161. For an overview of the fault-lines on the issue of clinical teaching, see Damerow, *Über die relative Verbindung,* 191–229 and Kaspar Max Brosius, "Über Irrenanstalten und deren Weiterentwicklung in Deutschland," *If* 10 (1868): 102–12.

162. Nasse was the director of the medical clinic in Bonn and editor of the somatically oriented but short-lived journal *Zeitschrift für psychische Ärzte* (1818–1822).

163. Friedrich Nasse, "Über das Bedürfniß," *Zeitschrift für psychische Ärzte* 2 (1819): 332. Even those fellow academicians such as Ideler, who detested Nasse's somaticism, could agree with him that it was imperative to impress upon medical students through clinical demonstration the interaction of body and mind. For Ideler, however, the chief purpose of clinical education was to demonstrate to students that emotions were the chief cause ("causa proxima") of madness and to refute "materialist pathogenesis." Ideler, "Über psychiatrische Klinik," 99.

164. See Brosius, "Über Irrenanstalten," 102–6.

165. Nasse, "Über das Bedürfniß," 342.

166. Ibid., 349 and idem, "Keine Irren in die klinischen Anstalten?" *Zeitschrift für psychische Ärzte* 5, no. 3 (1822): 191.

167. Idem, "Über das Bedürfniß," 337.

168. Nasse's clinic was never built in Bonn. See Medical Faculty Circular, 14 November 1842, UAB, MF 1102.

169. This position was held by Roller, Flemming, and to a degree also by Jacobi. However, Jacobi's close relationship with Nasse led him to support calls for academic clinics as well. C[arl] Flemming and M[aximilian] Jacobi, "Über die Errichtung einer Irrenanstalt im Großherzogthum Baden," *ZBHkS* 1 (1838): 728–42, especially 741, and Jacobi, "Irrenanstalten," 180.

170. On the dispute, see Hans Dieter Middelhoff, "C. F. W. Roller und die Vorgeschichte der Heidelberger Psychiatrischen Klinik," in *Psychologie als Grundlagenwissenschaft,* ed. Werner Janzarik, Klinische Psychologie und Psychopathologie, ed. Helmut Remschmidt, vol. 8 (Stuttgart: Enke, 1979), 33–50; Karl Wilmanns, "Die Entwicklung der badischen Irrenfürsorge mit besonderer Berücksichtigung der Universitäts-Kliniken," *AfPN* 87 (1929): 1–23; and Engstrom, "The Birth," 104–8. Cf. also Roller, *Grundsätze,* 31–57; *Psychiatrische Zeitfragen,* 185–202; and Georg Heermann, "Über das Studium der psychischen Medicin auf Universitäten, als das nächste Erforderniss ihrer Förderung," *Medicinische Annalen* 3 (1837): 443–96.

171. Roller, *Grundsätze,* 32.

172. See Adolf Albrecht Erlenmeyer, "Die Versammlung in Carlsruhe," *CblDGPgP* 5 (1858): 164. Other advocates included Reil, Ideler, Nostitz und Jänckendorf, and the editors of the *Correspondenzblatt.*

173. Leupoldt, 58.

174. Damerow, *Über die relative Verbindung,* 208.

175. Jetter, *Zur Typologie,* 124–5. See also Michael Viszánik, *Die Irrenheil- und Pflegeanstalten Deutschlands, Frankreichs* (Vienna: Gerold, 1845), 285. On Sonnenstein see G. A. E. von Nostitz und Jänckendorf, *Beschreibung der königl. Sächsischen Heil- und Pflegeanstalt Sonnenstein,* 3 vols. (Dresden: Walther, 1829). Also see *Geschichte der Heil- und Pflegeanstalt Pirna-Sonnenstein (1811–1939),* vol. 1 of *Sonnenstein: Beiträge zur Geschichte des Sonnensteins und der Sächsischen Schweiz,* ed. Kuratorium Gedenkstätte Sonnenstein (Lampertswalde: Stoba, 1998).

176. See Jetter, *Zur Typologie,* 136 for a list of Jacobi's visitors and assistants. On Jacobi's method of clinical teaching see Ludwig Snell, "Zur Erinnerung an Maximilian Jacobi," *AZP* 28 (1872): 417–19. On Siegburg itself, see Ingrid Kastner, "Die Geschichte der Versorgung psychisch Kranker im Rheinland" (Med. diss., University of Cologne, 1977), 30–72 and Dirk Blasius, *Umgang mit Unheilbarem* (Bonn: Psychiatrie-Verlag, 1986), 39–56.

177. Jetter, *Grundzüge,* 41. On the asylum in Illenau, see Wolfgang Gerke, "Die Reformanstalt Illenau" (Med. diss., University of Freiburg, 1995); Clemens Beck, "Die Geschichte der 'Heil- und Pflegeanstalt Illenau unter Chr. Fr. W. Roller (1802–1878)" (Med. diss., University of Freiburg, 1984); Cheryce Kramer, "A Fools Paradise: The Psychiatry of Gemüth in a Bidermeier Asylum" (Ph.D. Dissertation, University of Chicago, 1998); and Jetter, *Zur Typologie,* 151–60.

178. For an extensive list of assistants in Illenau, see Jetter, *Zur Typologie,* 158.

179. For details and exact citations on the following universities, see Engstrom, "The Birth," 112–17.

180. See the class roles at GStA PK, IHA, Rep. 76VIIID, Nr. 119.

181. See SMIKSA to Staatsministerium des königlichen Hauses und des Äußern, 18 September 1859, BHStA, MK 11158.

182. See the ministerial resolution of 1835 cited in Carl Friedrich Flemming, "Gesetze und Verordnungen in Deutschland betreffs Geisteskranken," *AZP* 19, supplement (1862): 14. See also August Solbrig, "Blicke auf die Entwickelung des Irrenanstaltswesens in Bayern im Laufe des letzten Decenniums," *AZP* 12 (1855): 401–24; "Die Irrenanstalten in Bayern," *Ärztliches Intelligenz-Blatt,* 2 (1855): 458–60; Julius Kollmann, "Zur Geschichte der Irrenpflege in Bayern," *Friedreich's Blätter für gerichtliche Medicin und Sanitätspolizei* 51 (1900): 340–56.

183. See Reinhold Köhler, "Die Psychiatrie als Gegenstand des medicinischen Unterrichts in Deutschland," *MCblWAL* 32 (1862): 292 and "Aus Bayern," *AZP* 15 (1858): 151.

184. See *CblDGPgP* 8 (1861): 340. Strictly speaking, psychiatry was still not included in the university examinations; it became, however, part of the state examinations required of every prospective general practitioner. Admission to the state examinations followed the successful completion of the academic examinations as well as a year of practical training. At the student's discretion, that training could include work in a mental asylum. See "Offizieller Erlass," *Ärztliches Intelligenz-Blatt* 5 (1858): 349–55, especially § 40. See also Christiane Scherg-Zeisner, "Die ärztliche Ausbildung an der königlich-bayerischen Julius-Maximilians-Universität Würzburg, 1814–1872" (Diss. med., University of Würzburg, 1973), 109–16.

185. On Solbrig's teaching, see Engstrom, "The Birth," 117–18, notes 334 and 335.

186. "Bericht über die Versammlung deutscher Irrenärzte zu Eisenach am 12. und 13. September 1860," *AZP* 17 (1860): 19.

187. August Solbrig, "Über psychiatrisch-klinischen Unterricht," *AZP* 18 (1861): 807–11.

188. Laehr, "Bericht über die Versammlung deutscher Irrenärzte in Frankfurt," 16.

189. Köhler, "Die Psychiatrie," 290.

Chapter 3

1. Cf. Pauleikhoff, vol. 2, 233 and Rudolf Thiele, "Über Griesingers Satz: 'Geisteskrankheiten sind Gehirnkrankheiten,'" *MschrPN* 63 (1927): 294–313.

2. Klaus Dörner has spoken of Griesinger's paradigmatic status and of a renaissance of his ideas in *Bürger und Irre,* 288 and 292. See also Güse and Schmacke, 40–1 and Gerald Detlefs, *Wilhelm Griesingers Ansätze zur Psychiatriereform* (Pfaffenweiler: Centaurus 1993), 79ff.

3. See for example A[lice] Rössler, "Zur Geschichte der Universitäts-Nervenklinik Erlangen," in *Psychiatrie in Erlangen,* ed. E. Lungershausen and R. Baer (Erlangen: perimed, 1985), 260 as well as Güse and Schmacke, 39.

4. For a survey of the literature and issues see Huppert and Brosius, "Über Irrenanstalten."

5. Laehr, *Fortschritt? — Rückschritt,* vol. 1.

6. Brosius, "Über Irrenanstalten," 115 and "'Der Umschwung,'" 34.

7. Laehr, "Bericht über die psychiatrischen Versammlungen zu Dresden im September 1868," *AZP* 25, supplement (1868): 66; Roller, *Psychiatrische Zeitfragen,* 26.

8. See Laehr, "Bericht über die psychiatrischen Versammlungen zu Dresden," 7–15 and 64–8, "Die psychiatrische Sektion auf der 42. Naturforscher-Versammlung zu Dresden," *Vierteljahrsschrift für Psychiatrie* 2 (1868): 238, and *AfPN* 1 (1868): 740–1. Cf. also Alexander Mette, *Wilhelm Griesinger,* vol. 26 of Biographien hervorragender Naturwissenschaftlicher, Techniker und Mediziner (Leipzig: BSB B. G. Teubner Verlagsanstalt, 1976), 73–4.

9. See "Zur Charakteristik der psychiatrischen Section der Naturforscherversammlung zu Dresden," *BKW* 5 (1868): 447–8 and "Die psychiatrische Sektion." An even sharper denunciation of the section's treatment of Griesinger and of alienists' "blind orthodoxy" and "mindless cliquishness" appeared in *CblDGPgP* 15 (1868): 337–41.

10. "Drei Nekrologe und einige Anschuldigungen," *AZP* 26 (1869): 268; Brosius, "Über Irrenanstalten," 81–123.

11. See Mette, 25, 48–51, 70–3; Carl August Wunderlich, *Wilhelm Griesinger* (Leipzig: Otto Wigand, 1869), 26–8.

12. See Laehr, *Fortschritt? — Rückschritt!,* vol. 1, 22–3, 75–7, and 87; Brosius, "'Der Umschwung in der Psychiatrie,'" 26; and Bonhoeffer, *Die Geschichte der Psychiatrie,* 17.

13. Medical Faculty to MgUMA, 23 February 1864, UAHUB Medical Faculty 238, Bl. 40–1. That academic psychiatry in Berlin not fall under the sway of alienists appears to have influenced the rejection of the alternate candidates, Heinrich Neumann and Heinrich Laehr. See Medical Faculty to MgUMA, 23 February 1864, GStA PK, IHA, Rep. 76Va, MgUMA, Sect. 2, Tit. IV, Nr. 46, Bd. III, Bl. 157–9 and Heinz-Peter Schmiedebach, "Wilhelm Griesinger," in *Berlinische Lebensbilder: Mediziner,* ed. Wolfgang Treue and Rolf Winau, vol. 60 of *Einzelveröffentlichungen der historischen Kommission zu Berlin* (Berlin: Colloquium, 1987), 126.

14. Griesinger, "Vorwort," iii.

15. Brosius, "'Der Umschwung in der Psychiatrie,'" 21, 32. See likewise "Aus der Provinz," *AZP* 24 (1867): 834 and Huppert, 335.

16. See Carl Friedrich Flemming, review of *Zur Kenntniss der heutigen Psychiatrie in Deutschland*" by W[ilhelm] Griesinger, *AZP* 25 (1868): 364–6. Although its editors successfully defended its autonomy, the *AZP* lost its long-time publisher August Hirschwald to Griesinger's *Archiv* and appeared after 1870 in the publishing house of Georg Reimer.

17. Indeed, contemporary accounts are often at a loss to explain the vehemence of the dispute. See Gerhart Zeller, "Von der Heilanstalt zur Heil- und Pflegeanstalt," *Fortschritte der Neurologie und Psychiatrie* 49 (1981): 125.

18. By contrast, the Swiss reception of his ideas was generally favorable. See "Fünfte Jahresversammlung des Vereins schweizerischer Irrenärzte," *AZP* 26 (1869): 231–43.

19. This analysis consciously ignores other important issues in the debate (such as family care and asylum organization) which do not touch directly on the emergence of university clinics.

20. Wilhelm Griesinger, "Über Irrenanstalten und deren Weiter-Entwicklung in Deutschland," *AfPN* 1 (1868): 8–43.

21. Ibid., 33–43.

22. Ibid., 33, 26.

23. Ibid., 29.

24. Ibid., 16.

25. They were to be amalgams of an infirmary and Parchappe's *division à surveillance continue*. See Jean-Baptiste-Maximilian Parchappe de Vinay, *Des principes à suivre dans la fondation et la construction des asiles d'aliénés* (Paris: Masson, 1853), 92.

26. Griesinger, "Über Irrenanstalten," 18. The importance of academic training in Griesinger's reform program has also been stressed by Heinz-Peter Schmiedebach, "Mensch, Gehirn und wissenschaftliche Psychiatrie," in *Vom Umgang mit Irren,* ed. Johann Glatzel, Steffan Haas and Heinz Schott (Regensburg: S. Roderer, 1990), 92–4.

27. Griesinger, "Über Irrenanstalten," 19.

28. Ibid., 22.

29. Wilhelm Griesinger, "Weiteres über psychiatrische Cliniken," *AfPN* 1 (1868): 500–4.

30. Roller, *Psychiatrische Zeitfragen,* 26.

31. On the book's favorable reception see Engstrom, "The Birth," 135, note 43 and Bodamer, 526–7.

32. Griesinger first formulated his ideas on reflex action in "Über psychische Reflexactionen," in *Gesammelte Abhandlungen,* ed. C. A. Wunderlich, vol. 2 (Berlin: Hirschwald, 1872), 3–45. On the mechanist content and philosophical context of Griesinger's ideas, see Verwey, 37–155.

33. For a history of the term 'unitary psychosis,' see Michael Schmidt-Degenhard, "Einheitspsychose: Begriff und Idee," in *Für und Wider der Einheitspsychose,* ed. C[hristoph] Mundt and H[ans-Martin] Saß (Stuttgart: Thieme, 1992), 1–11 and G[erman] E. Berrios and D[ominic] Beer, "The Notion of Unitary Psychosis," *HP* 5 (1994): 13–36.

34. Pauleikhoff, 2:231, 235, and 242. On the relationship between Griesinger and Zeller, see also Verwey, 140–51, who argues the case for Zeller as a somaticist.

35. Witness for example the debates in the AZP and GDNÄ. Griesinger himself recognized that polemics against moralism in the profession were no longer necessary. See Griesinger, *Die Pathologie und Therapie,* 11.

36. The same conclusion is reached by Verwey, 110.

37. To which might also be added a nosological advantage. According to Kahlbaum, Griesinger's ordering of psychiatric diseases satisfied the needs of two otherwise divergent nosological traditions: empiricists and dialectitions. Kahlbaum, *Die Gruppierung,* 46.

38. Such energetic models also influenced Karl Wernicke, Friedrich Jolly, Sigmund Freud, and Eugen Bleuler. See Leibbrand and Wettley, *Der Wahnsinn,* 555ff, 597ff. See also Anson Rabinbach, *The Human Motor* (New York: Basic Books, 1990).

39. See Roller, *Psychiatrische Zeitfragen,* 23.

40. Otto Marx has suggested that Griesinger was unaware of this dilemma. But in fact Griesinger was only too aware of the difficulties facing alienists. His reform program deftly exploited their weaknesses in an effort to advance the cause of clinical research and education. Compare Griesinger, "Weiteres," 503 and also Marx, "Wilhelm Griesinger," 541.

41. Roller, *Psychiatrische Zeitfragen,* vii, 57.

42. Laehr, "Bericht über die Versammlung deutscher Irrenärzte zu Frankfurt," iv.

43. Griesinger, "Weiteres," 503.

44. For a description of diverse range of the mechanical restraints employed in asylums in the early nineteenth century see Jacobi, "Irrenanstalten," 155–65.

45. John Conolly, *Die Behandlung der Irren ohne mechanischen Zwang,* trans. M[ax] Brosius (Lahr: M. Schauenburg, 1860). On the reception of Conolly's non-restraint in Germany, see Cor-

dula Geduldig, "Die Behandlung von Geisteskranken ohne physische Zwang" (Med. diss., University of Zurich, 1975).

46. Ludwig Meyer, "Das Non-Restraint und die Deutsche Psychiatrie," *AZP* 20 (1863): 542–81. On Meyer see Elisabeth Burkhart, "Ludwig Meyer (1827–1900): Leben und Werk" (Med. diss., Free University of Berlin, 1991).

47. Griesinger, *Die Pathologie und Therapie*, 2d ed., 506.

48. Griesinger, "Die freie Behandlung," in *Gesammelte Abhandlungen*, 317–31, 317.

49. Griesinger, "Über Irrenanstalten," 26.

50. Ibid., 33.

51. Compare *CblDGPgP* 5 (1858): 3–4, 11–12 and Damerow in "Ein Blick."

52. Neumann, "Zum Non-Restraint," *AZP* 28 (1872): 678, 679.

53. It would, however, be a mistake to overdraw the battle lines in the debate on non-restraint. There were several alienists at the forefront of the non-restraint effort, including Max Brosius, the translator of Conolly's monograph and an outspoken critic of Griesinger's urban asylums.

54. Laehr, *Fortschritt?—Rückschritt!*, 1:iv.

55. Griesinger, "Die freie Behandlung," in *Gesammelte Abhandlungen*, 330–1.

56. Idem, "Über Irrenanstalten," 23.

57. Laehr, *Fortschritt?—Rückschritt!*, 1:iv.

58. Carl Westphal, "Nachrichten von der psychiatrischen Clinik zu Berlin," *AfPN* 1 (1868): 233.

59. Westphal, "Psychiatrische Klinik," *CA* 1 (1874): 458.

60. Friedrich Jolly, *Bericht über die Irren-Abteilung des Juliusspitals* (Würzburg: Stahel'schen Buch- und Kunsthandlung, 1873), 25. Cf. also Scull, *Masters*, 152.

61. Thus Hermann Dick as cited in Roller, *Psychiatrische Zeitfragen*, 80.

62. Griesinger, *Pathologie und Therapie*, 3d ed., 507.

63. Griesinger, *Gesammelten Abhandlungen*, 1:324–6. Before accepting the position in Berlin, Griesinger made sure he would be able to hire and fire hospital personnel as he saw fit. MgUMA to Charité Director Esse, 16 December 1864, UAHUB, Charité Direktion, 1058, Bl. 1. On Griesinger's later efforts to reorganize the personnel, see his correspondence with Esse, 9 June 1865, 17 October 1866, and 16 December 1866, UAHUB Charité Direktion 1033, Bl. 59–67 and 93–100.

64. Max Seige, "Erinnerungen an Otto Binswanger," *Wissenschaftliche Zeitschrift der Friedrich-Schiller-Universität Jena, Mathematisch-Naturwissenschaftliche Reihe* 4 (1954–5): 374.

65. Emil Kraepelin, *Lebenserinnerungen* (Berlin: Springer, 1983), 14. See also Wolfgang Gudden, "Bernhard von Gudden: Leben und Werk" (Med. diss., University of Munich, 1987), 209–21.

66. Griesinger, *Gesammelte Abhandlungen*, 330. See likewise Meyer, "Das Non- Restraint," 581.

67. Griesinger, *Pathologie und Therapie*, 3d ed., 507. See also Dannemann, *Die psychiatrische Klinik zu Giessen*, 87. Other alternatives included temporary isolation, chemical restraint, tactics of diversion and translocation, and balneology. See Kaspar Max Brosius, "Soll man noch isolieren," *If* 15 (1873): 44–8 and Neumann, "Zum Non-Restraint," 689.

68. Wilhelm Griesinger, *Zur Kenntniss der heutigen Psychiatrie in Deutschland.* (Leipzig: Otto Wigand, 1868), 36.

69. Griesinger, "Über Irrenanstalten," 16–7. Compare also Griesinger, *Zur Kenntniss*, 5. For German perspectives on Parchappe, see Brosius, "Über Irrenanstalten," 100–101 and K[oloman] Pándy, *Irrenfürsorge in Europa*, edited by E. Engelken (Berlin: Georg Reimer, 1908), 391. See also Huppert, 335–6.

70. See ibid., 339 and Engstrom, "The Birth," 151–2, note 94.

71. Griesinger, *Pathologie und Therapie*, 3d ed., 478; Griesinger, "Über Irrenanstalten," 16.

72. Meyer, "Das Non-Restraint," 546. This was also the view of Conolly. See Scull, *Masters*, 66. Carl Westphal also claimed that non-restraint was a precondition to the observation of certain morbid conditions. Westphal, *Psychiatrie und psychiatrischer Unterricht*, 15–6.

73. This has also been suggested by Geduldig, 109 and Georg B. Gruber, "Zur Geschichte der Psychiatrie in Göttingen," *Sudhoffs Archiv* 40 (1956): 354–5.

74. Flemming, "Über Notwendigkeit," 706 and Laehr, *Über Irrsein und Irrenanstalten*, 115.

75. The rescript is published in Unger, 214–5; see also *AZP* 17 (1860): 804–5. The government was only marginally successful in achieving the aims of the rescript. See Engstrom, "The Birth," 154, note 103.

76. Arndt, 3 and 12–13.

77. Eric J. Engstrom and Volker Hess, eds. *Zwischen Wissens- und Verwaltungsökonomie,* in *Jahrbuch für Universitätsgeschichte* 3 (2000).

78. See Esse to MgUMA, 4 September 1860, UAHUB, Charité Direktion 242, Bl. 1–4 and the ministry's response on 22 September 1860, Bl. 5. On Esse see Hess, "Der Verwaltungsdirektor."

79. The medical faculty had attempted precisely that just two-and-a-half weeks earlier. See Medical Faculty to Bethmann Hollweg, 16 August 1860, UAHUB Medical Faculty 238, Bl. 26–7.

80. Ibid. and Esse to MgUMA, 30 October 1860, UAHUB, Charité Direktion 242, Bl. 8.

81. MgUMA to Esse, 22 September 1860, UAHUB, Charité Direktion 242, Bl. 5.

82. Two petitions to the ministry, one in August 1860 and another in October 1862, both failed to reassert the medical faculty's influence over the psychiatric ward. See UAHUB, Medical Faculty 238, Bl. 26–7 and 32–3.

83. For additional details see Kai Sammet, *Über Irrenanstalten und deren Weiterentwicklung in Deutschland,* Hamburger Studien zur Geschichte der Medizin, vol. 1 (Hamburg: Lit, 2000), 12–41.

84. Medical Faculty to MgUMA, 23 February 1864, GStA PK, IHA, Rep. 76Va, MgUMA, Sect. 2, Tit. IV, Nr. 46, Bd. III, Bl. 157–9.

85. "Dissenting vote in the matter concerning the chair in psychiatry," UAHUB, Medical Faculty 238, 24 February 1864, Bl. 43–4.

86. MgUMA to August Solbrig, 12 March 1864, GStA PK, IHA, Rep. 76Va, MgUMA, Sect. 2, Tit. IV, Nr. 46, Bd. III, Bl. 164. On the ministry's concerns, see its response to the recommendations of the medical faculties on Bl. 157–9. On Prussian perceptions of Solbrig and Bavarian psychiatry, see Heinrich Laehr to Academic Senate of the University of Berlin, 27 June 1862 and O. Heurmann to MgUMA, 30 March 1864, both GStA PK, IHA, Rep. 76Va, MgUMA, Sect. 2, Tit. IV, Nr. 46, Bd. III, Bl. 45 and Bl. 167 respectively.

87. August Solbrig, "Memorandum den psychiatrisch-klinischen Unterricht in Berlin betreffend," 31 May 1864, GStA PK, IHA, Rep. 76Va, MgUMA, Sect. 2, Tit. VII, Nr. 16, Bl. 24–7.

88. August Solbrig to MgUMA, 31 May 1864, GStA PK, IHA, Rep. 76Va, Sect. 2, Tit. IV, Nr. 46, Bd. III, Bl. 172–3. Solbrig was rewarded for his loyalty to Bavaria with a full chair in psychiatry at the university in Munich.

89. Officially the faculty objected to Westphal on the grounds of his inexperience and the great prestige of the position. Medical Faculty to MgUMA, 27 October 1863, UAHUB Medical Faculty 238, Bl. 34. Although the ministry was not unsympathetic to Westphal, it also deemed him still too inexperienced for the post. See the internal note in response to Medical Faculty to MgUMA, 10 October 1862, GStA PK, IHA, Rep. 76Va, MgUMA, Sect. 2, Tit. IV, Nr. 46, Bd. III, Bl. 40.

90. Charité Directorate to MgUMA, 14 July 1864, GStA PK, IHA, Rep. 76Va, MgUMA, Sect. 2, Tit. IV, Nr. 46, Bd. III, Bl. 243–6.

91. See MgUMA to Medical Faculty, 27 June 1864, GStA PK, IHA, Rep. 76Va, MgUMA, Sect. 2, Tit. VII, Nr. 16, Bl. 28.

92. MgUMA to Wilhelm Griesinger, 1 November 1864, GStA PK, IHA, Rep. 76Va, MgUMA, Sect. 2, Tit. IV, Nr. 46, Bd. III, Bl. 204. On the negociations, see Engstrom, "The Birth," 161–2 and Sammet, 26–7.

93. See Reichert to Medical Faculty, 1 December 1864, UAHUB, Medical Faculty 238, Bl. 50–1.

94. MgUMA to Medical Faculty, 1 February 1865, UAHUB Medical Faculty 238, Bl. 53.

95. Laehr, "Rundschau in Preussen," 327.

96. Thus Solbrig's earlier formulation that the "advanced science of psychiatry . . . makes fun-

damentally and wholly different demands on the knowledge of the physician." Solbrig, "Über psychiatrisch-klinischen Unterricht," 805–6.

97. *AZP* 21 (1864): 354–5.

98. See Flemming, "Über einige der nächsten Aufgaben der Psychiatrie," 51, 58.

99. Griesinger, *Zur Kenntniss*, 10.

100. Griesinger, "Über Irrenanstalten," 20.

101. With the growth in the number of psychiatric institutions came more detailed and rigorous admissions procedures. See Dörner, *Bürger und Irre*, 230 and Doris Kaufmann, " 'Irre und Wahnsinnige,' " in *Verbrechen, Strafen und soziale Kontrolle*, ed. Richard van Dülmen, (Frankfurt/M: Fischer, 1990), 181. For examples of slow admission procedures, see Engstrom, "The Birth," 165, note 139.

102. Griesinger, "Über Irrenanstalten," 13; also see his "Weiteres," 502.

103. The order is reprinted in *AZP* 21 (1864): 701–4.

104. See Heinrich Laehr, "Über die Aufnahmebedingungen in Irrenanstalten," *AZP* 22 (1865): 348.

105. For the subsequent debates at the VdI meetings in Heppenheim (1867) and Dresden (1868), see C. F. W. Roller, "Über Aufnahme-Bestimmungen in Irrenanstalten und Anstalts-Statuten Überhaupt," *AZP* 24 (1867): 642–60, 716–20; and see "Bericht über die psychiatrischen Versammlungen zu Dresden," 9–11, 23–35. For a summary of the arguments consult Roller, *Psychiatrische Zeitfragen*, 130–53.

106. Laehr, "Bericht über die psychiatrische Versammlungen zu Dresden," 29.

107. Peter Willers Jessen, "Vorschläge zu gesetzlichen Bestimmungen in Beziehung auf die Aufnahme von Geisteskranken in Irrenanstalten," *AZP* 24 (1867): 659. Jessen encountered very stiff resistance from Ludwig Meyer and Hermann Dick. In the end, after having sent the issue to commission in 1865 and having postponed it in 1867, alienists failed to reach a consensus in Dresden in 1868, whereafter the issue was dropped altogether.

108. "Every asylum is nothing other than a hospital for patients suffering from brain diseases." Griesinger, *Pathologie und Therapie*, 3d ed., 529.

109. See Griesinger, "Über Irrenanstalten," 34. As late as 1867 he had not made this distinction. See Griesinger, *Pathologie und Therapie*, 3d ed., 528–9, 536.

110. Damerow had argued the case in "Über Irrenpflegeanstalten," *Medicinische Zeitung* 2 (1833): 220. Even early advocates of university clinics thought that "incurable [patients] are just as valuable to research as curable ones." Heermann, 454.

111. Griesinger, "Über Irrenanstalten," 21.

112. Neumann, *Gedanken*, 6. Flemming, "Gesetze und Verordnungen," 29. For this reason, it is something of a mischaracterization to see Griesinger as the father of deinstitutionalization. Certainly, his program sought to deinstitutionalize certain patients living in large state asylums; but it simultaneously tried to institutionalize others residing beyond its walls.

113. Griesinger, "Über Irrenanstalten," 12–3 and the footnote on page 25.

114. Griesinger, "Weiteres," 501. The need not just for acute, but also "fresh" cases became one of the more ubiquitous arguments of academicians and of course lent added weight to the dogma of early admission. For two later examples of the same argument, see Flechsig, *Die Irrenklinik*, 51 and Ludwig Meyer, "Die psychiatrische Klinik der Königlichen Georg-August-Universität in Göttingen," *Klinisches Jahrbuch* 1 (1889): 212–3.

115. Cramer, "Die preußischen Universitätskliniken," 190.

116. Griesinger, "Über Irrenanstalten," 21.

117. Earlier Nasse tried to turn this handicap into an advantage, arguing that the hundreds of patients in the asylums would simply "squander the interest [of students] on mere curiosity without providing them with a solid foundation of knowledge." By contrast, in a small clinic students could better "interact" with patients. Draft letter of the Medical Faculty to University Curator, n.d. [ca. February 1848], UAB, MF 1102.

118. Heinrich Laehr, review of *Das Projekt des Neubaues einer zweiten Heil- und Pflege-Anstalt im Großherzogtum Baden, vor den Landständen und den beiden medicinischen Facultäten*, by Roller and Fischer, *AZP* 24 (1867): 220. And indeed, Griesinger conceived of the asy-

lum not in organic terms, but rather as a well-oiled, "silent" and "very complicated mechanism." Griesinger, *Pathologie und Therapie,* 535.

119. Eduard Hitzig, "Neubau der psychiatrischen und Nervenklinik für die Universität Halle a. S.," *Klinisches Jahrbuch* 2 (1890): 386.

120. On the development of nineteenth-century hospitals see Alfons Labisch and Reinhard Spree, *'Einen jeden Kranken in einem Hospitale sein eigenes Bett'* (Frankfurt/M: Campus, 1996); Reinhard Spree, "Krankenhausentwicklung und Sozialpolitik in Deutschland während des 19. Jahrhunderts," *Historische Zeitschrift* 260 (1995): 75–105; Spree, "Sozialer Wandel im Krankenhaus während des 19. Jahrhunderts," *Medizinhistorisches Journal* 33 (1998): 245–291; and Beate Witzler, *Großstadt und Hygiene,* Medizin, Gesellschaft und Geschichte, ed. Robert Jütte, vol. 5 (Stuttgart: Steiner, 1995). On hospitals in Berlin see Manfred Stürzbecher, "Allgemeine und Spezialkrankenhäuser, insbesondere Privatkrankenanstalten im 19. Jahrhundert in Berlin," in *Studien zur Krankenhausgeschichte im 19. Jahrhundert,* ed. Hans Schadewaldt, Studien zur Medizingeschichte im 19. Jahrhundert (Göttingen: V&R, 1976), 105–120." Specifically on Berlin's Charité hospital, see Eric J. Engstrom and Volker Hess, eds., *Zwischen Wissens- und Verwaltungsökonomie* and Peter Schneck and Hans-Uwe Lammel, eds., *Die Medizin an der Berliner Universität und an der Charité zwischen 1810 und 1850,* Abhandlungen zur Geschichte der Medizin und der Naturwissenschaften (Berlin: Matthiesen, 1995).

121. After 1880 national health and accident insurance comprised a growing percentage of hospital income. On hospital financing, see Spree, "Krankenhausentwicklung."

122. Alfons Labisch, "Stadt und Krankenhaus: Das Allgemeine Krankenhaus in der kommunalen Sozial- und Gesundheitspolitik des 19. Jahrhunderts," in *'Einem jeden Kranken in einem Hospitale sein eigenes Bett,'* ed. Alfons Labisch and Reinhard Spree (Frankfurt/M: Campus, 1996), 256.

123. On the laws and their wider context, see Reinhart Koselleck, *Preußen zwischen Reform und Revolution,* 3d ed. (Munich: DTV, 1981), 621–37; Florian Tennstedt, *Sozialgeschichte der Sozialpolitik in Deutschland* (Göttingen: V&R, 1981), 39–47, 92–103; Wehler, vol. 2, 293–6; and Hermann Beck, "The Social Policies of Prussian Officials: The Bureaucracy in a New Light," *JMH* 64 (1992): 274–85.

124. Passages of the law relevant to psychiatric issues can be found in Unger, 8–15 and Eulenberg, *Das Medicinalwesen,* 49–56.

125. On these machinations see Tennstedt, *Sozialgeschichte der Sozialpolitik,* 46–7 and Wehler, 3:31.

126. As early as the 1820s the Charité was struggling to cope with an influx of non-residents in search of free medical care. See Münch, 182–3.

127. Ibid., 97.

128. On the complex and contested legal relationship between the Charité and the city of Berlin, see A. Förster, *Denkschrift* (Berlin: Reichsdruckerei, 1892).

129. The cabinet order followed from a large-scale reorganization of the Charité's administration which had begun in 1828. On the Charité's administration see Eric Hilf, "Zur Geschichte der Charitédirektion im 19. Jahrhundert," in *Zwischen Wissens- und Verwaltungsökonomie,* ed. Eric J. Engstrom and Volker Hess, *Zeitschrift für Universitätsgeschichte* 3 (2000): 49–68. On the order of 1835, see Förster, 27–48; Carl Heinrich Esse, "Geschichtliche Nachrichten über das königliche Charité-Krankenhaus zu Berlin," *Annalen des Charité-Krankenhauses zu Berlin* 1 (1850): 31–3; Oskar Scheibe, "Zweihundert Jahre des Charité-Krankenhauses zu Berlin," *Charité-Annalen* 34 (1910): 129.

130. Charité Directorate to MgUMA, 2 December 1853, UAHUB Charité Direktion 1033, Bl. 25.

131. Scheibe, 128–9. See also Münch, 65–6.

132. Disputes over the residency status of patients were not unique to Berlin or Prussia. See the case of Saxony cited in Flemming, "Gesetze und Verordnungen," 160–2.

133. See Charité Directorate to MgUMA, 16 May 1862, UAHUB, Charité Direktion 1033, Bl. 278–85.

134. Armendirektion to Charité Directorate, 13 April 1874, UAHUB Charité Direktion 1034.

135. On the *Irrenverpflegungsanstalt,* see Karl Ludwig Ideler, "Geschichtliche Entwicklung der städtischen Irrenpflege," in *Die Städtische Irren-Anstalt zu Dalldorf,* by the Berlin Magistrate (Berlin: Springer, 1883), 8–12 and Johannes Rigler, *Das medicinische Berlin* (Berlin: Elwin Staude, 1873), 226–7.

136. Armendirektion to Charité Directorate, 27 March 1865, UAHUB Charité Direktion 1034, Bl. 46.

137. At issue in these court proceedings was the exact legal status of the cabinet order of 1835 and what impact it had on the long-standing rights of the city to have its poor treated in the Charité. On the subtle legal issues involved, see Förster. See also the records in UAHUB Charité Direktion 2152.

138. A manuscript copy of the agreement of 21 April 1863 is at UAHUB, Charité Direktion 1034, Bl. 269–71.

139. For accounts of Esse's impact on civic officials, see Engstrom, "The Birth," 182, note 186. On the city's neglect of hospital construction, see Manfred Stürzbecher, "Aus der Geschichte des städtischen Krankenhauses Moabit," in *1872–1972: Städtisches Krankenhaus Moabit,* ed. Bezirksamt Tiergarten (Berlin: n.p., 1972), 15.

140. See Charité Directorate to MgUMA, 24 April 1874, UAHUB, Charité Direktion 1034, Bl. 215. Westphal later attributed the decline to the police delivering prospective patients directly to the *Verpflegungsanstalt.* Westphal to the Charité Directorate, 19 April 1873, UAHUB, Charité Direktion 1034, Bl. 174.

141. See "Aus Berlin," *AZP* 22 (1865): 191 and "Aus Berlin," *AZP* 27 (1871): 653. Ideler, "Geschichtliche Entwicklung," 10. Between 1864 and 1868, the male population of the *Irrenverpflegungsanstalt* alone rose by nearly two-thirds from 156 to 246.

142. Ibid., 12.

143. Although Griesinger too was involved in this search, no satisfactory site was found. See Griesinger, *Zur Kenntniss,* 46–9.

144. Franz Richarz, "Thesen," *If* 10 (1868): 78–80.

145. Griesinger, *Zur Kenntniss,* 39–56.

146. Griesinger, "Über Irrenanstalten," 9.

147. Calls for the Charité to be separated from the system of public welfare dated back to the early nineteenth century. See Münch, 55–6. In 1823 Nasse too had appealed for broad-based public health care not conditional upon public welfare. Friedrich Nasse, *Von der Stellung der Ärzte im Staate* (Leipzig: Cnobloch, 1823), 292–305, cited likewise in Münch, 70.

148. For a critique of the *Stadtasyl*'s inability to segregate and classify patients, see also Huppert, 336–7.

149. Damerow, "Ein Blick," 152.

150. Gunnar Stollberg, "Zur Geschichte der Pflegeklassen in deutschen Krankenhäusern," in '*Einem jeden Kranken in einem Hospitale sein eigenes Bett,*' ed. Alfons Labisch and Reinhard Spree (Frankfurt/M: Campus, 1996) 378–81, 385–6.

151. Stollberg speaks of the "interpenetration of social stratification and internal differentiation [*Binnendifferenzierung*]" of the hospital. Ibid., 375.

152. Brosius, "Über Irrenanstalten," 90–1.

153. Bonhoeffer, *Die Geschichte der Psychiatrie,* 17.

154. As early as 1848 Nasse too believed that an institution with the name '*Klinik*' could attract wealthier patients, whose families were otherwise reluctant to place them in large asylums. Draft of Nasse's proposal, n.d. [ca. January 1848], UAB, MF 1102.

155. Cf. §§ 4 and 5 of the *Freizügigkeitsgesetz* of 1 November 1867 and § 3 of the *Reichswahlgesetz* of 31 May 1869.

156. Heermann, 481.

157. August Solbrig, "Denkschrift," BHStA, MK 11488.

158. Westphal, *Psychiatrie und psychiatrischer Unterricht,* 24.

159. Cramer, "Die preussischen Universitätskliniken," 190.

160. Damerow, "Ein Blick," 155.

161. See *Vossische Zeitung,* 16 June 1865 and "Aus Berlin," *AZP* 22 (1865): 192–3.

162. *Vossische Zeitung,* 16 June 1865.

163. See "Aus Berlin," *AZP* 42 (1886): 548–9.

164. Jolly, *Bericht,* 17 and 18. Gudden too appealed to the city magistrate in Munich to allow him to use the patients and lecture hall of the city hospital for his clinical instruction. Ibid., 17.

165. Griesinger, "Über Irrenanstalten," 13, 25.

166. Griesinger, "Weiteres," 502.

167. See the cases of Halle and Marburg. Of course, relations with city officials were not immune to similar problems. Disagreements in Breslau led to the wholesale collapse of clinical psychiatric training there in 1900. On the case of Breslau see GStA PK, IHA, Rep. 76Va, MgUMA, Sect. 4, Tit. X, Nr. 41, Bd. II and III.

168. See Carl Wernicke, "Stadtasyle und psychiatrische Kliniken," *Klinisches Jahrbuch* 2 (1890): 188–93.

169. Laehr, review of *Das Projekt,* 222.

170. Laehr, "Die Bedeutung der Psychiatrie für den ärztlichen Unterricht," *BKW* 34 (1897): 62. Laehr, *Fortschritt? — Rückschritt!,* 2:42.

171. Ibid., vol. I, 1–9.

172. On gendered spatial division and regulation in the nineteenth century see Karin Hausen, "Frauenräume," in *Frauengeschichte — Geschlechtergeschichte,* ed. Karin Hausen and Heide Wunder (Frankfurt/M: Campus, 1992), 22.

173. Griesinger's surveillance ward [*Wachabteilung*] conjured up visions of "chaos" and memories of the "madhouse" for Brosius, "Über Irrenanstalten," 89.

174. See Labisch, "Stadt und Krankenhaus," 272–3; Hermann Vezin, *Ueber Krankenhäuser* (Münster: Theissing, 1858); and Norbert Störmer, *Innere Mission und geistige Behinderung* (Münster: Lit, 1991). On these developments in Berlin, see Elm and Loock. For the case of Catholic assistance, see Nobert Klinkenberg, "Die sozialpolitische Isolierung des Krankenhauses," *Historia Hospitalium* 15 (1983–4): 213–25. On confessional nursing care, see Engstrom, "The Birth," 197, note 239.

175. Vezin, 7, 62.

176. On these plans, see Laehr, *Fortschritt? — Rückschritt!,* 2:20–33 and Griesinger, *Zur Kenntniss,* 51–56.

177. Flemming, "Ein Blick," 159. Government officials in Westphalia in the 1880s removed wealthy patients from asylums in Düren, Bonn, and Merzig. Stollberg, 379–80.

178. This was precisely the service which the private asylum of a certain Dr. Edel provided for the town of Charlottenburg near Berlin. See Caesar Heimann, *Bericht über Sanitätsrath Dr. Karl Edel's Asyl für Geisteskranke zu Charlottenburg 1869–1894* (Berlin: Hirschwald, 1895).

179. Rigler, 226–7; Armendirektion to Charité Directorate, 14 April 1874, UAHUB, Charité Direktion, 1034, Bl. 210; Heimann. Between 1880 and 1890 the number of patients in private institutions and homes nearly doubled to 1206. See Ideler, "Geschichtliche Entwicklung," 11 and *ZblNP* 13 (1890): 43.

180. See Friedrich Engelken, "Über die Prophylaxis der Geistesstörungen," *AZP* 10 (1853): 353–95. A review of the first ten volumes of the AZP confirms Engelken's viewpoint.

181. Griesinger, *Pathologie und Therapie,* 2d ed., 475.

182. As prophylactic measures Griesinger advocated marriage restrictions, a proper diet, avoiding mental strain, counteracting florid imaginations or excessive sexual drive, and "getting used to accepting objective circumstances." Ibid.

183. Griesinger also stressed the "demoralizing influence of large cities . . . , the decline of matrimony, and the fluctuating attitude toward religion" as operative factors. Ibid., 142–3.

184. Johanna Bleker has argued that physicians were mimicking the prejudices of popular opinion rather than relying on statistical evidence linking urban life and disease. Johanna Bleker, "Die Stadt als Krankheitsfaktor," *Medizinhistorisches Journal* 18 (1983): 118–36.

185. Dörner, *Bürger und Irre,* 299.

186. Ibid., 56.

187. See Christoph Sachße and Florian Tennstedt, *Geschichte der Armenfürsorge in Deutsch-*

land, (Stuttgart: Kohlhammer, 1988), 2:9; Alfons Labisch and Florian Tennstedt, *Der Weg zum 'Gesetz über die Vereinheitlichung des Gesundheitswesens vom 3. Juli 1934* (Düsseldorf: Akademie für öffentliches Gesundheitswesen, 1985), note 72.

188. Ibid., 27–35.

189. Cf. Heinrich Schipperges, *Utopien der Medizin* (Salzburg: Müller, 1968), 53–62.

Chapter 4

1. Laehr, *Über Irrsein und Irrenanstalten,* 115.

2. On the eclectic array of skills required of the alienist see Friedrich Wilhelm Hagen, "Psychiatrie und Anatomie," *AZP* 12 (1855): 3. Reference here is to alienists practicing in curative and not in custodial institutions. Throughout the nineteenth century most state officials and alienists—including Langermann, Damerow—did not uniformly believe that full-time medical supervision of custodial institutions was necessary. See Damerow, "Über Irrenpflegeanstalten," 219 and his *Über die relative Verbindung,* 245, as well as *Offizieller Bericht* (Berlin: Fischer's Medizinische Buchhandlung, 1903), 51.

3. In assuming the role of actors, alienists often engaged in an "artificial" therapeutic dialogue with their patients. See Müller, *Die Irrenanstalt,* 148–9. More generally on the "dramaturgical power" of general practitioners, see Jens Lachmund and Gunnar Stollberg, "The Doctor, his Audience, and the Meaning of Illness," *MGG* supplement 1 (1992): 53–65.

4. On Griesinger's early career, see Bettina Wahrig-Schmitt, *Der junge Wilhelm Griesinger im Spannungsfeld zwischen Philosophie und Physiologie* (Tübingen: Günther Narr, 1985) and Mette, 25–7.

5. On the terms *Neuropathologie, Nervenheilkunde,* and *Neurologie* and their largely synonymous usage around the turn of the century, see Gustav W. Schimmelpennig, "Alfred Erich Hoche," in *Berichte aus den Sitzungen der Joachim Jungius-Gesellschaft der Wissenschaften e.V., Hamburg,* vol. 8, no. 3. (Göttingen: V&R, 1990), 19, note 69.

6. Although Griesinger rejected as premature the outright merger of psychiatry and "brain-pathology," knowledge of the nervous system's anatomy, physiology, and pathology were for him essential prerequisites for every psychiatrist. See Griesinger, *Pathologie und Therapie,* 3d ed., 9–10.

7. Bonhoeffer, *Die Geschichte der Psychiatrie,* 27.

8. See Griesinger's opening lecture in 1865 in which he stressed psychiatry's proximity to medicine and the natural sciences. Wilhelm Griesinger, "Vortrag zur Eröffnung der Klinik für Nerven- und Geisteskrankheiten in der König[lichen] Charité in Berlin," in *Gesammelte Abhandlungen,* ed. C. A. Wunderlich (Berlin: Hirschwald, 1872 [1865]), 1:107–51. See also the review in *BKW* 2 (1865): 216.

9. To this list might also be added a number of other names, such as Friedrich Jolly, Karl Fürstner, Hermann Emminghaus, and Rudolf Arndt.

10. Bodamer, 520.

11. The term "scientific medicine" is drawn from the literature of the period, in particular, from Johannes Müller's journal, *Archiv für Anatomie, Physiologie und wissenschaftliche Medicin,* first published in 1834. See also Rudolf Virchow's programmatic article, "Über die Standpunkte in der wissenschaftlichen Medicin," *Archiv für Pathologische Anatomie und Physiologie und für klinische Medizin* 1 (1847): 3ff.

12. On nineteenth century experimental physiology, see William Coleman and Frederic L. Holmes, *The Investigative Enterprise* (Berkeley: University of California Press, 1988) and Eulner, *Die Entwicklung,* 46–65.

13. Heinz Schröer, *Carl Ludwig,* vol. 33 of *Grosse Naturforscher,* ed. Heinz Degen (Stuttgart: Wissenschaftliche Verlagsgesellschaft, 1967), 282.

14. Emil du Bois-Reymond, "Der physiologische Unterricht sonst und jetzt" [1877], in *Reden,* ed. Estelle Du Bois-Reymond, 2d ed. (Leipzig: Veit & Comp., 1912), 1:640.

15. On Johannes Müller, see Michael Hagner and Bettina Wahrig-Schmidt, *Johannes Müller und die Philosophie* (Berlin: Akademie, 1992), Brigitte Lohff, "Johannes Müller (1801–1858) als

akademischer Lehrer" (Med. Diss., University of Hamburg, 1977) as well as Verwey, 52–60 and Manfred Stürzbecher, "Zur Berufung Johannes Müllers an die Berliner Universität," *Jahrbuch für die Geschichte Mittel- und Ostdeutschlands* 21 (1972): 184– 226.

16. Cited in Ewald Harndt, "Die Stellung der medizinischen Fakultät," *Jahrbuch für die Geschichte Mittel- und Ostdeutschlands* 20 (1971): 134–160.

17. Eulner, *Die Entwicklung*, 95–112. More extensively on Virchow, see Constantin Goschler, *Rudolf Virchow: Mediziner, Anthropologe, Politiker* (Cologne: Böhlau, 2002).

18. For the motives of the Prussian minister of education von Altenstein, see Theodor Billroth, *The Medical Sciences in the German Universities* (New York: Macmillan, 1924), 114–5. After German unification the respective states were granted the authority to license physicians. See Eulenberg, *Das Medicinalwesen,* 322–5, 310, 330.

19. See Hans-Günter Wenig, "Medizinische Ausbildung im 19. Jahrhundert" (Med. diss., University of Bonn, 1969), 94–6.

20. See Eulenberg, *Das Medizinalwesen,* 302–8.

21. Eulner, *Die Entwicklung,* 43, 49, 65. For an in-depth case study of these developments at the university of Heidelberg see Arleen M. Tuchman, "From the Lecture to the Laboratory," in *The Investigative Enterprise,* ed. William Coleman and Frederic L. Holmes (Berkeley: University of California Press, 1988), 65–99.

22. Scherg-Zeisner, 104–5.

23. Drees, 108.

24. Abraham Flexner, *Medical Education in Europe* (Boston: Merrymount Press, 1912), 59; similarly Billroth, 74.

25. Ernst von Leyden, "Die innere Klinik und die innere Medicin in den letzten 25 Jahren," *DMW* 26 (1900): 2. It has more generally been argued that scientific medicine "made its first appearance in the world of medical practice on the diagnostic front, not in the realm of etiology or therapeutics." Coleman and Holmes, 11.

26. Oscar Hertwig, *Der anatomische Unterricht* (Jena: Fischer, 1881), 14. See also Billroth, 44–6.

27. According to Billroth, 59: "Modern physiology has grown almost entirely out of the more delicate, microscopic study of anatomy."

28. Richard L. Kremer, "Building institutes of physiology in Prussia, 1836–1846," in *The Laboratory Revolution in Medicine,* ed. Andrew Cunningham and Perry Williams (Cambridge: Cambridge University Press, 1992), 108.

29. Johann Purkyně, "Mikroskop," in *Handwörterbuch der Physiologie,* ed. Rudolf Wagner (Braunschweig: Vieweg, 1844), 413.

30. Hermann Reinhard, *Das Mikroskop und sein Gebrauch für den Arzt,* 2d ed. (Leipzig: Winter, 1864), 42–3.

31. Johann Christian Jüngken, "Promemoria," *BKW* 9 (1872): 35.

32. For a cursory survey of different techniques of cutting and staining, see Gudden, "Bernhard von Gudden," 232–4. On Gudden's microtome, see August Forel, *Rückblick auf mein Leben* (Zurich: Europa Verlag, 1935), 73–4.

33. Bruno Latour, *Science in Action* (Cambridge: Harvard University Press, 1987), 68.

34. In Breslau, Purkyně and his associates were constructing apparatus for microscopic photography in the early 1840s. See William Coleman, "Prussian Pedagogy: Purkyně at Breslau, 1823–1839," in *The Investigative Enterprise,* ed. William Coleman and Frederic L. Holmes (Berkeley: University of California Press, 1988), 24 and Joseph Gerlach, *Die Photographie als Hülfsmittel mikroskopischer Forschung* (Leipzig: Engelmann, 1863).

35. Reinhard, 75.

36. Hagen, 17.

37. See Forel, 64.

38. Purkyně, 411.

39. More generally, on the application of Foucault's ideas on power and discipline to laboratory situations, see Joseph Rouse, *Knowledge and Power* (Ithaca: Cornell University Press, 1987), 220–6.

40. Philipp Franz von Walther, *Über klinische Lehranstalten in städtischen Krankenhäusern* (Freiburg i.Br.: Herder, 1846), 20.

41. Johannes Orth, "Die Entwicklung des Unterrichts in der pathologischen Anatomie und allgemeinen Pathologie an der Berliner Universität," *BKW* 47 (1910): 1870.

42. Thus Adolf Bardeleben in the "Verhandlungen des XIX. deutschen Aerztetages zu Weimar am 22. und 23. Juni 1891," *Aerztliches Vereinsblatt* 18 (1891): 345.

43. Huerkamp, *Der Aufstieg der Ärzte*, 90; Billroth, 79. Compare also the situation in Heidelberg described by Otto Weber, *Das akademische Krankenhaus in Heidelberg* (Heidelberg: Mohr, 1865), 10–11.

44. Berlin is an especially instructive case in this regard. See Cay-Rüdiger Prüll, "Zwischen Krankenversorgung und Forschungsprimat," in *Zwischen Wissens- und Verwaltungsökonomie* ed. Eric J. Engstrom and Volker Hess, *Zeitschrift für Universitätsgeschichte* 3 (2000): 87–109. Flexner, 95–7. At times, anatomic institutes drew on the corpses of local hospitals. See Orth, "Die Entwicklung," 1870.

45. Billroth, 58–9.

46. Cited in Orth, "Die Entwicklung," 1869.

47. J. Grober, "Wissenschaftliche und Unterrichtsräume in Krankenanstalten," in *Ergebnisse und Fortschritte des Krankenhauswesens*, ed. E. Dietrich and J. Grober, vol. 3 (Jena: Fischer, 1920), 37; Weber, *Das akademische Krankenhaus*, 16; Walther, *Über klinische Lehranstalten*, 60.

48. Hertwig, 7.

49. Timothy Lenoir, "Science for the Clinic," in *The Investigative Enterprise*, ed. Colemann and Holmes (Berkeley: University of California Press, 1988), 143.

50. Tuchman, "From the Lecture to the Laboratory," 72–5 and 89–95; Timothy Lenoir, "Laboratories, Medicine and Public Life in Germany, 1830–1849," in *The Laboratory Revolution in Medicine*, ed. Andrew Cunningham and Perry Williams (Cambridge: Cambridge University Press, 1992), 48–50; Wilhelm Waldeyer, "Der Unterricht in den anatomischen Wissenschaften an der Universität Berlin im ersten Jahrhundert ihres Bestehens," *BKW* 47 (1910): 1864; Orth, "Die Entwicklung," 1869; Theodor Puschmann, *Geschichte des medizinischen Unterrichts* (Leipzig: Veit, 1889), 466–7; Eulenberg, *Das Medicinalwesen*, 311–2.

51. Michael Kutzer, "Der pathologisch-anatomische Befund und seine Auswertung in der deutschen Psychiatrie der ersten Hälfte des 19. Jahrhunderts," *Medizinhistorisches Journal* 26 (1991): 214–35.

52. Ibid., 231.

53. Damerow, *Über die relative Verbinding*, 186–91.

54. Ibid., 188.

55. Griesinger, *Pathologie und Therapie*, 3d ed., 416.

56. Ibid., 418.

57. Otto Binswanger, "Die Lehraufgaben der psychiatrischen Klinik," *Klinisches Jahrbuch* 4 (1892): 53.

58. Ludwig Wille, "Vortrag zur Eröffnung der psychiatrischen Klinik in Basel im Sommersemester 1877," *AZP* 34 (1878): 396.

59. Adolf Albrecht Erlenmeyer, "Bericht über die 51. Versammlung deutscher Naturforscher und Aerzte zu Cassel," *ZblNP* 1 (1878): 258.

60. Ewald Hecker, "Zur Begründung des klinischen Standpunktes in der Psychiatrie," *Archiv für pathologische Anatomie und Physiologie und für klinische Medizin* 52 (1871): 209.

61. At Erlenmeyer's urging in 1878 the psychiatric section appended "*Nervenkrankheiten*" to its name and after 1886 psychiatry was subordinated to neurology in its new name "*Section für Neurologie und Psychiatrie*".

62. Schmiedebach, *Psychiatrie und Psychologie*, 16–7.

63. "7. Versammlung des südwestdeutschen psychiatrischen Vereins am 2. und 3. Mai 1874 zu Heppenheim," *AZP* 31 (1875): 465.

64. The result was two psychiatric societies in Baden after 1878: Roller's psychiatrically oriented *Versammlung Südwestdeutsche Irrenärzte* (founded in 1867 and holding various names)

and its neurological offspring, the *Wanderversammlung der Südwestdeutschen Neurologen und Irrenärzte,* which from May of 1876 met annually in Baden-Baden.

65. This research comprised what one observer has called the "cerebral paradigm in psychiatry." See Klaus Wiese, "Vom hirnpsychiatrischen Paradigma zu einer humanwissenschaftlichen Psychiatrie," *Wissenschaftliche Zeitschrift der Karl-Marx-Universität Leipzig, Mathematisch-Naturwissenschaftliche Reihe* 31 (1982): 139.

66. Eduard Hitzig, *Untersuchungen über das Gehirn. Abhandlungen physiologischen und pathologischen Inhaltes* (Berlin: Hirschwald, 1874).

67. Carl Wernicke, *Der aphasische Symptomencomplex* (Breslau: Cohn & Weigert, 1874).

68. Theodor Meynert, *Zur Mechanik des Gehirnbaues* (Vienna: Braumüller, 1874); Bernhard von Gudden, *Gesammelte und hinterlassene Abhandlungen,* ed. Hubert Grashey (Wiesbaden: Bergman, 1889); and Paul Flechsig, *Die Leitungsbahnen im Gehirn und Rückenmark des Menschen* (Leipzig: Engelmann, 1876).

69. Emil Kraepelin, *Die Richtungen der psychiatrischen Forschung* (Leipzig: Vogel, 1887), 11.

70. For examples see Engstrom, "The Birth," 238.

71. Cited in Kraepelin, *Die Richtungen,* 8.

72. Westphal, *Psychiatrie und psychiatrischer Unterricht,* 27.

73. Ibid., 6–7.

74. Otto Binswanger, "Zum Andenken an Carl Westphal," *DMW* 16 (1890): 207.

75. Bernhard Naunyn, *Erinnerungen, Gedanken und Meinungen* (Munich: Bergmann, 1925), 84.

76. Ziehen, "Die Entwicklung," 1883.

77. Wernicke, "Zweck und Ziel," 221.

78. Paul Samt, *Die naturwissenschaftliche Methode in der Psychiatrie* (Berlin: August Hirschwald, 1874). On the putative "paradigmatic" status of Samt's work, see Schmiedebach, *Psychiatrie und Psychologie,* 108–11; and his "Zum Verständniswandel der 'psychopathischen' Störungen am Anfang der naturwissenschaftlichen Psychiatrie in Deutschland," *Nervenarzt* 56 (1985): 140–45.

79. Du Bois-Reymond, "Über die Grenzen des Naturerkennens," in *Reden,* 441–64.

80. Samt, *Die naturwissenschaftliche Methode,* 29.

81. Ibid., 59. Samt also constructed a hierarchy of proof that subordinated developmental and comparative anatomy below pathological anatomy or experimental physiology.

82. In 1878, however, he was dismissed from his position because of sexual misconduct and forced into private practice in Berlin, where he remained until moving to Breslau in 1885. On Wernicke's dismissal, see Engstrom, "The Birth," 242, note 135.

83. Pauleikhoff, 281. For an account of Wernicke's work see Mario Lanczik, *Der Breslauer Psychiater Carl Wernicke,* Schlesische Forschungen, vol. 2 (Sigmaringen: Thorbecke, 1988).

84. Carl Wernicke, "Über den wissenschaftlichen Standpunkt in der Psychiatrie," *Tageblatt der 53. Versammlung deutscher Naturforscher und Aerzte in Danzig 1880* 53 (1880): 132.

85. Wernicke's (and Hitzig's) enthusiasm for cerebral physiology was not shared by all. Bernhard von Gudden was far more reserved when it came to assessing physiology's achievements. Gudden, *Gesammelte und hinterlassene Abhandlungen,* 210. Compare also Theodor Meynert, "Naturexperimente am Gehirn," *Jahrbücher für Psychiatrie* 10 (1892): 171.

86. For examples, see Engstrom, "The Birth," 245–46.

87. One of the founding fathers of German psychiatry, Johann Langermann, had conducted very extensive experiments on animals and indeed headed the school of veterinary medicine in Berlin. Carl Wilhelm Ideler, "Necrolog," *Medicinische Zeitung* 1 (1832): 67.

88. See Forel, *Rückblick* and Julius Wagner von Jauregg, *Lebenserinnerungen* (Wien: Springer, 1950), 5, 11, 25–7.

89. On the method see Gudden, "Bernhard von Gudden," 234–42. Gudden's experimental methods were also practiced by his successor Anton Bumm. Thomas Schwarz, "Anton Bumm (1849–1903)" (Med. diss., University of Munich, 1982), 54.

90. Gudden, *Gesammelte und hinterlassene Abhandlungen,* iv.

91. Gudden, "Bernhard von Gudden," 123.

92. Kraepelin, *Lebenserinnerungen,* 16. On Gudden's work see also Laehr's eulogy in *AZP* 43 (1886): 177–87.

93. Carl Westphal, "Über künstliche Erzeugung von Epilepsie bei Meerschweinchen," *BKW* 8 (1871): 460–3. Cf. also Heinrich Obersteiner, "Zur Kenntnis einiger Hereditätsgesetze," *Wiener Medizinische Jahrbücher* (1875): 179–88; Eduard Hitzig, "Über Produktion von Epilepsie durch experimentelle Verletzung der Hirnrinde," in *Physiologische und klinische Untersuchungen über das Gehirn,* (Berlin: Hirschwald, 1904 [1874]), 63–72. For a summary of the state of the research on epilepsy, see Carl Wernicke, *Lehrbuch der Gehirnkrankheiten für Ärzte und Studierende* (Kassel: Theodor Fischer, 1881), 1:237–49 and Carl Spamer, "Beobachtungen über Erblichkeit, besonders bei Psychosen und Neurosen," *BKW* 18 (1881): 203.

94. Emanuel Mendel, "Über paralytischen Blödsinn bei Hunden," *Sitzungsberichte der preussischen Akademie der Wissenschaften, math.-nat.wiss. Klasse* 20 (1884): 393–5. See also his "Syphilis und Dementia paralytica," *BKW* 22 (1885): 549 and *AfPN* 15 (1884): 867–9.

95. Gudden, "Über die Frage der Localisation," in *Gesammelte und hinterlassene Abhandlungen,* 205–6.

96. Sigmund Kornfeld, "Geschichte der Psychiatrie," in *Handbuch der Geschichte der Medizin,* ed. Max Neuburger and Julius Pagel (Jena: Fischer, 1905), 3:719.

97. Emil Kraepelin, "Über die Einwirkung einiger medicamentöser Stoffe auf die Dauer einfacher psychischer Vorgänge," *Philosophische Studien* 1 (1883): 417–62, 573–605 and Emil Kraepelin to Ina Schwabe, 3 April 1882, MPI-K5, and 3 January 1883, MPI-K6.

98. Konrad Rieger, "Konrad Rieger," in *Die Medizin der Gegenwart in Selbstdarstellungen,* vol. 8, ed. L. R. Grote (Leipzig: Felix Meiner, 1929), 125–74.

99. *BKW* 19 (1882): 623. His Royal Highness signed his name in the role and heard reports on "modern psychiatric care."

100. Before diagnosing a patient incurable, Ideler observed them "much longer than is presently the case, often as long as an entire year." Charité Directorate to MgUMA, 24 April 1874, UAHUB, Charité Direktion 1034, Bl. 215.

101. Brosius, " 'Der Umschwung in der Psychiatrie,' " 26.

102. Hagen, 6.

103. Konrad Alt, "Videant consules!" *PNW* 7 (1905/6): 389–91, 397–400, 410–414. Cf. also Karl Jaspers, "Der Arzt im technischen Zeitalter," in *Wahrheit und Bewahrung* (Munich: Piper, 1983), 79.

104. Adolf Dannemann, *Bau, Einrichtung und Organization psychiatrischer Stadtasyle* (Halle: Carl Marhold, 1901), 19, 27.

105. See Hitzig, "Rede," 120–1 and the dispute pitting Max Fischer against Emil Sioli at the annual meeting of the *Verein* in 1900 at *ZblNP* 23, n.s. 11 (1900): 297ff.

106. See Albert Van Helden and Thomas L. Hankins, *Instruments,* Osiris, vol. 9 (Chicago: University of Chicago Press, 1994), 1–6; they claim that microscopes constructed bridges between natural science and popular culture.

107. Laehr, "Rundschau in Preussen," 324.

108. Wilhelm Griesinger, "Psychiatrische Congresse und Versammlungen," *AfPN* 1 (1868): 197.

109. Kahlbaum, *Die Gruppierungen,* 59–60.

110. Hagen, 59.

111. Solbrig, *Verbrechen und Wahnsinn,* 17–20. Roller, *Psychiatrische Zeitfragen,* 56.

112. Martin Schrenk, *Über den Umgang mit Geisteskranken* (Berlin: Springer, 1973), 143. See for example Heinrich Schüle, *Sektionsergebnisse bei Geisteskranken* (Leipzig: Duncker u. Humblot, 1874).

113. For Karl Jaspers, although Krafft-Ebing worked in academic environs, he remained very much an alienist. Karl Jaspers, "Historisches über Psychopathologie als Wissenschaft," in *Allgemeine Psychopathologie* (Berlin: Springer, 1948), 709.

114. Heinrich Kreuser, "Ernst v. Zeller," *MCblWAL* 72 (1902): 778. More likely than not, however, Zeller's microscope was used to pursue his great interest in parasitic worms rather than brain specimens.

115. GStA PK, IHA, Rep. 76Va, MgUMA, Sect. 6, Tit. X, Nr. 18, Bd. 1, August Cramer to MgUMA, 7 May 1907. The laboratories were considered "exemplary" by Johannes Bresler, *Ausgewählte Kapitel der Verwaltung öffentlicher Irrenanstalten* (Halle: Carl Marhold, 1910), 122–6. More generally on the asylum in Uchtspringe, see Heinz Trollenburg, "Die Entwicklung des Bezirkskrankenhauses für Neurologie und Psychiatrie Uchtspringe" (Med. diss., University of Leipzig, 1970).

116. Robert Wollenberg, *Erinnerungen eines alten Psychiaters* (Stuttgart: Enke, 1931), 56.

117. L. M. Kötscher, *Unsere Irrenhäuser* (Berlin: Langenscheidt, 1912), 64–7.

118. C. K. Clarke, "Notes on Some of the Psychiatric Clinics and Asylums of Germany," *The American Journal of Insanity* 65 (1908–9): 364.

119. See the debate unfolding on the heels of the article by Johannes Bresler, "Der wissenschaflichen Betrieb der öffentlichen Irrenanstalten," *PNW* 11 (1909–10): 223–6, 263–6, 370–2, 385–6, 434–5, 457–8, especially the controversy between Dobrick and Weber in *PNW* 12 (1910/11): 383, 393, 437, 465.

120. This remedy had been debated at the annual meeting of the *Verein* in Giessen in 1907. See *DMW* 33 (1907): 1120. At the initiative of the university clinic in Munich, the exchange of assistants between the clinic and the new asylum in Eglfing had been discussed and implemented in 1906. See SMIKSA to Verwaltungsausschuß der Ludwig-Maximilians-Universität, 24 May 1906, Nr. 8439, BHStA, MK 11245.

121. Bresler, "Der wissenschaftlichen Betrieb," 224.

122. See Obersteiner, "Grundzüge," 2 and Flechsig, *Die Irrenklinik,* 59. On internal medicine and its efforts to stem the tide of specialization, see Friedrich Theodor Frerichs, "Einleitung," *Zeitschrift für klinische Medicin* 1 (1880): i–viii and Johanna Bleker, "Medical Students—to the Bed-side or to the Laboratory?" *Clio Medica* 21 (1987/8): 43.

123. For a history of the literature on progressive paralysis, see Otto Mönckemöller, "Zur Geschichte der progressiven Paralyse," *ZgNP* 5 (1911): 500–90. On the theoretical debates, see Jörg Grefe, "Die Vorstellungen zur Ätiologie der Progressiven Paralyse in der Allgemeinen Zeitschrift für Psychiatrie 1884–1913" (Diss. med., University of Heidelberg, 1991) as well as Pauleikhoff, 2:299–306. On the importance of progressive paralysis in the United States, see Elizabeth Lunbeck, *The Psychiatric Persuasion* (Princeton: Princeton University Press, 1994), 49ff.

124. Carl Ludwig Ideler, "Mitteilungen über die Bewegung an der städtischen Irrenanstalt von Berlin für das Jahr 1875," *AZP* 34 (1878): 244. The same held true in Dalldorf after 1880 according to Heinz Schulze and Christian Donalies, "100 Jahre Psychiatrie und Neurologie," *Wissenschaftliche Zeitschrift der Humboldt Universität zu Berlin, Math.-Nat. Series* 17 (1968): 7; see also *BKW* 17 (1880): 463.

125. Emanuel Mendel, "Über Hirnbefunde bei der progressiven Paralyse der Irren," *BKW* 20 (1883): 249 and his *Die Progressive Paralyse der Irren: Eine Monographie* (Berlin: Hirschwald, 1880), iii. Bodamer has described progressive paralysis as the "cradle of neurology" and the "*Leitmotiv*" of the clinical psychiatry of Kahlbaum and Kraepelin. Bodamer, 533.

126. Wernicke, "Zweck und Ziel," 221. Clinicians were especially eager to see patients who were suffering from progressive paralysis admitted to their institutions. Carl Fürstner valued the fact that "post mortem [they] supplied a wealth of important material for clinical instruction." Fürstner, *Über Irrenkliniken,* 6.

127. Wernicke, "Zweck und Ziel," 222. Wernicke's ideal was the neurological ward in the Charité. Ibid., 221.

128. Kornfeld, 711 and 722.

129. Carl Westphal, "Ueber Erkrankungen des Rückenmarks bei der allgemeinen progressiven Paralyse der Irren," *Archiv für pathologische Anatomie und Physiologie und für klinische Medicin* 39 (1967): 90–115, 353–423, 592–606; 40 (1867): 226–82.

130. Binswanger, "Die Lehraufgaben," 47. See also his "Zum Andenken," 207.

131. See the remarks of Ewald Hecker, "Die Hebephrenie," *Archiv für pathologische Anatomie und Physiologie und für klinische Medizin* 52 (1871): 395.

132. Griesinger, *Pathologie und Therapie,* 3d ed., 408–9.

133. See the remark of Wilhelm Sander at the meeting of the Berlin Society for Psychiatry and Nervous Diseases, 12 January 1880, *BKW* 17 (1880): 464.

134. In all of Prussia, patients suffering from progressive paralysis were five times as likely to be male as female, according to Albert Guttstadt at a meeting of the Berlin Psychiatric Society, *AZP* 34 (1878): 244. Pauleikhoff, 2:306, cites Kahlbaum's claim that the disease was found exclusively in men.

135. Westphal, *Psychiatrie und psychiatrischer Unterricht*, 33–5. Westphal also emphasized psychiatry's usefulness in judging military fitness and exposing "simulators." Ibid., 31–3. See also Arndt, 17–22.

136. Westphal, *Psychiatrie und psychiatrischer Unterricht*, 34.

137. Arndt, 55.

138. GStA PK, IHA, Rep. 76Va, MgUMA, Sekt. 2, Tit. X, Nr. 43, Bd. I, Bl. 256–67.

139. See the meeting of the *Versammlung des psychiatrischen Vereins zu Berlin, AZP* 28 (1872): 342.

140. In response to the Franco-Prussian war, many psychiatrists had called for better training of military physicians. For some of their arguments, see the remarks of the director of the asylum Marsberg in Westphalia, Friedrich Koster, "Militaria," *If* 13 (1871): 5–12, 24–29, 43–48. 47–8. See also Koster's petition to the ministry of war in *AZP* 29 (1873): 466–7. On military psychiatry in general, see Martin Lengwiler, *Zwischen Klinik und Kaserne* (Zurich: Chronos, 2000).

141. For details on these issues, see Engstrom, "The Birth," 266, note 220.

142. "Versammlung des psychiatrischen Vereins zu Berlin," *AZP* 28 (1872): 340.

143. Ibid., 338.

144. On Hitzig, see Caoimhghin S. Breathnach, "Eduard Hitzig, neurophysiologist and psychiatrist," *HP* 3 (1992): 329–338; Erwin H. Ackerknecht, "Gudden, Huguenin, Hitzig: Hirnpsychiatrie im Burghölzli 1869–1879," *Gesnerus* 35 (1978): 66–78; Robert M. Young, "Fritsch and Hitzig and the Localized Electrical Excitability of the Cerebral Hemispheres," in *Mind, Brain and Adaptation in the Nineteenth Century* (Oxford: Clarendon Press, 1970), 224–33; Hans-Heinz Eulner, "Eduard Hitzig (1838–1907)," *Wissenschaftliche Zeitschrift der Martin-Luther-Universität Halle Wittenberg,* Mathematisch-Naturwissenschaftliche Reihe, 6, no. 5 (1957): 709–12; Manfred Bleuler, "Geschichte des Burghölzlis und der psychiatrischen Universitätsklinik," in *Züricher Spitalgeschichte,* by Canton Zürich, vol. 2 (Zurich: Berichthaus Zürich, 1951), 410–13; Gabriel Anton, "Nachruf auf E[duard] Hitzig anlässlich der Aufstellung des Hitzig-Denkmales in der Hallenser Klinik für Geistes- und Nervenkranke," *AfPN* 54,1 (1914): 1–7; Robert Wollenberg, "Eduard Hitzig," *AfPN* 43 (1907): iii–xiv; Fritz Kalberlah, "Eduard Hitzig," *ZblNP* 30 (1907): 765–8; Hagner, *Homo cerebralis,* 273–9.

145. On Hitzig's relationship with Althoff, see their extensive correspondence in GStA PK, IHA, Rep. 92 Althoff B, Nr. 73, Bd. 2 and Kretschmann, 148–82.

146. Siemerling as cited by Kretschmann, 150; Naunyn, 149; Wollenberg, *Erinnerungen,* 85.

147. Kretschmann, 161; Kalberlah, 767.

148. Bleuler, 410–3; Forel, 88–9, 99–100; Wollenberg, *Erinnerungen,* 83.

149. Hitzig to MgUMA, 30 March 1888, GStA PK, IHA, Rep. 76Va, MgUMA, Sect. 8, Tit. X, Nr. 17, Bd. II, Bl. 224. Hitzig's troubled relations with the doctors in his clinic continued until his retirement. See Curator of the University of Halle to MgUMA, 13 May 1904, GStA PK, IHA, Rep. 76Va, MgUMA, Sect. 8, Tit. XV, Nr. 26, Bd. I.

150. Kretschmann, 149.

151. Eulner, *Die Entwicklung,* 28; Kalberlah, 768.

152. On the significance of Hitzig's work in the history of neurology, see Young.

153. On Flourens, see Edwin Clarke and L. Steven Jacyna, *Nineteenth-Century Origins of Neuroscientific Concepts* (Berkeley: University of California Press, 1987), 267–85; Malcolm Macmillan, "Experimental and Clinical Studies of Localisation before Flourens," *Journal of the History of the Neurosciences* 4 (1995): 139–54.

154. Eduard Hitzig [and Gustav Fritsch], "Über die elektrische Erregbarkeit des Grosshirns" [1870], in *Physiologische und klinische Untersuchungen über das Gehirn* (Berlin: Hirschwald,

1904), 34; see likewise Eduard Hitzig, "Über den heutigen Stand der Frage von der Localisation im Grosshirn," *Sammlung Klinischer Vorträge* 112 (1876): 966.

155. Hitzig and Fritsch, 26.

156. By the mid-1880s Hitzig was already diagnosing brain tumors and having them operated on. Ackerknecht, "Gudden, Huguenin, Hitzig," 73; Wollenberg, *Erinnerungen,* 84; Wilhelm Tönnis, "Die Entwicklung der Neurochirurgie an der Freidrich-Wilhelms-Universität zu Berlin von der Reichsgründung bis 1945," in *Studium Berolinense,* ed. Hans Leussink, Eduard Neumann, and Georg Kotowski (Berlin: Walter de Gruyter, 1960), 281–4.

157. See Samt, 38.

158. Hitzig and Fritsch, 27–9.

159. Ibid., 14.

160. Eduard Hitzig, "Weitere Untersuchungen zur Physiologie des Gehirn," *BKW* 9 (1872): 504. Hagner has noted the significance of the confluence of experimental research and clinical observations for localization theory. See Hagner, *Homo cerebralis,* 272, 276.

161. See Wollenberg, *Erinnerungen,* 84 and Hitzig and Fritsch, 27.

162. Hitzig, "Über die beim Galvanisiren des Kopfes entstehenden Störungen der Muskelinnervation und der Vorstellungen vom Verhalten im Raume," *Archiv für Anatomie, Physiologie und wissenschaftliche Medizin* 5 (1871): 716–770; 6 (1872): 771ff. The article was reprinted in Hitzig, *Physiologische und klinische Untersuchungen,* pt. 1 (Berlin: Hirschwald, 1904), 339–385.

163. Eduard Hitzig, "Über den relativen Werth elektrischer Heilmethoden," *Tageblatt der 45. Versammlung deutscher Naturforscher und Ärzte in Leipzig* 45 (1872): 161–4.

164. Eduard Hitzig to MgUMA, 12 August 1872, UAHUB, Charité Direktion 850, Bl. 43.

165. Ibid.

166. MgUMA to Charité Directorate, 10 September 1872, UAHUB, Charité Direktion 850, Bl. 47. In the 1870s many young academics proposed similar electrotherapeutic wards. See Billroth, 80.

167. Westphal intervened both at the ministerial and faculty level. See his letters to MgUMA and the dean of the medical faculty (Virchow), 6 and 14 January 1873, UAHUB, Medizinische Fakultät 238, Bl. 64–7.

168. MgUMA to Eduard Hitzig, 24 January 1873, GStA PK, IHA, Rep. 76Va, MgUMA, Sect. 2, Tit. X, Nr. 43, Bd. I, Bl. 45.

169. On the dispute, see Hagner, *Homo cerebralis,* 281–3.

170. Naunyn, 150.

171. Hitzig could, in effect, admit whomever he chose and this practice set the standard for future psychiatric clinics in Prussia and elsewhere. Cramer, "Die preußischen Universitätskliniken," 191, 197; Hitzig, *Bericht über die Wirksamkeit,* 16.

172. On the disputes and Hitzig's petitions for a new psychiatric clinic, see GStA PK, IHA, Rep. 76Va, MgUMA, Sect. 8, Tit. X, Nr. 17, Bd. I, especially Bl. 103–44, 161–70, and 173–4 as well as his "Vorläufiges Program für den Neubau einer Irren- und Nervenklinik zu Halle" of 3 August 1885, in Bd. II, Bl. 61–8. See also University Curator to Medical Faculty, 24 September 1883, UAHa, Med. Fak. I, Rep. 29, Nr. 196, Bl. 13.

173. On the ministerial debates on financing the clinic, see GStA PK, IHA, Rep. 76Va, MgUMA, Sect. 8, Tit. XIX, Nr. 26, Bd. I. For the parliamentary debates on building the clinic, see *Stenographische Verhandlungen des Haus der Abgeordneten,* 14 March 1889, 34th Session, 1037–42.

174. While the psychiatric and neurological wards of the Charité had been joined, neither Griesinger nor Westphal had effective control over admissions. The clinic in Leipzig, however, was administratively autonomous and combined psychiatric and neurological wards. The Leipzig clinic had opened in 1882 and was headed by Paul Flechsig who, like Hitzig, was a neuropathologist. For an overview of the status of psychiatric clinics in German speaking lands in 1890, see Eduard Hitzig to Friedrich Althoff, 1 January 1890, GStA PK, IHA, Rep. 76Va, MgUMA, Sect. 2, Tit. X, Nr. 43, Bd. I, Bl. 224–8.

175. Hitzig, "Rede," 113. Accordingly, Hitzig justified the clinic's construction on the

grounds that it was inappropriate to separate diseases of the central nervous system from those of the brain. Ibid., 126.

176. Ibid., 126–7.

177. See also Engstrom, "Disciplin."

178. Medical Faculty to MgUMA, 18 November 1889, GStA PK, IHA, Rep. 76Va, MgUMA, Sect. 2, Tit. X, Nr. 43, Bd. I, Bl. 230.

179. Ibid., Bl. 231.

180. Carl Westphal to MgUMA, 5 August 1871, UAHUB, Charité Direktion 850, Bl. 30–1.

181. Ibid.

182. Ibid., Bl. 33. Shortly before Westphal's death, the psychiatric polyclinic held office hours two days a week, on Monday and Wednesday mornings. See GStA PK, IHA, Rep. 76Va, MgUMA, Sect. 2, Tit. X, Nr. 43, Bd. I, Bl. 256.

183. Scheibe, 95.

184. Griesinger to Esse, 19 June 1865, UAHUB, Charité Direktion 1058, Bl. 10.

185. Berlin City Magistrate to Charité Directorate, 13 March 1879 and 30 July 1879, UAHUB, Charité Direktion 1034, Bl. 243 and 255–6, here Bl. 243. Westphal was essentially able to dictate the terms of the agreement with the city, demanding that Dalldorf admit transit patients from the Charité without delay. See UAHUB, Charité Direktion 1034, Bl. 247 and Charité Directorate to Berlin City Magistrate, 31 March 1879, UAHUB, Charité Direktion 1034, Bl. 249.

186. Between 1879 and 1880 admissions to the psychiatric ward more than doubled, jumping from 301 to 693. *CA* 6 (1881): 8; 7 (1882): 10. In 1879 the city estimated the prospective patient volume to be ca. 153 patients per month. City magistrate to Charité directorate, 13 March 1879, UAHUB, Charité Direktion 1034, Bl. 243. No sooner had Dalldorf opened than Westphal was complaining about rising admissions and appealing for more expeditious transfer. Westphal to MgUMA, 18 May 1880, GStA PK, IHA, Rep. 76Va, MgUMA, Sect. 2, Tit. X, Nr. 43, Bd. I, Bl. 151; Westphal to Dalldorf Directorate, 27 June 1881, UAHUB, Charité Direktion 1034, Bl. 289.

187. Westphal to Charité directorate, 19 May 1873, UAHUB, Charité Direktion 1034, Bl. 173.

188. See Engstrom, "Disziplin," 167–70.

189. Bardeleben to members of the Medical Faculty, 28 June 1874, UAHUB, Medizinische Fakultät 1380, Bl. 85; *CblDGPgP* 20 (1874): 122, 118.

190. On the revival of plans for a new clinic in the wake Westphal's call to Leipzig, see MgUMA to Medical Faculty, 18 July 1874; UAHUB, Medizinische Fakultät 238, Bl. 82; and Westphal to Adolf Bardeleben, 25 July 1874, Bl. 83.

191. Westphal to MgUMA, 22 July 1874, GStA PK, IHA, Rep. 76Va, MgUMA, Sect. 2, Tit. X, Nr. 43, Bd. I, Bl. 75–8. See also the earlier correspondence of MgUMA to Charité directorate, 7 May 1874, UAHUB, Charité Direktion 1034, Bl. 219. Westphal was also promoted to full professor according to MgUMA to Medical Faculty, 27 August 1874, UAHUB, Medizinische Fakultät 1380, Bl. 89.

192. On Frerichs's arguments, see his letter to the Charité Directorate, 18 June 1875, UAHUB, Charité Direktion 850, Bl. 119. Frerichs was supported by the hospital administration. See Charité Directorate to MgUMA, 19 April 1875, UAHUB, Charité Direktion 850, Bl. 109–12.

193. See UAHUB, Charité Direktion 1034, Bl. 224; Engstrom, "Disziplin," 175.

194. See the note in UAHUB, Charité Direktion 1034, Bl. 224 and MgUMA to MFin, 19 August 1874, GStA PK, IHA, Rep. 76Va, MgUMA, Sect. 2, Tit. X, Nr. 43, Bd. I, Bl. 79–80.

195. Between 1872 and 1875, the number of cadavers at the Charité had fallen by over a quarter from 2353 to 1736. Medical Faculty to MgUMA, 1 August 1877, UAHUB, Charité Direktion 850, Bl. 229–31. See also Charité Directorate to MgUMA, 22 June 1875, UAHUB, Charité Direktion 850, Bl. 121 and, more generally on the economy of cadavers at the Charité, Prüll, "Zwischen Krankenversorgung."

196. MgUMA to Medical Faculty, 29 November 1877, UAHUB, Charité Direktion 850, Bl. 266.

197. Medical Faculty to MgUMA, 26 February 1878, UAHUB, Charité Direktion 850, Bl. 271.

198. The medical faculty hoped "that mildly sick patients and convalescing acute patients be sent to Moabit in order to make room [in the Charité] for new, severely ill patients." Not surprisingly, the city showed little inclination to cooperate. See UAHUB, Charité Direktion 850, Bl. 289.

199. Konrad Rieger, "Die Psychiatrie in Würzburg seit dreihundert Jahren," *Verhandlungen der physikalisch-medizinischen Gesellschaft zu Würzburg*, vol. 29 (Würzburg: Stahel'sche Verlags-Anstalt, 1898), 98; Dannemann, *Die psychiatrische Klinik zu Giessen*, 97.

200. Flechsig, *Die Irrenklinik*, 55.

201. Gerd Busse, "Schreber und Flechsig," *Medizinhistorisches Journal* 24 (1989): 291–3.

202. Flechsig, *Die Irrenklinik*, 35.

203. Eduard Hitzig, "Vorläufiges Program für den Neubau einer Irren- und Nervenklinik in Halle," 3 August 1885, GStA PK, IHA, Rep. 76Va, MgUMA, Sect. 8, Tit. X, Nr. 17, Bd. II, Bl. 61–8.

204. A draft of the contract is in UAM, Sen 307/1.

205. Medical Faculty to MgUMA, 18 November 1889, GStA PK, IHA, Rep. 76Va, MgUMA, Sect. 2, Tit. X, Nr. 43, Bd. I, Bl. 232 where the official wrote in the margin: "The third med[ical] clinic?"

206. See Eduard Hitzig to Friedrich Althoff, 1 January 1890, GStA PK, IHA, Rep. 76Va, MgUMA, Sect. 2, Tit. X, Nr. 43, Bd. I, Bl. 224–8 and the report "Gutachten betreffend die Frage der Verbindung des akademischen Unterrichts in der Psychiatrie und Neuropathologie an den preußischen Universitäten," 29 December 1889, Bl. 233–53. See Engstrom, "Eduard Hitzigs."

207. MgUMA to Medical Faculty, 16 January 1890, GStA PK, IHA, Rep. 76Va, MgUMA, Sect. 2, Tit. X, Nr. 43, Bd. I, Bl. 254.

208. See Engstrom, "Disziplin."

Chapter 5

1. Nasse, "Über das Bedürfniß," 344.

2. Flemming, *Pathologie und Therapie*, 281–2. Compare also Erwin Risak, *Der klinische Blick* 2d ed. (Vienna: Springer, 1938), 1, 9, 10.

3. Solbrig, "Über psychiatrisch-klinischen Unterricht," 810.

4. Binswanger, "Die Lehraufgaben," 49.

5. See Verwey, xvi, 34–6, 139. Verwey's thesis of methodological continuity does, however, ignore differences in clinical practice.

6. Kieser, *Elemente der Psychiatrik*, 385–6.

7. Griesinger, *Gesammelte Abhandlungen*, 125.

8. Hoche, *Jahresringe*, 139.

9. Binswanger, "Die Lehraufgaben," 45–6.

10. Robert Gaupp, "Die Psychiatrie als Lehr- und Prüfungsgegenstand," *MMW* 50 (1903): 1738–9.

11. Leibbrand and Wettley, *Der Wahnsinn*, 547. Wernicke's eulogist described his work as "eminently impractical" and "grandiosely one-sided." Hugo Liepmann, *Über Wernickes Einfluss auf die klinische Psychiatrie* (Berlin: S. Karger, 1911), 3; also see his article, "Carl Wernicke," *ZblNP* 16 (1905): 571.

12. Rieger, "Konrad Rieger," 158.

13. Paul Julius Möbius, *Über die Behandlung von Nervenkrankheiten und die Errichtung von Nervenheilstätten* (Berlin: Karger, 1896), 20, 30. Möbius's critique was also aimed at the psychological experiments conducted by Kraepelin, Sommer, and others.

14. At issue in the controversy was the cellular structure of the ganglion. On the details of the controversy see Gerd Udo Jerns, "Die neurologisch-psychiatrischen Vorträge" (Med. diss., Free University Berlin, 1991), 46–53.

15. To mention but two of the more prominent publications, August Forel's book *Der Hypnotismus, seine Bedeutung und seine Handhabung* (Stuttgart: Enke, 1889) saw twelve editions through 1923 and Albert Moll's *Der Hypnotismus mit besonderer Berücksichtigung der gerichtlichen Medizin* (Berlin: Fischer, 1889) saw five editions through 1924.

16. On some of the issues of the debate after the turn of the century, see Schindler, 124–7.

17. Wilhelm Erb, "Rückblick und Ausblick auf die Entwicklung und die Zukunft der deutschen Nervenpathologie," *Deutsche Zeitschrift für Nervenheilkunde* 35 (1908): 11–12. Carl Fürstner claimed that Griesinger's ideal of uniting neurologists and psychiatrists had never really been achieved. See Karl Fürstner, "Neuropathologie und Psychiatrie," *AZP* 38 (1904): 895–907 and Friedrich Schultze, "Neuropathologie und innere Medizin," *MMW* 51 (1904): 1301–3.

18. Ludwig Mann, "Bericht über die am 16. und 17. September 1898 zu Bonn abgehaltene Jahressitzung des Vereins der deutschen Irrenärzte," *MschrPN* 4 (1898): 339–41.

19. Martin Reichardt, *Über die Untersuchung des gesunden und kranken Gehirns mittels der Waage,* Arbeiten aus der Königlichen psychiatrischen Klinik zu Würzburg (Jena: Fischer, 1906), 1:2.

20. Ernst Siemerling, *Zur Erinnerung an Friedrich Jolly* (Berlin: Hirschwald, 1904), 13; Schindler, 58–63; A. H. A. C. Bakel, " 'Über die Dauer einfacher psychischer Vorgänge,' " in *Objekte, Differenzen und Konjunkturen,* ed. Michael Hagner, Hans-Jörg Rheinberger and Bettina Wahrig-Schmidt (Berlin: Akademie Verlag, 1994), 83–105; Eric J. Engstrom, "Kulturelle Dimensionen von Psychiatrie und Sozialpsychologie," in *Idealismus und Positivismus,* ed. Gangolf Hübinger, Friedrich Wilhelm Graf, and Rüdiger vom Bruch (Stuttgart: Steiner, 1997), 164–189. For a rather generous interpretation of Wundt's influence on Kraepelin's system of disease classification, see Helmut Hildebrandt, "Der psychologische Versuch in der Psychiatrie," *Psychologie und Geschichte* 5 (1993): 5–30. On Robert Sommer's work and the laboratories in Giessen, see Bresler, *Ausgewählte Kapitel,* 127–31 and Dannemann, *Die psychiatrische Klinik zu Giessen,* 65–8.

21. Robert Sommer, "Die Ausführung des Griesinger'schen Programms," *ZblNP* 16 (1893): 599.

22. Not the least as a consequence of their efforts, by the end of the century it again became easier to advance an idealistic attack on the materialist and mechanist precepts underpinning pathological anatomy. In Würzburg, Wilhelm Weygandt defended an experimental-psychological position in psychiatry, while at the Charité in Berlin Theodor Ziehen established a special laboratory for experimental psychology in the Wundtian tradition. See Wilhelm Weygandt, "Zur Frage der materialistischen Psychiatrie," *ZblNP* 24 (1901): 409–15; also see B. Luther, I. Wirth and C. Donalies, "Zur Entwicklung der Neurologie/Psychiatrie in Berlin, insbesondere am Charité-Krankenhaus," *Charité-Annalen,* n.s., 2 (1982): 284.

23. On this second generation, see chapter 7 below. One manifestation of their growing influence was the heated polemical exchange between Otto Juliusburger and Wilhelm Weygandt. Wilhelm Weygandt, "Psychologie und Hirnanatomie," *DMW* 26 (1900): 657–61 and Otto Juliusburger, "Materialistische Psychiatrie," *MschrPN* 9 (1901): 21–30.

24. Nor did Kraepelin shy away from directly letting Friedrich Althoff know his opinions. On this and Kraepelin's views on the relationship between psychiatry and neurology in general see Kraepelin, *Lebenserinnerungen,* 77; Clarke, "Notes," 358–9; and Neumärker, *Karl Bonhoeffer* (Berlin: Springer, 1990), 54–5.

25. Kraepelin, *Die Richtungen,* 16. On Snell, see Michael Schmidt-Degenhard, "Ludwig Snell (1817–1892)," *Jahrbuch für Stadt und Stift Hildesheim* 60 (1989): 83–98. On Kraepelin's work in Dorpat see Wolfgang Burgmair, Eric J. Engstrom, and Matthias Weber, eds., *Kraepelin in Dorpat, 1886–1891* (Munich: Belleville, 2003).

26. Kraepelin, *Die Richtungen,* 18.

27. Robert Gaupp, *Wege und Ziele psychiatrischer Forschung* (Tübingen: H. Laupp, 1907), 7.

28. Flechsig, *Die Irrenklinik,* 58–61; Weygandt, "Psychologie und Hirnanatomie," 659. On animosity between Flechsig and Kraepelin, see Holger Steinberg, *Kraepelin in Leipzig* (Bonn: Ed. das Narrenschiff, 2001).

29. Jolly, "Vorwort," *AfPN* 22 (1891): vii. The emphasis is Jolly's.

30. Ibid. Jolly's emphasis.

31. Carl Wernicke, "Tagesfragen," *MschrPN* 1 (1897): 5. Wernicke's and Ziehen's critique was directed at Flechsig's highly publicized rectorial address *Gehirn und Seele* (Leipzig: Veit, 1894). There, in the phrenological tradition of Franz Joseph Gall, Flechsig outlined his views on

the morphology of the human brain and claimed to have located numerous anatomically well de-fined cognitive centers or *"Associationscentren."* For a summary of the state of "modern phrenol-ogy," see Weygandt, "Psychologie und Hirnanatomie," 657–61.

32. Wernicke, "Tagesfragen," 5.

33. Binswanger, "Lehraufgaben," 56ff.

34. Karl Fürstner, *Über Irrenkliniken*, 16.

35. Ramaer, "Übersicht der Theorien der Psychiatrie," *Tageblatt* (Cassel: Baier & Lewalter, 1878), 280.

36. Leibbrand and Wettley, *Der Wahnsinn*, 556.

37. See Bleuler, 399 and Emminghaus as cited in Janzarik, "Die klinische Psychopathologie," 55.

38. See the account of Friedrich Jolly in Siemerling, *Zur Erinnerung*, 18.

39. Franz Tuczek, *Die wissenschaftliche Stellung der Psychiatrie* (Marburg: N. G. Elwert, 1906), 8.

40. Wille, "Vortrag," 397.

41. On the efforts and publications of these alienist clinicians, see Bodamer, 532–3.

42. Ludwig Snell, "Über Monomanie als primäre Form der Seelenstörung," *AZP* 22 (1865): 368–81. For Bodamer, Snell represented nothing less than the "beginnings of clinical research in psychiatry." Bodamer, 530. On Snell see also Schmidt-Degenhardt, "Ludwig Snell" and Erich Gerstenberg, "Nekrolog," *AZP* 49 (1893): 320–9.

43. See Karl Kahlbaum, *Klinische Abhandlungen über psychische Krankheiten* (Berlin: Hirschwald, 1874) and Hecker, "Die Hebephrenie." For a succinct overview of Kahlbaum's noso-logical position in the 1870s, see Kahlbaum, "Die klinisch-diagnostischen Gesichtspunkte."

44. Hecker, "Zur Begründung," 205–6.

45. Ibid., 209. By way of sharp contrast, Johann Langermann had dismissed the need for ei-ther a classification of psychiatric disorders or medical reports which delved into the history of the patient's illness. See Leibbrand and Wettley, *Der Wahnsinn*, 499–501.

46. Of the 14 patients used in his clinical study of hebephrenia, Hecker had post-mortem data on only one of them, and he altogether refused to speculate on the significance of even that limited data. Hecker, "Die Hebephrenie," 421–2.

47. See Bodamer, 534 and Ewald Hecker, "Zur klinischen Diagnostik und Prognostik der psy-chischen Krankheiten," *AZP* 33 (1877): 602–620. Hecker also pointed to the unique course of progressive paralysis as further proof of his clinical methods. Hecker, "Die Hebephrenie," 395.

48. Ibid., 396.

49. The problem of adequate anamnestic information was especially acute in state institu-tions, largely because contact with relatives was so tenuous there. In private institutions it was far easier to reconstruct the family history and ensure "observation over the entire course of the dis-ease." See *BKW* 18 (1881): 58.

50. Janzarik, "Die klinische Psychopathologie," 54–5.

51. Verwey, 139, where he cites Ey approvingly.

52. For an illustration of how strongly diagnostic procedures could be influenced by the use of instruments, see Robert Sommer, "Die klinische Untersuchung der Geisteskrankheiten," in *Die deutsche Klinik am Eingange des zwanzigsten Jahrhunderts*, ed. Ernst v. Leyden and Felix Klem-perer (Berlin: Urban, 1906), 1–58.

53. On the history of these and other clinical instruments, see Stanley Joel Reiser, *Medicine and the Reign of Technology* (Cambridge: Cambridge University Press, 1977).

54. See the remarks of Schroeter *AZP* 25 (1868): 305 and the paper given to the Psychiatric Association of Berlin, *AZP* 25 (1868): 850–1.

55. Karl Westphal, "Einige Beobachtungen," *AfPN* 1 (1868/69): 337–86; Eduard Hitzig, "Über subnormale Temperaturen bei Paralytiker," *BKW* 21 (1884): 537–40. More generally, see Volker Hess, *Der wohltemperierte Mensch* (Frankfurt/M: Campus, 2000).

56. On these and other diagnostic instruments, see Robert Sommer, *Diagnostik der Geis-teskrankheiten für praktische Aerzte und Studierende* (Vienna: Urban-Schwarzenberg, 1894).

57. Paul Näcke, "Über den Wert der sog. Kurven-Psychiatrie," *AZP* 61 (1904): 280–95.

58. On these methods, see Bakel; Hildebrandt; and Engstrom, "Die kulturelle Dimensionen."

59. Kraepelin, *Die Richtungen,* 14.

60. On the strict discipline governing the conduct of assistants, see Clarke, "Notes," 361 and Käte Frankenthal, *Jüdin, Intellektuelle, Sozialistin* (Frankfurt/M: Campus, 1985), 36.

61. "Instruktion für den Oberwärter der psychiatrischen und Nervenklinik," 10 May 1899, UAHa, Rep. 6, Nr. 1091, Bl. 9.

62. Rinecker to Head Nursing Office of the Julius Hospital, 14 July 1877, AJW 3963.

63. On these and other responsibilities of the head male-nurse at the clinic in Halle, see the "Instruktion für den Oberwärter der psychiatrischen und Nervenklinik," 10 May 1899, UAHa, Rep. 6, Nr. 1091.

64. Griesinger, "Über Irrenanstalten," 16–18 and 22. For details on the *Wachabteilung* in Berlin see Engstrom, "Disziplin" and "The Birth," 312, note 73.

65. Viszánik, 332.

66. See Bernhard von Gudden, "Über die Einrichtung von sogenannten Überwachungsstationen," *AZP* 42 (1886): 454–8; Jean Paul Friedrich Scholz, "Über Wachabteilungen in Irrenanstalten," *AZP* 45 (1889): 235–48; Albrecht Paetz, "Über die Einrichtung von Überwachungsstationen," *AZP* 44 (1888): 424–33.

67. Unger, 203. See also the report of Karl Haardt in *DMW* 27 (1901): 323.

68. For examples, see Engstrom, "The Birth," 313 and Pándy, 391.

69. Dannemann, *Die psychiatrische Klinik zu Giessen,* 90.

70. Quoted respectively in ibid., 111, 93, and 74.

71. Scholz, 236. On bed therapy, see Clemens Neisser, "Die Bettbehandlung der Irren," *BKW* 27 (1890): 863–66 and also "Noch einmal die Bettenbehandlung der Irren," *AZP* 50 (1894): 447–64; Hugo Hoppe, "Über einige Fortschritte in der Behandlung der Geisteskranken," *Therapeutische Monatshefte* 20 (1906): 228–38, 282–91. On the explicitly sedative function of bed therapy, see Emil Kraepelin, *Psychiatry: A Textbook for Students and Physicians,* ed. Jacques M. Quen, trans. Helga Metoui and Sabine Ayed (Canton: Watson Publishing International, [1899] 1991), 1:228.

72. Neisser, "Die Bettbehandlung," 863.

73. Friedrich Panse et al., *Das psychiatrische Krankenhauswesen,* Schriftenreihe aus dem Gebiete des öffentlichen Gesundheitswesens, ed. Josef Stralau and Bernhard Zoller (Stuttgart: Thieme, 1964), 19:39–41. By some accounts, the reception of bed therapy was slow and skeptical in alienist circles. See Otto Klinke, "Zur Geschichte der freien Behandlung und der Anwendung der Bettruhe bei Geisteskranken," *AZP* 49 (1893): 680–1 and Feger, 89.

74. The same effect was also obtained by wrapping patients in wet sheets. On the effects of hydrotherapy, see Kolb, *Sammel-Atlas,* 31–2; Scholz, 242–3; Oscar Maria Graf, *Wir sind Gefangene: Ein Bekenntnis* (Munich: DTV, 1978), 201.

75. See Panse, 41–3, and the doubts expressed by Karl Fürstner at the annual meeting of Southwest German Alienists in 1892. The merits of hydrotherapy were also discussed at length at the annual meeting of the VdI in Bonn in 1898. For a report on the debate seen *MschrPN* 4 (1898): 332–3.

76. Scholz, 243.

77. Clarke, "Notes," 361.

78. Hitzig, "Neubau," 397–8; Robert Sommer, "Die Wärterfrage," *ZblNP* 16 (1893): 606–7.

79. Dannemann, *Die psychiatrische Klinik zu Giessen,* 52.

80. Carl Pelman, *Erinnerungen eines alten Irrenarztes* (Bonn: Friedrich Cohen, 1912), 113.

81. Konrad Rieger, "Die neue psychiatrische Klinik der Universität Würzburg," *Klinisches Jahrbuch* 5 (1894): 152.

82. On the dispute, see chapter 2 above.

83. Werner Janzarik, "Hundert Jahre Heidelberger Psychiatrie," in *Psychologie als Grundlagenwissenschaft,* vol. 8 of *Klinische Psychologie und Psychopathologie,* ed. Helmut Remschmidt (Stuttgart: Enke, 1979), 3. Franz Nissl could speak of the clinic as a rural asylum *"en miniature."* Franz Nissl, "Die psychiatrische Klinik" TMs, 1, UAH, H III-682/1.

84. Reinhard Riese, *Die Hochschulen auf dem Wege zum wissenschaftlichen Großbetrieb,* Industrielle Welt, ed. Werner Conze (Stuttgart: Ernst Klett, 1977), 19:226.

85. Max Fischer, "Die Irrenfürsorge in Baden," *PNW* 4 (1902/3): 89–92, 102–4, 111–6. See also Kraepelin, *Lebenserinnerungen*, 116–8.

86. The great importance attached to the capacity to work as a criteria of admission was reflected in the fact that it was written into the statutes of Emmendingen and Pforzheim and reinforced by a special order of the Ministry of the Interior on 10 November 1890. Arnsperger, "Über Irrenversorgung in dem Grossherzogthum Baden," *Ärztliche Mitteilungen aus und für Baden* 45 (1891): 137.

87. On overcrowding in Baden see Fischer, "Die Irrenfürsorge" and Eric J. Engstrom, "Die Heidelberger psychiatrische Universitätsklinik am Ende des 19. Jahrhunderts," *Jahrbuch für Universitätsgeschichte* 1 (1998): 49–68.

88. Typhus broke out in the Heidelberg clinic itself in 1881, in the general hospital in 1886, in Emmendingen in 1900, and in Pforzheim in 1902. See the various letters in PKUH VIII/4.

89. Kraepelin, *Lebenserinnerungen*, 67–8; Wilmanns, 18; Janzarik, "Hundert Jahre," 4.

90. For detailed references see Engstrom, "The Birth," 322–35. For similar reforms in other clinics, see Annette Braunsdorf, "Leben und Werk Otto Binswangers, Jena 1882–1919" (Med. diss., University of Jena, 1988), 16–8.

91. Directorate of the Psychiatric Clinic Heidelberg [Kraepelin] to the MdJKU, 26 December 1891, Nr. 2000, PKUH, VIII/4.

92. Directorate of the Heidelberg Clinic to MdJKU, 26 December 1891, Nr. 2000, PKUH VIII/4.

93. MdJKU to Directorate of the Heidelberg Clinic, 8 June 1892, Nr. 6902, PKUH VIII/4.

94. Access to such files was, of course, also important for educational reasons. After the dispute over the admission files had been resolved, Kraepelin sought permission to reproduce excerpts from the files for his students. See the inspection report of Dr. Arnsperger, 31 January 1895, 6, GLA 235-30375.

95. See Emil Kraepelin, "Über die Wachabteilung der Heidelberger Irrenklinik," *AZP* 51 (1895): 1–21. On Kraepelin's use of psychological experiments see Bakel and Engstrom, "Kulturelle Dimensionen."

96. Directorate of the Psychiatric Clinic to MdJKU, 29 November 1892, Nr. 2715/2786, GLA 235-3571.

97. Ibid. The state inspector remarked that Kraepelin's renovations had serious adverse effects on patients. See the reports of Dr. Arnsperger, 13 January 1893 and March 1900, GLA 235-30375.

98. Kraepelin, "Über die Wachabteilung," 21.

99. Directorate of the Psychiatric Clinic Heidelberg to MdJKU, 4 June 1894, Nr. 1376, GLA 235-3563. Directorate of the Psychiatric Clinic Heidelberg to MdJKU, 24 October 1894, Nr. 2542, PKUH I/1.

100. See the quarterly reports of the clinic at GLA 235-746/7/8.

101. Emil Kraepelin, "Die Lage der Irrenfürsorge in Baden," *ZblNP* 20, n.s. 8 (1897): 661–2. It was not until 1910 and the promulgation of Baden's new law on psychiatric care that provision was made for self-admission.

102. Report of the Inspector Dr. Arnsperger, 13 January 1893, GLA 235-30375; City Council of Heidelberg to Directorate of the Psychiatric Clinic Heidelberg, 28 May 1894, GLA 235-3563; Ribstein Report, 5 March 1893, GLA 235-4858. See also Eric J. Engstrom, "Der Verbrecher als wissenschaftliche Aufgabe," in *Emil Kraepelin*, ed. Wolfgang Burgmair, Eric J. Engstrom, Matthias M. Weber (Munich: Bellville, 2001), 353–90.

103. According to an order of the MdJKU, 19 November 1892, Nr. 22888, GLA 235-3563, Kraepelin had admitted a patient for observation "without the necessary documentation." See also Kraepelin, *Psychiatry*, 1:247 where he claims that for years he had admitted his patients without supporting documents.

104. Kraepelin, *Lebenserinnerungen*, 117.

105. In 1887, under Fürstner's directorate, the clinic had already lost a portion of its admission district. Report of the Directorate of the Psychiatric Clinic in Heidelberg, 16 February 1887, Nr. 135, GLA 235-3565.

106. Directorate of the Psychiatric Clinic Heidelberg to MdJKU, 6 May 1897, Nr. 1045, 8, PKUH VIII/4.

107. Directorate of the Psychiatric Clinic Heidelberg to MdJKU, 22 June 1893, Nr. 868, PKUH VIII/4.

108. Emil Kraepelin to MdJKU, 20 June 1896, Nr. 1328, PKUH I/1.

109. Emil Kraepelin to MdJKU, 12 July 1896, Nr. 1577, PKUH VIII/4.

110. For details see Engstrom, "The Birth," 331, note 151.

111. Report of the grand-ducal *Verwaltungshof,* 8 September 1897, Nr. 36818, PKUH VIII/4.

112. Statement of the Medical Advisor for Psychiatric Affairs, 26 December 1896, PKUH VIII/4.

113. Finding of the grand-ducal Ministry of the Interior, 2 January 1897, Nr. 37593, PKUH VIII/4.

114. Emil Kraepelin to MdJKU, 6 May 1897, PKUH, VIII/4, 10.

115. Emil Kraepelin to MdJKU, 2 August 1899, PKUH, I/1. See also Wilmanns, 19.

116. See Engstrom, "The Birth," 335, note 168.

117. Kraepelin, *Lebenserinnerungen,* 67; and see his *Psychiatrie,* 5th ed. (Leipzig: J. A. Barth, 1896), v.

118. Kraepelin, *Lebenserinnerungen,* 49. Also see German E. Berrios and Renate Hauser, "The Early Development of Kraepelin's Ideas on Classification," *Psychological Medicine* 18 (1988): 815.

119. W. Mayer-Gross, "Die Entwicklung der klinischen Anschauungen Kraepelins," *AfPN* 87 (1929): 32.

120. In the preface to that textbook, he wrote that "this edition represented a decisive step from a symptomatic to a clinical view of insanity. The necessity of this shift in perspective was impressed upon me by practical needs and is illustrated above all in the delimitation and ordering of clinical cases (*Krankheitsbilder*). The importance of external clinical signs (*Krankheitszeichen*) has necessarily and everywhere been subordinated to considerations of the *conditions of origin,* the *course,* and the *terminus* which result from individual disorders. Thus, all purely 'symptomatic categories' (*Zustandsbilder*) have disappeared from the nosology." Kraepelin, *Psychiatrie,* v.

121. On the diagnostic cards, see Matthias Weber and Eric J. Engstrom, "Kraepelin's Diagnostic Cards," *HP* 8 (1997): 375–385.

122. Kraepelin, *Lebenserinnerungen,* 142.

123. Mayer-Gross, 34.

124. Kraepelin, *Lebenserinnerungen,* 67.

125. Although psychiatrists keenly desired reliable statistical categories, they notoriously disagreed over just what those categories should be. On the contentious debates in the VdI see Carl Westphal, "Vorschläge zur Abänderung der amtlichen Zählkarten für die Irrenanstalten," *AZP* 38 (1882): 717–9 and *AZP* 39 (1883): 612–6.

126. See Eulenberg, *Das Medicinalwesen,* 255; Guttstadt, "Die Geisteskranken."

127. See Engstrom, "The Birth," 336–40 and Weber and Engstrom, 377–8.

128. Kraepelin, *Lebenserinnerungen,* 117.

129. On the complex and ambiguous interrelationship of clinic size and patient frequency in relation to the clinical interests of research and teaching, see also Karl Wilmanns, "Die Psychiatrische Universitätsklinik in Heidelberg," 16–17, UAH HIII-682/1.

130. Kraepelin, *Lebenserinnerungen,* 67–8. Kraepelin had sought permission to visit Emmendingen and Pforzheim as early as 1894. See the report of inspector Arnsperger, 31 January 1895, GLA 235-30375.

131. Emil Kraepelin, "Ziele und Wege der klinischen Psychiatrie," *AZP* 53 (1897): 842.

132. Felix Plaut as cited in Kolle, *Kraepelin und Freud,* 23. Kraepelin described in detail the way in which he used patient cards to construct and delimit specific diseases in his "Ziele und Wege der psychiatrischen Forschung," *ZgNP* 42 (1918): 181–2.

133. Kraepelin, "Ziele und Wege der klinischen Psychiatrie," 842.

134. Ibid., 844.

135. Ibid., 845.

136. See MdJKU to Directorate of the Psychiatric Clinic Heidelberg, 14 April 1900, Nr. 11207 and Kraepelin's response of 17 April 1900, PKUH I/8. Psychiatrists in the Königsberg clinic acted along similar lines, although their motives appear to have been chiefly financial ones. See Burghardt, 154.

137. Kraepelin, *Lebenserinnerungen*, 119.

138. Robert Wollenberg, "Einweihungsfeier der Psychiatrischen- und Nervenklinik," *Strassburger Medizinische Zeitung* 8 (1911): 223.

139. Clarke, "Notes," 360. The same view was expressed by Siemens, "Die Errichtung," 730. On the clinic as transit station see also Kolb, *Sammel-Atlas,* 246–51.

140. Fürstner, *Über Irrenkliniken*, 5.

141. Wernicke, "Stadtasyle," 188. The transitory nature of admissions meant that the urban asylum served essentially as an "observation station." Ibid., 189.

142. Compare the case of Erlangen. Engstrom, "The Birth," 346, note 204.

143. Rieger, "Die neue psychiatrische Klinik," 148.

144. Wollenberg, *Erinnerungen*, 57.

145. See the "Vorlage 533 zur Verhandlungen der Stadtversammlung Berlin (Juni 1892)" and, in particular, "Vorlage Nr. 2146 FB II 92 betr. der Neuregelung der Aufnahme für Geisteskranke," 3 June 1892, UAHUB, Charité Direktion 1034, Bl. 391–5.

146. On transports to Dalldorf see Engstrom, "The Birth," 347, note 209.

147. The corollary to higher frequency was, of course, reduced lengths of stay and hence lower mortality rates. In 1873 the clinic in Vienna posted an average length of stay of only fifteen-and-a-half days. *CBlDGPgP* 21 (1875): 3.

148. Gaupp, "Die Psychiatrie," 1738.

149. It should be noted, however, that one of Kraepelin's harshest critics, Alfred Hoche, believed that many alterations from one edition of the textbook to the next had made psychiatric instruction more difficult. Hoche also objected to the clear delineation of disease categories, which he saw as inappropriate in the field of psychiatry and as a corruption the "facts." Alfred E. Hoche, "Eintheilung und Benennung der Psychosen mit Rücksicht auf die Anforderungen der ärztlichen Prüfung," *AfPN* 38 (1904): 1074.

Chapter 6

1. Compare Rose, 63 and Donald Light, *Becoming Psychiatrists* (New York: W. W. Norton, 1980), chapters 11 and 15.

2. On medical education, see Huerkamp, chapt. 2 and 3 in *Der Aufstieg der Ärzte*; Bleker, "Medical Students;" Eulner, *Die Entwicklung*, 185–201; Godelieve van Hetern, "Clinical Education in Nineteenth-Century Germany: A Theatre of Knowledge," *Bulletin of the Society for the Social History of Medicine* 41 (1987): 41–5; Thomas Neville Bonner, *Becoming a Physician* (New York: Oxford University Press, 1995); Hans H. Simmer, "Principles and Problems of Medical Undergraduate Education in Germany during the Nineteenth and early Twentieth Centuries," in *The History of Medical Education*, ed. C. D. O'Malley, UCLA Forum in Medical Sciences, vol. 12 (Berkeley: University of California Press, 1970), 173–200; Puschmann, *Geschichte des medizinischen Unterrichts*; Flexner; Billroth.

3. For an overview of regulations pertaining to medical education in Prussia, see Billroth, 112–27. Other German states followed suit. See Bonner, 187–90 and for the case of Württemberg Drees, 31–2, 50–9.

4. Huerkamp, *Der Aufstieg der Ärzte*, 48, 51.

5. Anon., "Zur Regelung der Prüfungen für die Aerzte," *Preußische Jahrbücher* 23 (1869): 230–3. On requirements in different German states, see Puschmann, *Geschichte des medizinischen Unterrichts*, 465–71 and for Württemberg Drees, 100–14.

6. Eulenberg, *Das Medicinalwesen*, 309–22, 331. Students were, however, required to have attended a university, passed the *tentamen physicum,* and have practiced in the surgical, medical, and gynecological clinic.

7. On these differences see Huerkamp, *Der Aufstieg der Ärzte,* 104–5, Drees, 111, 119,

304, and Heinrich Quincke, "Zur Reform des medizinischen Unterrichts und der Prüfungsordnung," *DMW* 17 (1891).

8. Billroth, 31–2, 65–8. For the emphasis on practice-based learning see Coleman, "Prussian
Pedagogy," 28–38 and Kathryn M. Olesko, *Physics as a Calling*, Cornell History of Science Series,
ed. L. Pearce Williams (Ithaca: Cornell University Press, 1991).

9. *Encyclopädisches Wörterbuch der medicinischen Wissenschaften,* 1839 ed., s.v. "Klinik,
medicinisch," 686.

10. Kieser, *Elemente der Psychiatrik,* 386. By the term *Psychiatrik* Kieser meant theoretical
psychiatry as opposed to *Psychiatrie* or practical psychiatry.

11. In light of this shift in the didactic intent of clinical instruction, it becomes more difficult
to maintain, as Verwey has, that there existed a fundamental continuity in clinical psychiatric research throughout the nineteenth century. Stressing differences in practical activity relativizes any
continuity in phenomenological approach. Verwey, 35–6, 138–51.

12. Huerkamp, *Der Aufstieg der Ärzte,* 46–7.

13. Compare the remarks of Billroth, 65. See also MgUMA to University Curators, 22 November 1872, cited in Eulenberg, *Das Medizinalwesen in Preussen,* 301 and Ernst Theodor
Nauck, *Zur Geschichte des medizinischen Lehrplans und Unterrichts der Universität Freiburg
i.Br.,* Beiträge zur Freiburger Wissenschafts- und Universitätsgeschichte, ed. Johannes Vincke, vol.
2 (Freiburg i. Br.: Eberhard Albert, 1952).

14. Hitzig, "Rede," 122.

15. Kraepelin, *Die königliche Psychiatrische Klinik,* 31.

16. For statistics on medical students and debates on overcrowding, see Huerkamp, *Der Aufstieg der Ärzte,* 62–5 and 110–18. And Franz Eulenburg, *Die Frequenz der deutschen Universitäten* (Leipzig: Teubner, 1904).

17. See the *Aerztliches Vereinsblatt* 17 (1890): 333–8 and Huerkamp, *Der Aufstieg der Ärzte,*
98–9.

18. Report of the Berlin Physician's Association in 1890 as cited in Arthur Hartmann, *Die Reform des medicinischen Unterrichtes* (Berlin: Fischer 1894), 2.

19. Dörner describes the *Wanderjahre* of young alienists as virtually "obligatory" between
1810 and 1870. Dörner, *Bürger und Irre,* 237.

20. Jastrowitz, "Über die Staatsaufsicht," 719.

21. Bresler, "Der wissenschaftlichen Betrieb." Symptomatic of this change was the appoint-
ment of Alexander Westphal in Bonn in 1904. See Alexander Westphal, Robert Schulze and A. H.
Hübner, "Die neue Klinik für psychisch und Nervenkranke der Universität Bonn," *Klinisches
Jahrbuch* 24 (1910): 230.

22. The first such chair had been created for Johann Christian Heinroth in Leipzig in 1819.
After 1819, Heinroth held a full chair for *psychische Heilkunde* and from 1827 for *psychische
Therapie.* The chair lapsed upon his passing in 1843. On Heinroth see Pauleikhoff, *Das Menschenbild,* 1:84–108 and Leibbrand and Wettley, *Der Wahnsinn,* 492ff. For a concise listing of
psychiatry's standing at different German universities, see Eulner, *Die Entwicklung,* 510, 670–80.

23. Such personal unions had been very widespread, existing at one time or another during the
nineteenth century in Jena, Bonn, Greifswald, Marburg, Breslau, Göttingen, Munich, and elsewhere.

24. Such was the case in Marburg in 1875. See Engstrom, "The Birth," 361, note 32.

25. See the case of Bonn in the late 1870s, as depicted in the Circulars of the Medical Faculty,
4 April and 2 May 1877, as well as the "Gutachterliche Äusserung über die dem Director der
Provincialirrenanstalt Dr. Nasse einzunehmende akademische Stellung," UAB, MF 1102. A manuscript copy of the contract is in UAB, Rektorat A 3,20.

26. MgUMA to Curator of the University of Halle, 31 March 1879, UAHa, Med. Fak. I, Rep.
29, Nr. 186, Bl. 70.

27. See chapter 2 above and Lachner, 190; Bresler, *Ausgewählte Kapitel,* 7; and Lessing's address to the VdI in Landau in 1861, *AZP* 18 (1861): 818ff. The topic also occupied the attention
of the Prussian parliament. See GStA PK, IHA, Rep. 76Va, MgUMA, Sect. 8, Tit. XIX, Nr. 26, Bd.
I and *Stenographische Verhandlungen des [preussischen] Hauses der Abgeordneten,* 34th Session,

14 March 1889, 1037–42. In Bonn, Carl Pelman was a convinced opponent of the fusion of alienist and academic posts. Pelman, *Erinnerungen,* 141.

28. For the case of Bavaria, see *ZblNP* 9 (1886): 736; *MMW* 42 (1895): 1136. And in Baden compare Emil Kraepelin to Alfons Bilharz, 23 February 1902, UBT, Md 939 22 and Emil Kraepelin, *Die psychiatrischen Aufgaben des Staates* (Jena: Fischer, 1900).

29. See Nasse, "Über das Bedürfniß," 332ff and Müller, 63.

30. See Eulenberg, *Das Medicinalwesen,* 278–83.

31. See the reports in the *Ärztliches Intelligenz-Blatt,* 1 (1854): 233–4, 7 (1860): 594 and 8 (1861): 151.

32. See Roller, *Psychiatrische Zeitfragen,* 64.

33. Laehr, Review of *Das Projekt,* 218.

34. See Obersteiner, "Grundzüge," 2; Valentin Wieczorek, "Die Nervenklinik Jena im 19. und zu Beginn des 20. Jahrhunderts," in *Jenaer Hochschullehrer der Medizin,* ed. Günther Wagner (Jena: Friedrich-Schiller-Universität, 1988), 67–8; and Gudden, "Bernhard von Gudden," 116–18.

35. MgUMA to MFin, 10 October 1884, GstA PK, IHA, Rep. 76Va, MgUMA, Sect. 8, Tit. X. Nr. 17, Bd. 1, Bl. 239–44.

36. Ibid. For more details, see Engstrom, "The Birth," 367, note 50 and Hitzig, *Bericht über die Wirksamkeit,* 7–10.

37. Fearing that a psychiatric clinic in Halle would open the floodgates at other Prussian universities, the ministry of finance tried to preempt this conclusion. See MFin to MgUMA, 17 October 1884, and MgUMA to MFin, 27 December 1884, GStA PK, IHA, Rep. 76Va, MgUMA, Sect. 8, Tit. X, Nr. 17, Bd. 1, Bl. 247 and 280 respectively.

38. On Binswanger, see Braunsdorf, "Leben und Werk."

39. For a listing of Binswanger's course offerings, see UAJ, L 230, Bl. 87.

40. Seige, 377.

41. Binswanger modeled his lecture courses on those of Ludwig Meyer and Carl Westphal. Binswanger, "Die Lehraufgaben," 51; Westphal, "Nachrichten."

42. Binswanger, "Die Lehraufgaben."

43. The above citations are from ibid., 49. Compare similarly Nasse, "Über das Bedürfniß," 327, 341–4, 354–5, 361 and the view of Ideler cited in Dannemann, *Die psychiatrische Klinik zu Giessen,* 23.

44. Binswanger, "Die Lehraufgaben," 53.

45. Ibid.

46. Compare similarly Hitzig, *Bericht über die Wirksamkeit,* 10.

47. For Damerow the chief purpose of clinical instruction was to advance the "art of anthropological healing." Damerow, *Über die relative Verbindung,* 210, 228.

48. Binswanger, "Die Lehraufgaben," 60. Compare the views of Nasse, for whom clinical instruction served to reduce admissions and not, as for Binswanger and his contemporaries, to deliver patients more quickly into urban asylums. Nasse, "Über das Bedürfniß," 336.

49. Ibid., 346. See likewise the views of W. A. F. Browne in Scull, *Masters,* 115.

50. Nasse, "Keine Irren?" 191–2.

51. Damerow, "Über Irrenpflegeanstalten," 220.

52. Fürstner, *Über Irrenkliniken,* 4–5; See also chapter 3 above.

53. Nasse, "Über das Bedürfniß," 347.

54. Rinecker to Medical Faculty, 25 February 1880, UAW, ARS 3293; Hitzig, *Bericht über die Wirksamkeit,* 28; Fürstner, *Irrenkliniken,* 35.

55. Directorate of the Heidelberg Psychiatric Clinic to MInn, 6 September 1878, GLA 235-3565.

56. Dean of the Medical Faculty to Rector of the University of Jena, 4 December 1913, UAJ, BA 1345.

57. Hartmann, 55. Compare also Clarke, "Notes," 375.

58. Meyer, "Die psychiatrische Klinik," 213.

59. See Braunsdorf, "Leben und Werk," 19 and Alt, 410.

60. Wernicke, "Zweck und Ziel," 223.

61. Consequently, in spite of rising medical student enrollments, psychiatric courses were rarely overcrowded and open positions were often difficult to fill. See Engstrom, "The Birth," 381–2, note 93.

62. On textbooks see Olesko's remarks in Coleman and Holmes, 315–6.

63. Remarking on his own textbook, Heinrich Neumann agreed with his critic Karl Kahlbaum that it would never become a standard work: "academic youth" would only purchase "prettily compiled, ordered, and systematic" textbooks and those, which, like Griesinger's, were full of "empty phrases and pretty rhetoric" and wholly devoid of original ideas. Cited in Henseler, 20–1.

64. Wille, "Vortrag," 395.

65. Flechsig, *Die Irrenklinik*, 59.

66. Wernicke, "Zweck und Ziel," 219.

67. For a bibliography of major textbooks of the period, see Kraepelin, *Psychiatry*, 2:7. Probably the most widely used textbook in the 1870s and 1880s was Richard von Krafft-Ebing's *Lehrbuch der Psychiatrie*. Through 1897, it was published in six editions. For an assessment of its significance, see Pelman's review in *DMW* 22 (1896): 126 and Oosterhuis.

68. Curator to MgUMA, 18 August 1900, GStA PK, IHA, Rep. 76Va, MgUMA, Sect. 6, Tit. X, Nr. 18, Bd. I.

69. Gustav Specht to Academic Senate of the University of Erlangen, 16 July 1903, UAE I/9/57.

70. Ortmann, 69.

71. Friedrich Jolly, *Vorgeschichte und gegenwärtige Einrichtung der psychiatrischen Klinik in Strassburg* (Strassburg: Karl Trübner, 1887), 21. A list of the instruments and teaching aids in the lecture hall in Bonn can be found in UAB, MF 1102.

72. Cf. Flechsig, "Die psychiatrische und Nervenklinik," 197–8.

73. Rieger, "Die neue psychiatrische Klinik," 150. In Tübingen beds were placed on wheels to facilitate demonstration. Ernst Siemerling, *Bericht über die Wirksamkeit der psychiatrischen Universitätsklinik in Tübingen* (Tübingen: Franz Pietzcker, 1901), 5.

74. Rinecker to Medical Faculty, 12 June 1875, UAW, ARS 3293.

75. Flechsig, *Die Irrenklinik*, 57.

76. Richard von Krafft-Ebing, *Der klinische Unterricht in der Psychiatrie* (Stuttgart: Enke, 1890), 32.

77. Ibid., 33. Of course, patients might also resist being demonstrated entirely and thereby throw the best laid pedagogical plans awry. Patients in Heidelberg took issue to participating in clinical demonstrations in the same room used for church services. Consult Sälzer to Directorate of the University Clinic of Heidelberg, 20 March 1894, GLA 235–7729.

78. Flexner, 175–6, 183–4.

79. Krafft-Ebing, *Der klinische Unterricht*, 33.

80. For specific references see Engstrom, "The Birth," 389–90.

81. See "Offizieller Erlass," *Aerztliches Intelligenz-Blatt* 5 (1858): 349–55 and Wilhelm Lexis, *Die Deutschen Universitäten* (Berlin: Asher, 1893), 2:322. According to Rudolf Arndt, psychiatry was also tested in the state of Nassau. Arndt, 58.

82. For the regulations in various German states see A. Guttstadt, "Das Civil-Medicinalwesen," in *Das deutsche Medizinalwesen*, ed. S. Guttmann (Leipzig: Thieme, 1887), 159–75 and Unger. Compare also Engstrom, "The Birth," 407–8.

83. See Arndt, 58 and Adolf Hoffmann, "Die neue Prüfungsordnung für Aerzte," *Aerztliches Vereinsblatt* 7 (1878): 93. In the words of one commentator, southern Germany was "yearning for the good old particularist days." *ZblNP* 16 (1893): 276. At the university of Erlangen, German unification had preempted plans for a chair in psychiatry. See Gustav Specht, "Geschichte der Entwicklung der Erlanger Psychiatrischen und Nervenklinik," TMs [ca. 1935], UAE I/9/57.

84. For the composition of the commission and its report, see *Aerztliches Vereinsblatt* 7 (1878): 169–70, 173–185, *BKW* 15 (1878): 603–5.

85. See *AZP* 39 (1883): 617–8, Guttstadt, "Das Civil-Medicinalwesen," and Unger, 215–23. The new regulations did take some account of psychiatry, but only in passing as a minor addendum to the examination in internal medicine and pharmacology. Otherwise, the regulations ex-

tended the required length of medical study from eight to nine semesters and placed greater emphasis on the pre-clinical, natural scientific aspect of the examinations.

86. Arndt, 12, 37–48. See also Huerkamp, *Der Aufstieg der Ärzte,* 106–7.

87. Karl Fürstner, "Die Psychiatrie in der neuen Prüfungsordnung," *BKW* 20 (1883): 477.

88. See *AfPN* 19 (1888): 557 and Forel, *Rückblick,* 139–40.

89. The issue of overcrowding had come to the fore at the *Aerztetage* in the latter half of the 1880s. On these and related debates see Huerkamp, *Aufstieg der Ärzte,* 60–1, 110–18, Drees, 112–20, Riese, 54–8, the "Verhandlungen des XIX. deutschen Aerztetages," 293, and finally the nationalist and anti-semitic views expressed in Billroth, 105–110.

90. See Dressler, "Das Studium der Medicin und die Examenordnung für Aerzte," *Aerztliche Mittheilungen aus und für Baden* 45 (1891): 183–8.

91. See Asch's remarks in the "Verhandlungen des XVIII. deutschen Aerztetages zu München am 23. und 24. Juni 1890," *Arztliches Vereinsblatt* 17 (1890), 308–9.

92. Ibid., 317.

93. The petition was published by Rieger, "Psychiatrie als Examensfach." It was addressed to the governments of Bavaria, Württemberg, Baden, Alsace Lorraine, and Hesse and had been submitted by the directors of the university clinics in Strassburg (Fürstner), Heidelberg (Kraepelin), and Würzburg (Rieger), as well as two leading alienists from Heppenheim (Ludwig) and Schussenried (Kreuser).

94. Compare similarly Arndt, 39–44.

95. Konrad Rieger, "Psychiatrie als Examensfach," *ZblNP* 16 (1893): 498.

96. Ibid.

97. See above, page 41.

98. The signatories included Friedrich Jolly (Berlin), Carl Pelman (Bonn), Carl Wernicke (Breslau), Anton Bumm (Erlangen), Hermann Emminghaus (Freiburg), Ludwig Meyer (Göttingen), Rudolf Arndt (Greifswald), Eduard Hitzig (Halle), Emil Kraepelin (Heidelberg), Otto Binswanger (Jena), Franz Meschede (Königsberg), Paul Flechsig (Leipzig), August Cramer (Göttingen), Hubert Grashey (Munich), Karl Fürstner (Strassburg), Ernst Siemerling (Tübingen), Konrad Rieger (Würzburg). The petition was published in Rieger, *Zusammenstellung einiger Begründungen,* 12–21; also UAJ, L236, Bl. 175–82.

99. Rieger, *Zusammenstellung* (Jena: Fischer, 1896), 15.

100. Ibid., 16.

101. See chapter 5 above.

102. See Laehr, "Die Bedeutung," 62.

103. The exchange between Schultze and Binswanger extended over three years and generated some six publications. In order of their publication they included Bernhard Sigmund Schultze, *Über den Plan"* ([Jena]: n.p., 1893); Otto Binswanger, *Die Psychiatrie* (Jena: Frommann, 1893); Bernhard Sigmund Schultze, *Die Psychiatrie* (Jena: Fischer, 1893); Bernhard Sigmund Schultze, *Mein Votum zur Revision der medizinischen Prüfungen* (Berlin: Mittler & Sohn, 1896); Otto Binswanger, *Zur Revision der medizinischen Prüfungen* (Jena: Pohle, 1896); Bernhard Sigmund Schultze, *Die Psychiatrie* (Jena: Fischer, 1896). The citations in this section are all taken from these publications. See also Ortmann, 167.

104. While the revisions of 1883 had extended the length of medical study from eight to nine semesters, the number of obligatory clinical semesters had remained unchanged at four. Schultze therefore suggested extending the length of clinical study to six semesters. Only then might one seriously consider adopting psychiatry into the state examinations.

105. Erlangen was one example. See Gustav Specht, "Geschichte der Entwicklung der Erlanger Psychiatrischen und Nervenklinik," TMs [ca. 1935], UAE I/9/57.

106. *ZblNP* 24 (1901): 460.

107. Tuczek, 6.

108. Ibid., 13.

109. See Unger, 229–30 and MgUMA to the Curator of the University of Halle-Wittenberg, 6 July 1897, UAHa, Rep. 6, Nr. 1084. Similar courses already existed in other fields as well and the work of the committee was modeled on the continuing education program for military doctors.

See August Paul Wassermann, "Die medizinische Fakultät," in *Die Universitäten im deutschen Reich,* ed. W. Lexis (Berlin: Ascher, 1904), 151–6 and Eva Heine, *Die Anfänge einer organisierten ärztlichen Fortbildung im Deutschen Reich,* Schriftenreihe der Münchener Vereinigung für Geschichte der Medizin, vol. 17 (Gräfelfing: Demeter-Verl., 1985).

110. Cf. Alzheimer, 858–9.

111. See *DMW* 27 (1901): 323 and Engstrom, "Der Verbrecher," 373–7.

112. See *DMW* 29 (1903): 152 and Schindler, 131–2.

113. See Reichardt to Medical Faculty, 13 July 1912, UAW, ARS 3294 and the review of M. Kauffmann, "Notwendigkeit psychiatrischer Ausbildung der Bahnärzte," *ZgNP* (1910): 160.

Chapter 7

1. Schrenk, *Über den Umgang,* 146. According to Schrenk, it was not until the rise of psychoanalysis that psychiatry (chiefly in Anglo-Saxon lands) again opened itself toward society.

2. See Radkau, *Das Zeitalter* and Andreas Steiner, *'Das nervöse Zeitalter'* (Zurich: Juris, 1964).

3. Tuczek, 15–16.

4. Gaupp, *Wege und Ziele,* 28.

5. Adolf Dannemann, "Psychologie und Psychotherapie im Polizeiwesen," *MMW* 55 (1908): 122. See also his "Zur Angelegenheit Scholz gegen Bodelschwingh," *ZblNP* 19 (1896): 56.

6. Alzheimer, 861.

7. Elsewhere—in England, the United States, and France—psychiatrists were likewise turning their attention to social questions. Andrew Scull has extended Charles Rosenberg's interpretation of a "crisis of psychiatric legitimacy" in the United States to England and France in the 1860s and 1870s, arguing that it prompted alienists toward greater social activism. Andrew Scull, "Psychiatry and Social Control in the Nineteenth and Twentieth centuries," *HP* 2 (1991): 158. For the United States, Elizabeth Lunbeck has argued that the expansion of psychiatry into everyday life was central to its professional authority, disciplining function, and normalizing power. Lunbeck, 70.

8. Nikolas Rose has spoken in this regard of psychological disciplines' eagerness to "give themselves away" by lending their vocabularies and explanations to other social groups. Rose, 33–4.

9. Among others, this generation included psychiatrists, such as Otto Binswanger, Konrad Rieger, Emil Kraepelin, Ernst Siemerling, August Cramer, Gustav Specht, Robert Wollenberg, Theodor Ziehen, Alfred E. Hoche, Robert Sommer, Ernst Schultze, and Karl Bonhoeffer.

10. On theories of degeneration, see Paul Weindling, *Health, Race, and German Politics between National Unification and Nazism* (Cambridge: Cambridge University Press, 1989); Peter Weingart, Jürgen Kroll and Kurt Bayertz, *Rasse, Blut, und Gene* (Frankfurt/M: Suhrkamp, 1992); Gunther Mann, "Dekadenz, Degeneration, Untergangsangst im Lichte der Biologie des 19. Jahrhunderts," *Medizinhistorisches Journal* 20 (1985): 6–35.

11. Dörner, "Wir verstehen," 80. See also Roelcke, *Krankheit und Kulturkritik.*

12. Dirk Blasius, *Der verwaltete Wahnsinn* (Frankfurt/M: Fischer, 1980), 95; Zeller, "Von der Heilanstalt," 126. The same has been said of general medicine following the introduction of natural scientific methods. Eulner, *Die Entwicklung,* 23.

13. Binswanger, "Die Lehraufgaben," 61.

14. Kraepelin, *Die psychiatrische Aufgaben.*

15. Obviously, hereditary theories were not the only font of a socially oriented psychiatry. Many other forms of what one can call social psychiatry, ranging from family care and agricultural colonies to patient aid organizations, existed on the periphery of German psychiatry in the late nineteenth century. See Thomas Beddies and Heinz-Peter Schmiedebach, "Die Diskussion um die ärztlich beaufsichtigte Familienpflege in Deutschland," *Sudhoffs Archiv* 85 (2001): 82–107. The point here is simply that mainstream psychiatry had socio-hygienic ambitions, albeit grounded firmly in somatic premises.

16. See Eulner, *Die Entwicklung,* 670–80. Gustav Schimmelpennig has pointed out this rupture around 1900, although his claim that nearly all chairs in psychiatry changed hands is overstated. In addition to Jena, Leipzig, and Würzburg, there was personal continuity in Marburg, Rostock, Giessen, and Erlangen from the mid-1890s through 1913, and with the exception of Rostock through World War One. From 1896 there was continuity in fully a third of the chairs. Schimmelpennig, "Alfred Erich Hoche," 13.

17. According to Klemens Dieckhöfer, the term 'anti-psychiatry' was not coined until 1909 by the *Psychiatrisch-Neurologischen Wochenschrift.* On anti-psychiatry in the 1890s in Germany, see Ann Goldberg, "The Mellage Trial and the Politics of Insane Asylums in Wilhelmine Germany," *JMH* 74 (2002): 1–32; Heinz-Peter Schmiedebach, "Eine 'antipsychiatrische Bewegung' um die Jahrhundertwende," in *Medizinkritische Bewegungen im deutschen Reich (ca. 1870 bis ca. 1933),* Medizin, Geschichte und Gesellschaft, ed. Martin Dinges, supplement no. 9 (Stuttgart: Steiner, 1996), 127–59; and Klemens Dieckhöfer, "Frühe Formen der Antipsychiatrie und die Reaktion der Psychiatrie," *Medizinhistorisches Journal* 19 (1984): 100–11. For an extensive survey of that literature from a psychiatric standpoint, see Bernhard Beyer, *Die Bestrebungen zur Reform des Irrenwesens* (Halle: Marhold, 1912). See also Niels Reisby, "An Anti-Psychiatry Debate of the 1890's," in *The Department of Psychiatry,* ed. Fini Schulsinger et al., Acta Psychiatrica Scandinavica, Supplementum 261 (Copenhagen: Munksgaard, 1975), 15–20.

18. Witzler, 159.

19. On the law, see Unger, 8–12, and Ursula Teuscher, "Die Irrenpflege in der Rheinprovinz im 19. Jahrhundert am Beispiel Aachens" (Med. diss., Rheinisch-Westphälische Technische Hochschule Aachen, 1979), 87–97.

20. For an account of these developments and the extent of state support for religious asylums, see Hans Kurella, "Das preussische Irrenwesen im Lichte des Processes Mellage," *ZblNP* 18 (1895): 337–44. For examples elsewhere see Engstrom, "The Birth," 427, note 41.

21. The revision of 1891 did not so much nullify existing contractual arrangements with private and charitable asylums as transfer the liability to the provinces. Rather than dissolving those contracts, provinces chose to extend and supplement them.

22. See Fritz Siemens and August Zinn, "Zur Frage der Reform des Irrenwesens in Deutschland, insbesondere in Preussen," *AZP* 52 (1896): 818–20.

23. At least this was the concern of Dannemann, *Bau,* 28–9.

24. On the strength and expansion of church run hospitals in Germany at the turn of the century, see Alfons Labisch and Florian Tennstedt, "Die Allgemeinen Krankenhäuser der Städte und der Religionsgemeinschaften Ende des 19. Jahrhunderts," in *'Einem jeden Kranken in einem Hospitale sein eigenes Bett',* eds. Alfons Labisch and Reinhard Spree (Frankfurt/M: Campus, 1996), 297–319.

25. On these social reform efforts, see Rüdiger vom Bruch, "Bürgerliche Sozialreform im deutschen Kaiserreich," in *Weder Kommunismus noch Kapitalismus,* ed. Rüdiger vom Bruch (Munich: Beck, 1985), 99–111 and Gerhard A. Ritter, *Sozialversicherung in Deutschland und England* (Munich: Beck, 1983), 23.

26. Thomas Nipperdey, *Deutsche Geschichte 1866–1918* (Munich: Beck, 1990), 1:499.

27. The questionnaire had been sent by activists involved with the *Innere Mission* (Bodelschwingh, Hafner, and Knodt). Later reports of the association were widely but secretly distributed. In early 1890, following the first conference of the association, Bodelschwingh and his supporters submitted a report to church officials complaining about the status of asylum clergy. See Fritz Siemens and August Zinn, "Psychiatrie und Seelsorge," in *Bericht,* by the Verein der deutschen Irrenärzte (Munich: Lehmann, 1893), 18. See Pieper, "Erwiederung gegen Pf[arrer] Hafner," *Evangelisches Gemeindeblatt für Rheinland und Westfalen* (No. 48, 1893), reprinted in *AZP* 50 (1894): 854–5.

28. *AZP* 50 (1894): 869.

29. On the *Wärterfrage* see Engstrom, "The Birth," 431–33.

30. Hugo Hoppe, "Die Wärterfrage," *ZblNP* 15 (1892): 531.

31. See Scheibe, 138; Ferdinand Karrer, "Zur Wärterfrage," *AZP* 53 (1897): 477–8; Danne-

mann, *Die psychiatrische Klinik zu Giessen,* 113; Hitzig to MgUMA, 19 July 1898, GStA PK, IHA, Rep 76Va, MgUMA, Sect. 8, Tit. X, Nr. 17, Bd. IV. Of course, the problem also plagued asylums, albeit to a lesser degree.

32. In early June, the Berlin police presidium had complained that a "dangerous" patient had been discharged from the Charité. The complaint led to an agreement by which the Charité reported to police before dismissing such patients. At the same time, the completion of the new asylum, Herzberge, led to debates on psychiatric care in Berlin city chambers and on 22 June the Prussian House of Representatives began debates on unlawful incarceration. On these issues see UAHUB Charité Direktion 1034, Bl. 379–86 and 391–5.

33. The article was republished widely in the medical press, among other places in the *Aerztliches Vereinsblatt* 19 (1892): 281–3.

34. On Stoecker, see Günter Brakelmann, Martin Greschat and Werner Jochmann, *Protestantismus und Politik: Werk und Wirkung Adolf Stöckers,* Hamburger Beiträge zur Social- und Zeitgeschichte, vol. 17 (Hamburg: Christians, 1982). Both before and after the appearance of the *Kreuzzeitung* article, Stoecker had raised the issue of unlawful detention in psychiatric hospitals on the floor of the Prussian house of representatives. On the debates there, see Beyer, 397–422. Beyer attributes the article to Stoecker, Eduard August Schröder, and possibly also von Oertzen. Ibid., 413.

35. On conservative populism, see David Blackbourn and Geoff Eley, *The Peculiarities of German History* (Oxford: Oxford University Press, 1984).

36. On the anti-Semitic motives behind the *Kreuzzeitung* article, see Schmiedebach, "Eine 'antipsychiatrische Bewegung.'" Carl Pelman considered the agitation of the editors of the *Kreuzzeitung* as a "symptom of the age like antisemitism." *AZP* 50 (1894): 348.

37. See August Zinn, as cited in Beyer, 426.

38. For example, in 1892 the province of Brandenburg acted to comply with the law of 11 July 1891. On the recommendation of the *Innere Mission,* it purchased two confessional asylums, infused them with capital, while retaining the hospitals' religious board of directors. *AZP* 48 (1892): 702–3.

39. The VdI had the papers of Siemens and Zinn published in a separate volume. See Siemens and Zinn, "Psychiatrie und Seelsorge," 1–37. Much of the literature and an extensive bibliography of the dispute was republished in *AZP* 50 (1893): 801–96.

40. Siemens and Zinn, "Psychiatrie und Seelsorge," 6.

41. Kurella, "Das preussische Irrenwesen," 341; Beyer, 427, 442.

42. Karl Fürstner, *Wie ist die Fürsorge für Gemütskranke von Aerzten und Laien zu Fördern?* (Berlin: Karger, 1900), 32.

43. On the resolution, see von Kirchenheim and Reinartz, *Zur Reform des Irrenrechts* (Barmen: Wiemann, 1895) and *AZP* 51 (1895): 845–6.

44. On the trial, see Linda Orth, et al., *Pass op, sonst küss de bei de Pelman* (Bonn: Grenzenlos, [1994]), 95–107. See also the contemporary reports in *AZP* 51 (1895): 458–75, *If* 36 (1895): 65–7, 97–8, and the running reports during 1894 in the *Ärztliches Vereinsblatt* (1892).

45. See the *Reichstag* debates of 1897, 1898, and 1902 in Beyer, 450–530, 539–79, 586–602 and Otto Juliusberger, "Psychiatrische Tagesfragen," *AZP* 69 (1912): 122. Most important among the associations was the *Irrenrechtsreformverein* and the *Bund für Irrenfürsorge und Irrenrechts-Reform* established in 1897 and 1909 respectively.

46. The case was widely reported on in the German press. See Goldberg, "The Mellage Trial"; Kurella, "Das preussische Irrenwesen"; Teuscher, 98–112; and the anonymous publication *Die empörenden Zustände in dem Alexianer-Kloster Mariaberg* (Berlin: Weichert, [1895]). One observer described the case as psychiatry's "savior [*Retter in der Noth*]." W. Zenker, "Irrenanstalten und die medizinische Fachpresse," *Ärztliches Vereinsblatt* 22 (1895), 640.

47. Hugo Hoppe, "Die Verhandlungen über das preussische Irrenwesen im Abgeordneten Hause am 25. Juni 1895," *ZblNP* 18 (1895), 523 and Kurella, "Das preussische Irrenwesen," 338.

48. *ZblNP* 18 (1895): 334. Compare also Adolf Dannemann, "Zur Angelegenheit Scholz gegen Bodelschwingh," *ZblNP* 19 (1896): 51–3.

49. Kurella, "Das preussische Irrenwesen," 341. See also the criticisms of Siemens and Zinn, "Zur Frage der Reform," 819–20. On earlier calls for better state supervision, see Jastrowitz and

Bernhard Ascher's articles "Über die staatliche Beaufsichtigung der öffentlichen Irrenanstalten," "Die staatliche Beaufsichtigung der Privatirrenanstalten in Preussen," "Vorschläge zur Verbesserung der staatlichen Beaufsichtigung der Irrenanstalten in Preussen," all in *ZblNP* 15 (1892): 193–201, 246–252, 385–96, respectively.

50. On the measures, see the circular of 20 September 1895 to the *Oberpräsidenten* in Unger, 82–93, and Hoppe, "Die Verhandlungen," 522–8. The orders of 1895 were revised in several subsequent orders. Unger, 94–100.

51. See *Augsburger Abendzeitung,* 2 June 1902, and especially the case of Hamburg cited in *Frankfurter Zeitung,* 9 July 1899.

52. See *Augsburger Zeitung,* 2 June 1902, *Kölnische Zeitung,* 15 May 1902 as well as Beyer, 450–530 and 539–79; Max Hackl, *Das Anwachsen der Geisteskrankheiten in Deutschland* (Munich: Seitz & Schauer, 1904), 84ff; and Hermann Ortloff, *Zur Irrengesetzgebung* (Weimar: Böhlaus, 1897), 121–2. In the early 1890s the issue had been revived by F. Kretzschmar, *Die Unvollkommenheit der heutigen Psychiatrie und die Mangelhaftigkeit der deutschen Irrengesetzgebung* (Leipzig: Uhlig, 1891).

53. See the correspondence of the Königlich Bayerisches Staatsministerium des königlichen Hauses und des äusseren to the Königliche Gesandtschaft Berlin, 3 April 1897, BHStA, MInn 62037. On the position of the professional groups see *Offizieller Bericht,* 27 and 42–3.

54. *Frankfurter Zeitung,* 28 June 1902. See also Reichskanzler to Königlich Bayerisches Staatsministerium des königlichen Hauses und des äusseren, 24 May 1902, BHStA, MInn 62037.

55. Compare the different views of Laehr, "Die Bedeutung der Psychiatrie," 62; Fürstner, *Wie ist die Fürsorge,* 9; and Konrad Rieger, *Die Julius-Universität und das Julius-Spital* (Würzburg: Curt Kabitzsch, 1916), 135.

56. See Juliusberger, "Psychiatrische Tagesfragen," and *AZP* 69 (1912): 121–48. This strategy paid some small dividends when the government created a special section for psychiatric affairs within the medical division of the ministry of culture. See Siemens and Zinn, "Zur Frage der Reform," 827–8. The position was filled by Karl Moeli.

57. See Fürstner, *Wie ist die Fürsorge,* 58–9.

58. See the recommendations of Siemens and Zinn, "Zur Frage der Reform," 839 and Friedrich Jolly, *Über Irrthum und Irrsinn* (Berlin: Hirschwald, 1893).

59. See Feger, 244.

60. Siemens and Zinn, "Zur Frage der Reform," 839.

61. On psychiatric expectations see the resolution of the VdI at *AZP* 52 (1896): 839–41.

62. Otto Binswanger, "Zur Reform der Irrenfürsorge in Deutschland," *Sammlung klinischer Vorträge,* n. s., 148 (1896): 536.

63. Compare for example Jolly's arguments in *Über Irrthum und Irrsinn.*

64. The traditional term *Irre* was, however, not without its own advocates. See the spirited defense mounted by Max Fischer, *Die Benennung der Krankenhäuser für Geisteskranke* (Halle: Carl Marhold, 1905), 21–23 and the remarks of Max Brosius, "Der Narr und der Irre," *If* 25 (1883): 129–30. For some, the name *Irrenanstalt* had become problematic much earlier. See Kieser, *Elemente der Psychiatrik,* 277–8 and Laehr, *Die Heil- und Pflegeanstalten,* iv.

65. See Franz Nissl to Medical Faculty of the University of Heidelberg, 6 December 1906, 8547, GLA 235–3565 and Busse, "Schreber und Flechsig," 290.

66. Hugo v. Keyserlingk, "Die Jenaer Nervenklinik im Wandel der Zeit," *Wissenschaftliche Zeitschrift der Friedrich-Schiller-Universität Jena, Mathematisch-Naturwissenschaftliche Reihe* 2 (1952–3): 17. Even before the asylum in Jena had been renamed, Binswanger reported how admissions had risen thanks to the favorable public image of the asylum as a *psychiatrische Klinik.* Otto Binswanger, "Bericht über die Grossherzoglich Sächsische Landes-Irren-Heilanstalt in Jena," *CblAVT* 19 (1892): 189.

67. Rieger, *Die Julius-Universität,* 62–3.

68. See Johannes Bresler, "Bemerkung zu dem Vorschlag des Herrn Kollegen Lomer," *PNW* 11 (1909/10): 179. Bresler also wanted to modify annual hospital reports to make them more useful for public relations purposes. See Bresler, "Der wissenschaftlichen Betrieb," 225.

69. See E. Ritterhaus, *Irrsinn und Presse* (Jena: Fischer, 1913); Schindler, 127ff and 141ff; and Dieckhöfer, 107–9.

70. *AZP* 50 (1894): 348.

71. See the conference report in *DMW* 33 (1907): 1120.

72. Georg Lomer, "Ein psychiatrisches Nachrichtenbüro?" *PNW* 11 (1909/10): 177–9.

73. See *AZP* 69 (1912): 569 as well as the remarks of Edel at the meeting of the Berlin Psychiatric Society in 1911, *AZP* 69 (1912): 145.

74. See Wernicke's report of 17 September 1904 on the situation in Halle in GStA PK, IHA, Rep. 76Va, MgUMA, Sect. 8, Tit. X, Nr. 17, Bd. VI, Bl. 44.

75. See Fürstner, *Wie ist die Fürsorge*, 3–4. Several years earlier at a meeting of the VdI, Pelman had also recommended a more aggressive public relations offensive. See *AZP* 50 (1894): 348.

76. Fürstner, *Wie ist die Fürsorge*, 21. Others also suggested that restrictions on visiting be liberalized. See *ZblNP* 19 (1896): 579–84.

77. Fürstner, *Wie ist die Fürsorge*, 4.

78. Rieger, *Zusammenstellung*, 5. See also Eugen Hallervorden, "Klinische Psychologie, die Vorstufe der Psychohygiene," *DMW* 22 (1896): 656 and Meschede's motion at the meeting of the *Verein für wissenschaftliche Heilkunde* in 1898, *DMW* 25 (1899): 118.

79. See *AZP* 50 (1894): 873; Dannemann, "Zur Angelegenheit," 55; and Sommer, "Die Wärterfrage," 607–8. By contrast, alienists tended to stress better pay rather than more intensive observation as the most viable solution to the *Wärterfrage*. See Hoppe, "Zur Wärterfrage."

80. An early draft of revised regulations was published in 1891 and did not included psychiatry. This heightened psychiatrists' sense of urgency in the anti-psychiatry debates. See Eulner, *Die Entwicklung*, 262; *ZblNP* 21 (1898): 188–90; and Heinrich Kreuser, "Geschichtlicher Überblick über die Entwicklung des Irrenwesens in Württemberg," *MCblWAL* 72 (1902): 755.

81. On the different types of polyclinic, see *Encyclopädisches Wörterbuch der medicinischen Wissenschaften*, 1839 ed., s.v. "Klinik, medicinisch," 688 and Engstrom, "The Birth," 453–6.

82. Walther, *Über klinische Lehranstalten*, 22.

83. Westphal to MgUMA, 5 August 1871, UAHUB, Charité Direktion 850, Bl. 30–1. Polyclinical facilities were not restricted to university psychiatric clinics. However, they were far more prevalent there than in asylums. In Illenau an "ambulatory clinic" existed for patients in nearby towns. Roller, *Psychiatrische Zeitfragen*, 67. Plans for a *Volksheilstätte für Nervenkranke* also existed as early as 1891. See *AZP* 59 (1902): 579–81.

84. Binswanger, "Zum Andenken," 231.

85. Hitzig, *Bericht über die Wirksamkeit*, 17; also see his "Rede," 129.

86. Jolly, *Vorgeschichte*, 20 and 22.

87. See Fürstner to MInn, 30 September 1879, GLA 235–3565.

88. See Cramer, "Die preußischen Universitätskliniken." Polyclinics were also established Jena (1896), Göttingen (1901), Freiburg (1903), Marburg (1904), Leipzig (1906), Bonn (1908), and Erlangen (1910). The newly built clinics in Kiel (1901), Munich (1904), Greifswald (1906), and Königsberg (1913) all had polyclinical office hours. See Directorate of the Psychiatric Clinic Freiburg (Hoche) to MdJKU, 19 October 1903, GLA 235–7731; Westphal, Schulze and Hübner, 232, 248; *Münchner Neueste Nachrichten*, 13 November 1904, Nr. 531; BHStA, MK 11287, vol. III. On some of the contentious issues surrounding their construction, see Kraepelin, *Lebenserinnerungen*, 48–9; UAJ, L 216, Bl. 115–7; and Director of the Psychiatric Clinic to SMIKSA, 2 June 1910, BHStA MK 11488.

89. Flechsig, "Die psychiatrische und Nervenklinik," 198.

90. See John C. Burnham, *Jeliffe* (Chicago: University of Chicago Press, 1983), 52. Alfred Grotjahn reported that, because of the large volume of patients, polyclinical treatment in Berlin involved "schematized prescription writing" and "electrotherapy en masse." Alfred Grotjahn, *Erlebtes und Erstrebtes* (Berlin: Herbig, 1932), 86.

91. Cramer, "Die preußischen Universitätskliniken," 213.

92. Binswanger, "Zur Reform," 537.

93. For a survey of these methods, see Jakob Kläsi, "Über psychiatrisch-poliklinische Behandlungsmethoden," *ZgNP* 36 (1917): 431–50.

94. See Albert Eulenberg, "Der gegenwärtige Stand der Elektrotherapie in Theorie und Praxis," *BKW* 23 (1886): 181–4, 202–7.

95. Hitzig to Friedrich Althoff, 23 September 1887, GStA PK, IHA, Rep. 92, Althoff B, Nr. 73, Bd. 2, Bl. 41–2.

96. Fürstner, *Wie ist die Fürsorge*, 55.

97. Dannemann, *Die psychiatrische Klinik zu Giessen*, 100, 106.

98. Citations quoted in ibid., 107–8.

99. Dannemann, *Bau, Einrichtung und Organisation*, 172.

100. On Weygandt's appeal for a polyclinic, see "Denkschrift betr. der Eröffnung einer poliklinischen Institution für psychisch-nervöse Erkrankungen im Anschluß an die psychiatrische Universitätsklinik," [ca. February 1903], UAW, ARS 3294. Compare also Administration Committee to Academic Senate, 19 February 1909, Nr. 183, UAW, ARS 3294.

101. Reichardt to Medical Faculty, 13 July 1912, Nr. 19142, UAW, ARS 3294.

102. Although backed by the medical faculty, Reichardt's project received only tepid support from the ministry in Munich. See Administrative Commission to Academic Senate, 6 August 1912, Nr. 906 and SMIKSA to Academic Senate, 21 August 1912, Nr. 19142, both UAW, ARS 3294.

103. On Cramer see H. Vogt, "August Cramer," *AfPN* 50,2 (1912): iii–xi.

104. August Cramer to Curator of the University of Göttingen, 28 April 1901, GStA PK, IHA, Rep. 76Va, MgUMA, Sect. 6, Tit. X, Nr. 18, Bd. I. On the deficiencies of clinical psychiatry in Göttingen, see Engstrom, "The Birth," 465, note 186.

105. August Cramer to Curator of the University of Göttingen, 28 April 1901, GStA PK, IHA, Rep. 76Va, MgUMA, Sect. 6, Tit. X, Nr. 18, Bd. I.

106. Ibid. A statistical study of patients admitted to the polyclinic in 1902/3 has shown that over 90 percent returned home after their visit. A majority (49.6 percent) came from the "lower middle class." Some 50.8 percent of the polyclinical patients were diagnosed with either neurasthenia, hysteria, or other forms of neurosis. Silvia Siadek, "Psychiatrische Gesamtversorgung" (Med. diss., University of Göttingen, 1987), 23.

107. August Cramer, "Die Heil- und Unterrichtsanstalten für psychische und Nervenkranke," *Klinisches Jahrbuch* 14 (1905): 3.

108. Ibid., 12.

109. August Cramer, "Die Prophylaxe in der Psychiatrie," *BKW* 40 (1903): 421–2.

110. Cramer, "Heil- und Unterrichtsanstalten," 6.

111. Within the provincial asylum Cramer also had at his disposal an observation ward for adolescents (as of 1907) and a detention house for asocial psychiatric patients.

112. In this, universities were hurrying to catch up with civic hospitals. Because city hospitals were less constrained by the *Direktorialprinzip*, they were administratively much more integrated than their academic counterparts. What Cramer did in Göttingen was by no means unique among psychiatrists. To varying degrees, such institutional diversification—spreading across the boundary between the psychiatric clinic and society—was attempted by many others as well.

113. See Neumärker, 61.

114. See the description of the polyclinic given by the MdJKU, 22 March 1913, GLA 235-7731.

115. See Fürstner, *Wie ist die Fürsorge*, 9.

116. Ludwig Snell, "Naturwissenschaftliche und ärztliche Standpunkte dem Unterrichtswesen unserer Zeit gegenüber," *AZP* 30 (1874): 689–96.

117. See the meetings of the VdI in 1880 and in Frankfurt in 1881.

118. In their report, they reached the conclusion that the issue had not yet evolved to the point at which definitive conclusions could be reached. See Carl Westphal, "Gutachten," *Vierteljahresschrift für gerichtliche Medizin*, n.s., 40 (1884): 351–82.

119. See the announcement of the Ministry of Culture in *ZblNP* 13 (1890): 94–5 and Jerns, 262–6.

120. Rieger, *Zusammenstellung*, 8.

121. Ritter, 28–41.

122. See Richard Wetzell, *Inventing the Criminal*, Studies in Legal History, edited by Thomas

A. Green and Hendrik Hartog (Chapel Hill: University of North Carolina Press, 2000), 79 and Engstrom, "The Birth," 472, note 210.

123. Binswanger, *Die Psychiatrie*, 4–6.

124. On alcoholism and the temperance movement in Germany, see James S. Roberts, *Drink, Temperance, and the Working Class in Nineteenth-Century Germany* (Boston: Allen & Unwin, 1984).

125. See the discussions at its annual meeting in Frankfurt in 1881 and Jolly's paper to the *Verein* in 1891. *ZblNP* 14 (1891): 428–9. Other regional associations had dealt with the question and petitioned the imperial government on numerous occasions. The issue was heatedly debated, for example, in the psychiatric association of Berlin, which finally resolved to petition the German Reichstag in 1903. See Feger, 185–201.

126. *AZP* 34 (1878): 707–13, here 712.

127. Bonhoeffer, *Die Geschichte der Psychiatrie*, 23. See also the letters of Westphal to Charité Directorate, 5 February 1883, 16 October 1883, and 4 February 1886 at UAHUB, Charité Direktion 1034, Bl. 321, 329, and 343–4 respectively.

128. Compare also the earlier effort of Ewald Hecker, "Über das Verhältnis zwischen Nerven- und Geisteskrankheiten in Bezug auf ihre Behandlung in getrennten Anstalten," *DMW* 7 (1881): 121–5, 137–41.

129. Fürstner, *Wie ist die Fürsorge*, 40–1.

130. Westphal, Schulze and Hübner, 248.

131. On Kraepelin's efforts, see Eric J. Engstrom, "Emil Kraepelin," *HP* 2 (1991): 117–18. One of the more curious recommendations in this context was a suggestion by Ackerknecht that "psycho-diagnostic offices" be built to supplement the "deficiencies of official public control." Ackerknecht, "Psychodiagnostische Ämter," *Dokumente des Fortschritts* 7 (1914): 401–5.

132. Robert Sommer, "Die öffentliche Schlaf- und Ruhehallen bei der Internationalen Hygiene-Ausstellung in Dresden," *PNW* 13 (1911): 202–5; also see his "Die weitere Entwicklung der öffentlichen Ruhehallen," *Klinik für psychisch und nervöse Krankheiten* 6 (1911): 368.

133. Calls for *Nervenheilanstalten* grew in the 1890s. The first such asylum was opened in Berlin in the early 1890s by Heinrich Laehr and given the name "*Haus Schönow.*" On *Haus Schönow* see Renate Ulrike Amberger, "Haus Schönow" (Med. diss., Free University Berlin, 2001).

134. See Theodor Benda, *Öffentliche Nervenheilanstalten?* (Berlin: Hirschwald, 1891); Friedrich Jolly, "Über Heilstätten für Nervenkranke," *Zeitschrift für Krankenpflege* 20 (1898): 94–8; Julius Schwalbe, "Heilstätten für minderbemittelte Nervenkranke," *DMW* 24 (1898): 211–12; and Möbius. See also the meeting of the Psychiatric Association of the Rhine Province in 1899, especially the reports of Joseph Peretti, "Über den Stand der Frage der Einrichtung von Nervenheilstätten und die Wege zu ihrer Lösung," *AZP* 56 (1899): 567–76 and August Hoffmann, "Über die Notwendigkeit und Einrichtung von Volksheilstätten für Nervenkranke," *AZP* 56 (1899): 577–94.

135. *Augsburger Abendzeitung*, 8 November 1904.

136. Bickel, 71 and 74.

137. Cramer, "Die preußischen Universitätskliniken," 190.

138. Ewald Stier, *Die Bedeutung der Psychiatrie für den Kulturfortschritt* (Jena: Fischer, 1911), 11.

139. See Max Brosius, "Zeichen des beginnenden Irreseines," *If* 2 (1860): 1–6.

140. See Forel, *Rückblick*, 131.

141. See for example Stier, 29.

142. On the early debates in the 1860s on free will and determinism, see Schmiedebach, *Psychiatrie und Psychologie*, 55–71; Schindler, 152–67; Jerns, 306–40. More generally, see Wetzell.

143. On Lombroso's influence in Germany see Mariacarla Gadebusch Bondio, *Die Rezeption der kriminalanthropologischen Theorien von Cesare Lombroso in Deutschland von 1880–1914*, Abhandlungen zur Geschichte der Medizin und der Naturwissenschaften, eds. Rolf Winau and Heinz Müller-Dietz, vol. 70 (Husum: Matthiesen Verlag, 1995).

144. See Emil Kraepelin, *Die Abschaffung des Strafmaßes* (Stuttgart: Enke, 1880).

145. August Cramer, *Gerichtliche Psychiatrie* (Jena: Fischer, 1908), 18.

146. For a survey of debates on *verminderte Zurechnungsfähigkeit*, see C. E. Rautenberg, *Verminderte Schuldfähigkeit*, Kriminologische Schriftenreihe, vol. 85 (Heidelberg: Kriminalistik Verlag, 1984), especially chapters four and five, as well as Wetzell.

147. *Verhandlungen des Siebenundzwanzigsten Deutschen Juristentages (Innsbruck 1904)* (Berlin: Guttentag, 1905).

148. On Kraepelin's criminological theories, see Engstrom, "Der Verbrecher" and Wetzell.

149. *Verhandlungen des Siebenundzwanzigsten Deutschen Juristentages)*, 410.

150. Ibid., 411.

151. Thus the opinion of v. Birkemeyer as cited in Rautenberg, 65.

152. Ibid., 68.

153. See Cramer, *Gerichtliche Psychiatrie*, 54.

Conclusion

1. See the general argument in Blasius, *'Einfache Seelenstörungen'*.

2. See Witzler, 159.

3. Sachße & Tennstedt, 44–5.

4. Ibid., 31. Sachße & Tennstedt are referring here to public health. The same shifts were occurring in other branches of social welfare, such as child welfare. See Edward Ross Dickenson, *The Politics of German Child Welfare* (Harvard: Harvard University Press, 1996), 59.

5. See Beddies and Schmiedebach, as well as Gustav Kolb, *Vorschläge für die Ausgestaltung der Irrenfürsorge und für die Organisation der Irrenanstalten* (Halle: Carl Marhold, 1908). In the 1920s these programs were in part implemented, only to be exploited and then disbanded under National Socialism. See H. Haselbeck, "Zur Sozialgeschichte der 'Offenen Irren-Fürsorge,'" *Psychiatrischer Praxis* 12 (1985): 171–9.

6. Juliusburger, "Psychiatrische Tagesfragen," 123.

7. Remarking on the purpose and goals of psychiatric clinics, Carl Wernicke noted that the medical treatment of patients began with the infringement of their personal freedom. Given the high premium placed upon personal freedom, Wernicke therefore reasoned that the responsibility of psychiatrists was enormous. In other words, by virtue of their carceral authority, psychiatrists had become the true guarantors of individual rights and of the rule of law. Wernicke, "Zweck und Ziel," 218.

8. On this view of the relationship of law and discipline, see Jan Goldstein, "Framing Discipline with Law," *AHR* 98 (1993): 372 and Foucault, *Discipline and Punish*, 222.

9. Rudy Koshar, "Foucault and Social History," *AHR* 98 (1993): 361.

10. Rose, 46.

Bibliography

List of Archives and Libraries

Berlin: Geheimes Staatsarchiv Pruessischer Kulturbesitz (GStA PK)
*Files of the Ministry of Culture (IHA, Rep. 76Va, MgUMA): Sect. 2
(University of Berlin), Tit. IV, Nr. 46, Bd. II-V; Tit. VII, Nr. 16; Tit. X,
Nr. 43, Bd. I; Sect. 6 (University of Göttingen), Tit. X, Nr. 18, Bd. I;
Sect. 7 (University of Greifswald), Tit. X, Nr. 21, Bd. I; Sect. 8 (Uni-
versity of Halle), Tit. X, Nr. 17, Bd. I-IX; Tit. XV, Nr. 26, Bd. I; Tit.
XIX, Nr. 26, Bd. I-IV; Sect. 12 (University of Marburg), Tit. X, Nr. 14,
Bd. I.*
*Papers of Friedrich Althoff (IHA, Rep. 92, Althoff): B 30, Bd. II; B 73,
Bd. II, B 197, Bd. I-II; B 83, Bd. I; B 99, Bd. II; B 13; B 143, Bd. I.*

Universitätsarchiv der Humboldt Universität (UAHUB)
*Files of the Charité Directorate: 242, 374, 457, 498, 506, 621, 752, 753,
828, 849, 850, 1033, 1034, 1058, 1180, 1191, 1324.*
Files of the Medical Faculty: 238, 1380.

Staatsbibliothek Preussischer Kulturbesitz (Haus 2) (SBB2)
Darmstaedter Papers.

Bonn: Universitätsarchiv (UAB)
Files of the University Rector (Rektorat): A 3,20.
Files of the Medical Faculty (MF): 1102.

Erlangen: Universitätsarchiv (UAE)
I/9/57, II/1/53, IV/7/72.

Universitätsbibliothek (UBE)
*Manuscript Collections (MS): 2523 2n, 2523 3b, 2523 4a, 2523 2m,
2606, 2616.*

Freiburg: Staatsarchiv (StF)
Files of the Hochbauamt: 1050, 1052, 1724.

Stadtarchiv (StadtAF)
Files of the City Council: C2/4/1, C2/4/1.

Universitätsarchiv (UAF)
Files of the University Clinics (B1): 3235, 3236, 3239, 3241, 3243, 3244, 3245, 3246, 3247.

Giessen: Universitätsarchiv (UAG)
Robert Sommer Papers.

Halle: Universitätsarchiv (UAHa)
Files of the University Psychiatric Clinic: Rep. 6, Nr. 499, 1084, 1091.
Files of the Medical Faculty (I): Rep. 29, Nr. 186, 196, 199, 206, 208.

Heidelberg: Psychiatrische Universitätsklinik (PKUH)
Files of the Hospital Administration: I/1, I/2, I/4, I/7, I/8, I/10, I/11, II/1, II/2, II/4, II/5, II/6, II/7, II/8, II/10, III/1, IV/1, V/1, V/5, V/6, V/7, V/8, VI/1, VII/1, VIII/2, VIII/3, VIII/4, VIII/5, VIII/6, IX/1, X/1, XII/1, XII/2, XIII/1, XV/4, XVI/1, XVI/3, XVI/4, XVI/5, XVIII/2.

Universitätsarchiv (UAH)
Files of the Medical Faculty: 1890/91 I, III, 4a, Nr. 136; 1892/93 I, III, 4a, Nr. 152; 1903/4 I, III, 4a, Nr. 174a and 174b; H III 682/1; XXXV/19, IX, 13, Nr. 99; XXXV/19a, IX, 13, Nr. 100.
Acta Personalia: A 219.

Jena: Universitätsarchiv (UAJ)
Files of the Medical Faculty: BA 15, BA 132, BA 420, BA 424, BA 425, BA 1345, C 390, L 121, L 200–3, L 216–19, L 230, L 232, L 236–9, L 400.

Karlsruhe: Badisches Generallandesarchiv (GLA)
Files of the Ministry of Justice, Culture, and Education (235–): 745, 746, 747, 748, 749, 750, 751, 3563, 3565, 3569, 3570, 3571, 3588, 3854, 3899, 3900, 3902, 4524, 4531, 4532, 4533, 4858, 7674, 7675, 7689, 7692, 7696, 7698, 7701, 7707, 7709, 7710, 7712, 7715, 7729, 7731, 30351, 30353, 30354, 30358, 30360, 30363, 30368, 30373, 30375.
Papers of Willy Hellpach (69 N Hellpach/): 123a, 155, 174, 204, 206, 240, 241, 277, 281, 282, 284, 285, 286, 287, 289, 292, 296.

Munich: Bayerisches Hauptstaatsarchiv (BHStA)
Files of the Ministry of Culture (MK): 11149, 11158, 11163, 11167, 11168, 11243, 11244, 11245, 11248, 11249, 11250, 11285, 11287, 11288, 11488, 15469, 17654, 17682, 17704, 17810, 17880, 17914, 19286, 19287, 39588, 39660, 39661, 40514.
Files of the Ministry of the Interior (MInn): 60633, 60800, 61378, 61380, 61955, 62037, 62041, 62042, 62043, 62044, 62045, 62046, 62053a, 62054, 62059, 62060, 62062, 73623.
Files of the Ministry of Justice (MJu): 16956.

Historisches Archiv des Max-Planck-Instituts für Psychiatrie (MPI)
Kraepelin Papers.

Staatsarchiv (StM)
Files of the Police Directorate (Pol. Dir.): 1328, 1362, 1832, 3524, 4342 I-IV, 4475, 4559, 4560, 4561, 4590, 4595, 4596, 5141.

Stadtarchiv (StadtAM)
Bürgermeister und Rat (BuR): 310/4, 867, 799, 865, 869, 908, 1063/1, 1063/2, 1436.

Universitätsarchiv (UAM)
Files of the Academic Senate: E II 621, E II N, Sen. 218, Sen. 307, Sen. 307a, Sen. 307/1.
Files of the University Administration (VA): AI 21c, AI 21d, AI 21f, AII 33.1, AII 33.5, AII 33.4, AII 33.8, AII 33.10, AII 33.11, AII 33.17.

Universitätsbibliothek (UBM)
Kuhn Papers.

Tübingen: Universitätsarchiv (UAT)
Papers of Max Wundt: 228/17.

Universitätsbibliothek (UBT)
Manuscript Collections: Md 939 22.

Würzburg: Archiv des Juliusspitals Würzburg (AJW)
Nr. 3963, Nr. 23072, Nr. 23566.

Universitätsarchiv (UAW)
Files of the Academic Senate (ARS): 166, 432, 497, 567, 738, 3292, 3293, 3294.

Primary Sources

Ackerknecht. "Psychodiagnostische Ämter." *Dokumente des Fortschritts* 7 (1914): 401–5.

Alt, Konrad. "Videant consules!" *PNW* 7 (1905/6): 389–91, 397–400, 410–414.

Alzheimer, A[lois]. "25 Jahre Psychiatrie: Ein Rückblick anlässlich des 25jährigen Jubiläums von Professor Dr. Emil Sioli als Direktor der Frankfurter Irrenanstalt." *AfPN* 52 (1913): 853–66.

Anonymous. "Zur Regelung der Prüfungen für die Aerzte." *Preußische Jahrbücher* 23 (1869): 230–3.

Anton, G[abriel]. "Nachruf auf E[duard] Hitzig anlässlich der Aufstellung des Hitzig-Denkmales in der Hallenser Klinik für Geistes- und Nervenkranke." *AfPN* 54,1 (1914): 1–7.

Arndt, Rudolf. *Die Psychiatrie und das medicinische Staats-Examen.* Berlin: Reimer, 1880.

Arnsperger. "Über Irrenversorgung in dem Grossherzogthum Baden." *Ärztliche Mitteilungen aus und für Baden* 45 (1891): 133–40.

Ascher, [Bernhard]. "Über die staatliche Beaufsichtigung der öffentlichen Irrenanstalten." *ZblNP* 15 (1892): 193–201.

——. "Die staatliche Beaufsichtigung der Privatirrenanstalten in Preussen." *ZblNP* 15
(1892): 246–252.

——. "Vorschläge zur Verbesserung der staatlichen Beaufsichtigung der Irrenanstalten
in Preussen." *ZblNP* 15 (1892): 385–96.

"Aus der Provinz." *AZP* 24 (1867): 829–35.

Benda, Theodor. *Öffentliche Nervenheilanstalten?* Berlin: Hirschwald, 1891.

"Bericht über die Versammlung deutscher Irrenärzte zu Eisenach am 12. und 13. September 1860." *AZP* 17 (1860): 3–19.

"Bericht über die Versammlung deutscher Irrenärzte zu Heppenheim im September."
AZP 24 (1867): 697–720.

"Bericht über die Versammlung in Landau und Speyer vom 11. bis 20. September
1861." *AZP* 18 (1861): 790–873.

"Bericht über die Versammlung des deutschen Vereins der Irrenärzte in Hildesheim im
September 1867." *AZP* 22 (1865): 331–51.

Beyer, Bernh[ard]. *Die Bestrebungen zur Reform des Irrenwesens. Material zu einem
Reichs-Irrengesetz für Laien und Ärzte.* Halle: Marhold, 1912.

Bickel, Adolf. *Wie studiert man Medizin? Der Bildungsgang des Arztes auf Grund der
Studienpläne und Prüfungsbestimmungen.* Stuttgart: Wilhelm Violet, 1906.

Billroth, Theodor. *The Medical Sciences in the German Universities. A Study in the
History of Civilization.* New York: Macmillan, 1924.

Binswanger, O[tto]. "Zum Andenken an Carl Westphal." *DMW* 16 (1890): 205–7,
227–31.

——. "Bericht über die Grossherzoglich Sächsische Landes-Irren-Heilanstalt in Jena für
die Jahre 1880–1890." *CblAVT* 19 (1892): 185–99.

——. "Die Lehraufgaben der psychiatrischen Klinik: Rede gehalten beim Antritte der
ordentlichen Professur in der Universitätsaula zu Jena." *Klinisches Jahrbuch* 4
(1892): 45–61.

——. *Die Psychiatrie als obligatorischer Unterrichts- und Prüfungsgegenstand. Sepa-
ratvotum zur Aufklärung und zur Widerlegung der Denkschrift des Herrn Geh.
Hofrath Prof. Dr. Schultze.* Jena: Frommann, 1893.

——. "Zur Reform der Irrenfürsorge in Deutschland." *Sammlung klinischer Vorträge,*
n. s., 148 (1896): 529–62.

——. *Zur Revision der medizinischen Prüfungen.* Jena: Pohle, 1896.

Birnbaum, Karl. "Geschichte der psychiatrischen Wissenschaft." In *Handbuch der
Geisteskrankheiten,* edited by Oswald Bumke, vol. 1, 11–49. Berlin: Springer, 1928.

Börner, Paul. "Die Zukunft der wissenschaftlichen Hygiene in Deutschland." *Preußische Jahrbücher* 56 (1885): 234–66.

Bonhoeffer, Karl. "Psychiatrische und Nervenklinik." In *Festschrift zur Feier des hun-
dertjährigen Bestehens der Universität Breslau,* edited by Georg Kaufmann.
2:319–22. Breslau: F. Hirt, 1911.

——. *Die Geschichte der Psychiatrie in der Charité im 19. Jahrhundert.* Berlin:
Springer, 1940.

Bopp. "Antrag des Geh.-Med.-Raths und Prof. Dr. Ritgen zu Giessen auf dem Grossh-
erz. Hessischen Landtage der Jahre 1835/1836 wegen Errichtung eines Hospitals für
heilbare Irre an der Landesuniversität." *Jahrbuch der gesammten Staatsarzneikunde*
3 (1837): 534–65.

Brandau. "Wie sind Geisteskranke in ihren häuslichen Verhältnissen zu behandeln." *If* 3 (1861): 38–43.

Bresler, [Johannes]. "Der wissenschaflichen Betrieb der öffentlichen Irrenanstalten." *PNW* 11 (1909–10): 223–6, 263–6, 370–2, 385–6, 434–5, 457–8.

——. "Bemerkung zu dem Vorschlag des Herrn Kollegen Lomer." *PNW* 11 (1909/10): 179.

——. *Ausgewählte Kapitel der Verwaltung öffentlicher Irrenanstalten.* Halle: Carl Marhold, 1910.

Brosius, [Kaspar Max]. "Über die Vorutheile gegen Irre und Irrenanstalten." *If* 1 (1859): 105–10.

——. "Zeichen des beginnenden Irreseins." *If* 2 (1860): 1–6.

——. "Wieder ein Wort über die Vorurtheile über die Irren-Anstalten." *If* 2 (1860): 9–19.

——. " 'Der Umschwung in der Psychiatrie' nach dem Vorworte zu Griesinger's Archiv für Psychiatrie und Nervenkrankheiten." *If* 10 (1868): 17–34.

——. "Über Irrenanstalten und deren Weiterentwicklung in Deutschland." *If* 10 (1868): 81–123.

——. "Soll man noch isolieren." *If* 15 (1873): 44–8.

——. "Der Narr und der Irre." *If* 25 (1883): 129–30.

Brunn, Walter. *Das deutsche Medizinische Zeitschriftenwesen seit der Mitte des 19. Jahrhunderts.* Berlin: Idra, 1925.

Buschan, [Georg]. Review of "Läßt sich eine Zunahme der Geisteskranken feststellen?" by L[udwig] W[ilhelm] Weber. In *ZgNP* 3 (1911): 109–110.

Clarke, C. K. "Notes on Some of the Psychiatric Clinics and Asylums of Germany." *The American Journal of Insanity* 65 (1908–9): 357–76.

Conolly, John. *Die Behandlung der Irren ohne mechanischen Zwang.* Translated by M[ax] Brosius. Lahr: M. Schauenburg, 1860.

Cramer, A[ugust]. *Über die ausserhalb der Schule liegenden Ursachen der Nervosität der Kinder.* Sammlung von Abhandlungen aus dem Gebiete der pädagogischen Psychologie und Physiologie, edited by H. Schiller and Th[eodor] Ziehen, vol. 2,5. Berlin: Reuther and Reichard, 1899.

——. "Die Prophylaxe in der Psychiatrie." *BKW* 40 (1903): 421–2.

——. *Über Gemeingefährlichkeit vom ärztlichen Standpunkte aus.* Halle: Marhold, 1905.

——. "Die Heil- und Unterrichtsanstalten für psychische und Nervenkranke in Göttingen unter besonderer Berücksichtigung des Sanatoriums 'Rasemühle.' " *Klinisches Jahrbuch* 14 (1905): 1–40.

——. *Die Nervosität, ihre Ursachen, Erscheinungen und Behandlung. Für Studierende und Ärzte.* Jena: Fischer, 1906.

——. *Gerichtliche Psychiatrie: Ein Leitfaden für Mediziner und Juristen.* Jena: Fischer, 1908.

——. "Die preußischen Universitätskliniken für psychische und Nervenkrankheiten." *Klinisches Jahrbuch* 24 (1910): 185–226.

——. "Die weitere Entwicklung der Anstalten für psychische und Nervenkrankheiten in Göttingen unter besonderer Berücksichtigung der Aufnahmestation, des Verwahrungshauses für unsoziale Geisteskranke und der neuen Villa für Patienten I. Klasse im Sanatorium Rasemühle," *Klinisches Jahrbuch* 22 (1910): 339–74.

——. "Bericht an das Landesdirektorium über die psychiatrisch-neurologische Untersuchung der schulentlassenen Fürsorgezöglinge im Frauenheim bei Himmelsthür vor Hildesheim, Magdalenium bei Hannover, Moorburg bei Freistadt, Stephansstift bei

Hannover, Kästorf bei Gifhorn und Kalandshof bei Rotenburg," *AZP* 67 (1910): 493–519.

Damerow, Heinrich. "Über Irrenheilanstalten." *Medicinische Zeitung* 2 (1833): 131–3.

——. "Über Irrenpflegeanstalten." *Medicinische Zeitung* 2 (1833): 217–20.

——. *Über die relative Verbindung der Irren-Heil- und Pflege-Anstalten in historisch-kritischer, so wie in moralischer, wissenschaftlicher und administrativer Beziehung. Eine staatsarzneiwissenschaftliche Abhandlung.* Leipzig: Otto Wigand, 1840.

——. "P[ro] M[emoria] An Deutschlands Irrenärzte, über die Herausgabe einer allgemeinen Zeitschrift für Psychiatrie, mit besonderer Berücksichtigung der Irrenanstalten und öffentlichen Irrenangelegenheiten." *Medicinische Zeitung* 10 (1841): 33–42.

——. "Einleitung." *AZP* 1 (1844): i–xlviii.

——. "Einladung an die Irrenanstalts-Directoren zur Benützung gemeinschaftlicher Schemata zu den tabellarischen Übersichten." *AZP* 1 (1844): 430–40.

——. "Die Zeitschrift: Ein Blick rückwärts und vorwärts." *AZP* 3 (1846): 1–32.

——. "Denkschrift der Zustand der Irren-Abtheilung in der Königl. Charité-Heil-Anstalt und die Nothwendigkeit des Neubaues einer Irren-Heil- und Pflege-Anstalt für die Residenzen Berlin und Potsdam betreffend." *AZP* 6 (1849): 49–78.

——. "Ein Blick über die Lage von Irrenanstaltsfragen der Gegenwart." *AZP* 19 (1862): 143–89.

Dannemann, Adolf. "Zur Angelegenheit Scholz gegen Bodelschwingh." *ZblNP* 19 (1896): 51–6.

——. *Die psychiatrische Klinik zu Giessen: Ein Beitrag zur praktischen Psychiatrie.* Berlin: S. Karger, 1899.

——. *Bau, Einrichtung und Organisation psychiatrischer Stadtasyle: Betrachtungen über eine zeitgemässe Verbesserung der Fürsorge für Geistes- und Nervenkranke.* Halle: Carl Marhold, 1901.

——. "Psychologie und Psychotherapie im Polizeiwesen." *MMW* 55 (1908): 122.

de Boor, Wolfgang. *Psychiatrische Systematik: Ihre Entwicklung in Deutschland seit Kahlbaum.* Berlin: Springer, 1954.

Die empörenden Zustände in dem Alexianer-Kloster Mariaberg: Ein ausführlicher Bericht über die soeben beendeten Gerichtsverhandlungen in Aachen. Berlin: Weichert, [1895].

"Die Irrenanstalten in Bayern." *Ärztliches Intelligenzblatt* 2 (1855): 458–60.

"Die psychiatrische Sektion auf der 42. Naturforscher-Versammlung zu Dresden." *Vierteljahrsschrift für Psychiatrie* 2 (1868): 238–9.

"Die Versammlung in Heppenheim." *AZP* 24 (1867): 826–9.

"Drei Nekrologe und einige Anschuldigungen." *AZP* 26 (1869): 265–70.

Dressler. "Das Studium der Medicin und die Examenordnung für Aerzte." *Aerztliche Mittheilungen aus und für Baden* 45 (1891): 183–8.

Du Bois-Reymond, Emil. *Reden.* Edited by Estelle Du Bois-Reymond, 2 vols. 2d ed. Leipzig: Veit & Comp., 1912.

Engelken, Friedrich. "Über die Prophylaxis der Geistesstörungen." *AZP* 10 (1853): 353–95.

Erb, Wilhelm. "Über die nächsten Aufgaben der Nervenpathologie." *Deutsche Zeitschrift für Nervenheilkunde* 1 (1891): 1–12.

——. "Rückblick und Ausblick auf die Entwicklung und die Zukunft der deutschen Nervenpathologie." *Deutsche Zeitschrift für Nervenheilkunde* 35 (1908): 1–17.

Erlenmeyer, A[dolf Albrecht]. *Die Verhandlungen der 'deutschen Gesellschaft für Psy-*

chiatrie und gerichtliche Psychologie' und der 'Sektion für Staatsarzneikunde und Psychiatrie.' Neuwied: Strüder, 1857.

——. "Die Versammlung in Carlsruhe." *CblDGPgP* 5 (1858): 161–7.

——. "Rechenschaftsbericht über die ersten 5 Jahre der Gesellschaft." *CblDGPgP* 5 (1858): 145–8.

——. "Bericht über die 51. Versammlung deutscher Naturforscher und Aerzte zu Cassel." *ZblNP* 1 (1878): 257–64.

Esse, [Carl Heinrich]. "Geschichtliche Nachrichten über das königliche Charité-Krankenhaus zu Berlin." *Annalen des Charité-Krankenhauses zu Berlin* 1 (1850): 1–45.

Eulenberg, A[lbert]. "Der gegenwärtige Stand der Elektrotherapie in Theorie und Praxis." *BKW* 23 (1886): 181–4, 202–7.

Eulenberg, Hermann. *Das Medicinalwesen in Preussen.* 3d ed. Berlin: Hirschwald, 1874.

Eulenburg, Franz. *Die Frequenz der deutschen Universitäten von ihrer Gründung bis zur Gegenwart.* Leipzig: Teubner, 1904.

Fischer, Max. "Die Irrenfürsorge in Baden." *PNW* 4 (1902/3): 89–92, 102–4 and 111–6.

——. *Die Benennung der Krankenhäuser für Geisteskranke.* Halle: Carl Marhold, 1905.

Flechsig, Paul. *Die Leitungsbahnen im Gehirn und Rückenmark des Menschen, auf Grund entwicklungsgeschichtlicher Untersuchungen dargestellt.* Leipzig: Engelmann, 1876.

——. *Die Irrenklinik der Universität Leipzig und ihre Wirksamkeit in den Jahren 1882–1886.* Leipzig: Veit & Comp., 1888.

——. *Gehirn und Seele.* Leipzig: Veit, 1894.

——. "Die psychiatrische und Nervenklinik." In *Festschrift zur Feier des 500 jährigen Bestehens der Universität Leipzig,* by the Rector and Senate [of the University of Leipzig], 3:189–200. Leipzig: Hirzel, 1909.

Flemming, [Carl Friedrich]. *Die Irren-Heil-Anstalt Sachsenberg bei Schwerin im Großherzogtum Mecklenberg: Nachrichten über ihre Entstehung, Einrichtung, Verwaltung und bisherige Wirksamkeit.* Schwerin: Kürschner, 1833.

——. "Über Prophylaxis der Geisteskrankheiten." *ZBHkS* 1 (1838): 293–310.

——. "Über Notwendigkeit, Nutzen und Benutzung der Irren-Heilanstalten." *ZBHkS* 1 (1838): 702–16.

——. "Was heisst Fortschritt in der Psychiatrie und welches ist sein Weg." *AZP* 16 (1859): 176–181.

——. *Pathologie und Therapie der Psychosen.* Berlin: Hirschwald, 1859.

——. "Gesetze und Verordnungen in Deutschland betreffs Geisteskranken." *AZP* 19, supplement (1862).

——. "Über einige der nächsten Aufgaben der Psychiatrie." *AZP* 21, supplement (1864): 49–58.

——. Review of *Zur Kenntniss der heutigen Psychiatrie in Deutschland. Eine Streitschrift gegen die Broschüre des Sanitätsraths Dr. Laehr in Zehlendorf "Fortschritt?–Rückschritt!"* by W[ilhelm] Griesinger. In *AZP* 25 (1868): 364–6.

Flemming, C[arl] and M[aximilian] Jacobi. "Über die Errichtung einer Irrenanstalt im Großherzogthum Baden." *ZBHkS* 1 (1838): 717–42.

Flexner, Abraham. *Medical Education in Europe: A Report to the Carnegie Foundation for the Advancement of Teaching.* Boston: Merrymount Press, 1912.

Förster, A. *Denkschrift über das zwischen dem Charité-Krankenhause und der Stadt Berlin bestehende Rechtsverhältniß.* Berlin: Reichsdruckerei, 1892.

Forel, August. *Rückblick auf mein Leben.* Zurich: Europa Verlag, 1935.

Frerichs, Fr[iedrich] Theod[or]. "Einleitung." *Zeitschrift für klinische Medicin* 1 (1880): i-viii.

Friedreich, J. B. *Systematische Literatur der ärztlichen und gerichtlichen Psychologie.* Berlin: Ensslin, 1833; reprint, Amsterdam: E. J. Bonset, 1968.

Fürstner, [Karl]. "Die Psychiatrie in der neuen Prüfungsordnung." *BKW* 20 (1883): 477–8.

———. *Über Irrenkliniken an der Hand eines Berichtes über den Betrieb der Universitäts-Irrenklinik zu Heidelberg während der Jahre 1878–1883.* Heidelberg: J. Hörning, 1884.

———. *Wie ist die Fürsorge für Gemütskranke von Aerzten und Laien zu Fördern?* Berlin: Karger, 1900.

———. "Neuropathologie und Psychiatrie." *AZP* 38 (1904): 895–907.

Gaupp, Robert. "Die Psychiatrie als Lehr- und Prüfungsgegenstand." *MMW* 50 (1903): 1738–9.

———. *Wege und Ziele psychiatrischer Forschung: Eine akademische Antrittsvorlesung.* Tübungen: H. Laupp, 1907.

Gerlach, Joseph. *Die Photographie als Hülfsmittel mikroskopischer Forschung.* Leipzig: Engelmann, 1863.

Gerstenberg, [Erich]. "Nekrolog." *AZP* 49 (1893): 320–9.

Griesinger, Wilhelm. *Die Pathologie und Therapie der psychischen Krankheiten.* 1st-3d ed.. Stuttgart: Krabbe, 1861; 3d ed. reprint, Amsterdam: Bonset, 1964.

———. "Vorwort." *AfPN* 1 (1868): iii-viii.

———. "Über Irrenanstalten und deren Weiter-Entwicklung in Deutschland." *AfPN* 1 (1868): 8–43.

———. "Psychiatrische Congresse und Versammlungen." *AfPN* 1 (1868): 182–99.

———. "Weiteres über psychiatrische Cliniken." *AfPN* 1 (1868): 500–4.

———. *Zur Kenntniss der heutigen Psychiatrie in Deutschland. Eine Streitschrift gegen die Broschüre des Sanitätsraths Dr. Laehr in Zehlendorf: 'Fortschritt?—Rückschritt!'* Leipzig: Otto Wigand, 1868.

———. *Gesammelte Abhandlungen.* Edited by C. A. Wunderlich. Berlin: Hirschwald, 1872.

Grober, J. "Wissenschaftliche und Unterrichtsräume in Krankenanstalten." In *Ergebnisse und Fortschritte des Krankenhauswesens: Jahrbuch für Bau, Einrichtung und Betrieb von Krankenanstalten,* edited by E. Dietrich and J. Grober, 3:33–44. Jena: Fischer, 1920.

Grotjahn, Alfred. *Erlebtes und Erstrebtes: Erinnerungen eines sozialistischen Arztes.* Berlin: Herbig, 1932.

Gudden, Bernhard. *Bernhard von Gudden's gesammelte und hinterlassene Abhandlungen.* Edited by H[ubert] Grashey. Wiesbaden: Bergman, 1889.

———. "Über die Einrichtung von sogenannten Überwachungsstationen." *AZP* 42 (1886): 454–8.

Guttstadt, Albert. "Die Geisteskranken in den Irrenanstalten während der Zeit von 1852 bis 1872 und ihre Zählung im ganzen Staat am 1. Dezember 1871, nebst Vorschlägen zur Gewinnung einer deutschen Irrenstatistik." *Zeitschrift des königlich preussischen statistischen Bureau* 14 (1874): 201–248h.

Guttstadt, A. "Das Civil-Medicinalwesen." In *Das deutsche Medizinalwesen,* edited by S. Guttmann, 138–43. Leipzig: Thieme, 1887.

Hackl, Max. *Das Anwachsen der Geisteskrankheiten in Deutschland.* Munich: Seitz & Schauer, 1904.

Hagen, F[riedrich] W[ilhelm]. "Psychiatrie und Anatomie." *AZP* 12 (1855): 1–63.

Hallervorden, Eugen. "Klinische Psychologie, die Vorstufe der Psychohygiene." *DMW* 22 (1896): 656–9.

Hartmann, Arthur. *Die Reform des medicinischen Unterrichtes: Gesammelte Abhandlungen.* Berlin: Fischer, 1894.

Hecker, Ewald. "Zur Begründung des klinischen Standpunktes in der Psychiatrie." *Archiv für pathologische Anatomie und Physiologie und für klinische Medizin* 52 (1871): 203–18.

——. "Die Hebephrenie: Ein Beitrag zur klinischen Psychiatrie." *Archiv für pathologische Anatomie und Physiologie und für klinische Medizin* 52 (1871): 394–429.

——. "Zur klinischen Diagnostik und Prognostik der psychischen Krankheiten." *AZP* 33 (1877): 602–620.

——. "Über das Verhältnis zwischen Nerven- und Geisteskrankheiten in Bezug auf ihre Behandlung in getrennten Anstalten." *DMW* 7 (1881): 121–5, 137–41.

Heermann, G[eorg]. "Über das Studium der psychischen Medicin auf Universitäten, als das nächste Erforderniss ihrer Förderung." *Medicinische Annalen* 3 (1837): 443–96.

Heimann, Caesar. *Bericht über Sanitätsrath Dr. Karl Edel's Asyl für Geisteskranke zu Charlottenburg 1869–1894.* Berlin: Hirschwald, 1895.

Heinroth, Johann Christian August. "Ein Wort über Irren-Anstalten." Afterword to *Über die Verrücktheit: ihren Sitz; ihre Zufälle; ihre Ursachen; ihren Gang und ihre Ausgänge; ihre Verschiedenheit vom hitzigen Delirium; ihre Behandlung; nebst Resultaten von Leichen-Oeffnungen,* by M. Georget, 410–18. Translated by Johann Christian August Heinroth. Leipzig: Weidmann, 1821.

Hertwig, Oscar. *Der anatomische Unterricht. Vortrag beim Antritt der anatomischen Professur an der Universität Jena am 28. Mai 1881.* Jena: Fischer, 1881.

Hess, Eduard. "Zum fünfzigjährigen Bestehen der Kahlbaum'schen Nervenheilanstalt zu Görlitz." *ZblNP* 28 (1905): 770–2.

Hitzig, Eduard. "Über den relativen Werth elektrischer Heilmethoden." *Tageblatt der 45. Versammlung deutscher Naturforscher und Ärzte in Leipzig* 45 (1872): 161–4.

——. "Weitere Untersuchungen zur Physiologie des Gehirn." *BKW* 9 (1872): 504–5.

——. *Untersuchungen über das Gehirn. Abhandlungen physiologischen und pathologischen Inhaltes.* Berlin: Hirschwald, 1874.

——. "Über Produktion von Epilepsie durch experimentelle Verletzung der Hirnrinde." In *Physiologische und klinische Untersuchungen über das Gehirn,* 63–72. Berlin: Hirschwald, 1904 [1874].

——. *Ziele und Zwecke der Psychiatrie.* Zurich: Orel Füssli, 1876.

——. "Über den heutigen Stand der Frage von der Localisation im Grosshirn." *Sammlung Klinischer Vorträge* 112 (1876): 963–78.

——. "Über subnormale Temperaturen bei Paralytiker." *BKW* 21 (1884): 537–40.

——. "Die neue Irren- und Nerven-Klinik in Halle a/S." *BKW* 22 (1885): 294.

——. *Bericht über die Wirksamkeit der Universitäts psychiatrischen und Nervenklinik zu Halle a.S. für die Jahre 1885/86 und 1886/87.* Halle: Gebauer-Schwetschke'sche Buchdruckerei, 1887.

——. "Neubau der psychiatrischen und Nervenklinik für die Universität Halle a. S." *Klinisches Jahrbuch* 2 (1890): 383–405.

——. "Rede gehalten zur Einweihung der Psychiatrischen und Nervenklinik zu Halle a.S." *Klinisches Jahrbuch* 3 (1891): 112–30.

——. *Physiologische und klinische Untersuchungen über das Gehirn.* Berlin: Hirschwald, 1904.

Hitzig, Eduard [and Gustav Fritsch]. "Über die elektrische Erregbarkeit des Grosshirns" [1870]. In *Physiologische und klinische Untersuchungen über das Gehirn,* 8–35. Berlin: Hirschwald, 1904.

Hoche, Alfred E. *Die Aufgaben des Arztes bei der Einweisung Geisteskranker in die Irrenanstalt.* Halle: Carl Marhold, 1900.

——. "Vorschläge zur Schaffung einer statistischen Centralstelle." *AZP* 59 (1902): 724–9.

——. "Eintheilung und Benennung der Psychosen mit Rücksicht auf die Anforderungen der ärztlichen Prüfung." *AfPN* 38 (1904): 1070–80.

——. *Jahresringe: Innenansicht eines Menschenalters.* Munich: Lehmann, 1934.

Hoffmann, Adolf. "Die neue Prüfungsordnung für Aerzte." *Aerztliches Vereinsblatt* 7 (1878): 93–9.

Hoffmann, August. "Über die Notwendigkeit und Einrichtung von Volksheilstätten für Nervenkranke." *AZP* 56 (1899): 577–94.

Hoppe, Hugo. "Die Wärterfrage." *ZblNP* 15 (1892): 529–40.

——. "Die Verhandlungen über das preussische Irrenwesen im Abgeordneten Hause am 25. Juni 1895." *ZblNP* 18 (1895): 522–8.

Huppert, Max. "Über die beste Art der öffentlichen Irrenfürsorge in Deutschland." *Schmidt's Jahrbücher* 144 (1869): 321–47.

Humboldt, Wilhelm von. "Über die innere und äussere Organisation der höheren wissenschaftlichen Anstalten in Berlin." In *Die Idee der deutschen Universität,* edited by Ernst Anrich, 375-86. Darmstadt: WBG, 1956 [1810].

Ideler, [Carl Wilhelm]. "Necrolog." *Medicinische Zeitung* 1 (1832): 67.

——. "Über psychiatrische Klinik." *Medicinische Zeitung* 2 (1833): 99–101.

——. "Über den Zweck der psychiatrischen Klinik." *CA* 1 (1850): 96–146.

——. "Über die Methode der psychiatrischen Klinik." *CA* 1 (1850): 391–435.

Ideler, C[arl Ludwig]. "Mitteilungen über die Bewegung an der städtischen Irrenanstalt von Berlin für das Jahr 1875." *AZP* 34 (1878): 243–5.

——. "Geschichtliche Entwicklung der städtischen Irrenpflege." In *Die städtische Irren-Anstalt zu Dalldorf,* edited by the Berlin Magistrate, 8–12. Berlin: Springer, 1883.

J[acobi, Maximilian]. "Irrenanstalten." In *Encyclopädisches Wörterbuch der medicinischen Wissenschaften,* edited by D. W. H. Busch et al. Berlin: Veit et Comp., 1839.

——. *Über die Anlegung und Einrichtung von Irren-Heilanstalten mit ausführlicher Darstellung der Irren-Heilanstalt in Siegberg.* Berlin: Reimer, 1834.

Jaspers, Karl. *Allgemeine Psychopathologie: Ein Leitfaden für Studierende, Ärzte und Psychologen.* Berlin: Springer, 1913.

——. "Historisches über Psychopathologie als Wissenschaft." In *Allgemeine Psychopathologie.* Berlin: Springer, 1948.

——. "Der Arzt im technischen Zeitalter." In *Wahrheit und Bewahrung: Philosophieren für die Praxis.* Munich: Piper, 1983.

Jastrowitz, [Moritz]. "Über die Staatsaufsicht über die Irrenanstalten, ihre Nothwendigkeit und Ausführungsart." *AZP* 34 (1878): 713–24.

Jessen, P[eter Willers]. "Über die in Beziehung auf Geistes- und Gemüthskranke herrschende Vorurtheile." In *Amtlicher Bericht über die 24. Versammlung deutscher Naturforscher und Aerzte in Kiel im September 1846,* edited by G. A. Michaelis and H. F. Scherk, 56–61. Kiel: Akademische Buchhandlung, 1847.

——. *Das Asyl Hornheim, die Behörden und das Publicum.* Kiel: Homann, 1862.

——. "Vorschläge zu gesetzlichen Bestimmungen in Beziehung auf die Aufnahme von Geisteskranken in Irrenanstalten." *AZP* 24 (1867): 659–60.

Jessen, P[eter Willers] and W[illers] Jessen. "Vorlagen für die vierte Versammlung deutscher Psychiater." *AZP* 20, 2d Supplement (1863): 1–33.

Jolly, Friedrich. *Bericht über die Irren-Abteilung des Juliusspitals zu Würzburg für die Jahre 1870, 1871 und 1872.* Würzburg: Stahel'schen Buch- und Kunsthandlung, 1873.

——. *Vorgeschichte und gegenwärtige Einrichtung der psychiatrischen Klinik in Strassburg: Rede zur Feier der Eröffnung des Neubaus der Klinik.* Strassburg: Karl Trübner, 1887.

——. "Vorwort." *AfPN* 22 (1891): iii–vii.

——. *Über Irrthum und Irrsinn. Rede gehalten zur Feier des Stiftungstages der militärärztlichen Bildungsanstalten.* Berlin: Hirschwald, 1893.

——. "Über Heilstätten für Nervenkranke." *Zeitschrift für Krankenpflege* 20 (1898): 94–8.

——. "Rede zur Eröffnung der Jahresversammlung des Vereins der deutschen Irrenärzte und zur Einweihung des Hörsaals der neuen psychiatrischen und Nervenklinik in der Königl. Charité am 22. April 1901." *AfPN* 34 (1901): 694–707.

——. "Erläuterungen zum Neubau der psychiatrischen und Nervenklinik der Kgl. Charité." *CA* 26 (1902): 336–47.

Juliusburger, Otto. "Materialistische Psychiatrie. Erwiderung auf den Aufsatz des Dr. Weygandt: Psychologie und Hirnanatomie, mit besonderer Berücksichtigung der modernen Phrenologie." *MschrPN* 9 (1901): 21–30.

——. "Psychiatrische Tagesfragen." *AZP* 69 (1912): 121–38.

Jüngken, [Johann Christian]. "Promemoria, die medicinischen Studien, medicinischen Prüfungen und die Stellung der Ärzte unter das neue Gewerbe-Gesetz betreffend." *BKW* 9 (1872): 35.

Kahlbaum, K[arl]. *Die Gruppierung der psychischen Krankheiten und die Einteilung der Seelenstörungen.* Danzig: A. W. Kafemann, 1863.

——. *Klinische Abhandlungen über psychische Krankheiten: Die Katatonie oder das Spannungsirresein.* Berlin: Hirschwald, 1874.

——. "Die klinisch-diagnostischen Gesichtspunkte der Psychopathologie." *Sammlung Klinischer Vorträge* 126 (1877): 1127–46.

Kalberlah, Fritz. "Eduard Hitzig." *ZblNP* 30 (1907): 765–8.

Karrer, [Ferdinand]. "Zur Wärterfrage." *AZP* 53 (1897): 455–82.

Kieser, D[ietrich] G[eorg]. "Psychiatrie oder Psychiaterie?" *AZP* 5 (1848): 136–8.

——. *Elemente der Psychiatrik: Grundlage klinischer Vorträge.* Breslau: Weber, 1855.

Kirchenheim and Reinartz. *Zur Reform des Irrenrechts: Elf Leitsätze zur Besserung der Irrenfürsorge und Beseitigung des Entmündigungsunfugs.* Barmen: Wiemann, 1895.

Kläsi, Jakob. "Über psychiatrisch-poliklinische Behandlungsmethoden." *ZgNP* 36 (1917): 431–50.

Klinke, Otto. "Zur Geschichte der freien Behandlung und der Anwendung der Bettruhe bei Geisteskranken." *AZP* 49 (1893): 669–87.

Koch, J[ulius] L[udwig] A[ugust]. *Zur Statistik der Geisteskrankheiten in Württemberg und der Geisteskrankheiten überhaupt.* Stuttgart: Kohlhammer, 1878.

Köhler, R[einhold]. "Die Psychiatrie als Gegenstand des medicinischen Unterrichts in Deutschland, im Besondern in Württemberg." *MCbWAL* 32 (1862): 289–93, 297–9.

Kolb, G[ustav]., ed. *Sammel-Atlas für den Bau von Irrenanstalten: Ein Handbuch für Behörden, Psychiater und Baubeamte,* Pt. A. Halle: Marhold, 1907.

———. *Vorschläge für die Ausgestaltung der Irrenfürsorge und für die Organisation der Irrenanstalten: Unter besonderer Berücksichtigung der bayerischen Verhältnisse.* Halle: Carl Marhold, 1908.

Kollmann, [Julius]. "Zur Geschichte der Irrenpflege in Bayern." *Friedreich's Blätter für gerichtliche Medicin und Sanitätspolizei* 51 (1900): 340–56.

Kornfeld, S[igmund]. "Geschichte der Psychiatrie." In vol. 3 of *Handbuch der Geschichte der Medizin,* edited by Max Neuburger and Julius Pagel, 601–728. Jena: Fischer, 1905.

Koster, [Friedrich]. "Militaria." *If* 13 (1871): 5–12, 24–29, 43–48.

Kötscher, L. M. *Unsere Irrenhäuser.* Berlin: Langenscheidt, 1912.

Kraepelin, Emil. *Die Abschaffung des Strafmaßes: Ein Vorschlag zur Reform der Strafrechtspflege.* Stuttgart: Enke, 1880.

———. "Über die Einwirkung einiger medicamentöser Stoffe auf die Dauer einfacher psychischer Vorgänge." *Philosophische Studien* 1 (1883): 417–62, 573–605.

———. *Die Richtungen der psychiatrischen Forschung: Vortrag, gehalten bei der Übernahme des Lehramtes an der kaiserlichen Universität Dorpat.* Leipzig: Vogel, 1887.

———. "Über die Wachabteilung der Heidelberger Irrenklinik." *AZP* 51 (1895): 1–21.

———. *Psychiatrie: Ein Lehrbuch für Studierende und Aerzte.* 5th ed. Leipzig: J. A. Barth, 1896.

———. "Ziele und Wege der klinischen Psychiatrie." *AZP* 53 (1897): 840–8.

———. "Die Lage der Irrenfürsorge in Baden." *ZblNP* 20, n.s. 8 (1897): 654–63.

———. *Die psychiatrischen Aufgaben des Staates.* Jena: Fischer, 1900.

———. *Die königliche Psychiatrische Klinik in München, Festrede zur Eröffnung der Klinik am 7. November 1904.* Leipzig: Barth, 1905.

———. "Das Verbrechen als soziale Krankheit." *MschrKS* 3 (1906/7): 257–79.

———. "Ziele und Wege der psychiatrischen Forschung." *ZgNP* 42 (1918): 169–205.

———. *Lebenserinnerungen.* Berlin: Springer, 1983.

———. *Psychiatry: A Textbook for Students and Physicians.* 1899. 2 vols. Edited by Jacques M. Quen. Translated by Helga Metoui and Sabine Ayed. Canton: Watson Publishing International, 1991.

Krafft-Ebing, [Richard] von. "Rede zur Eröffnung der psychiatrischen Klinik in Straßburg am 17. Mai 1872." *AZP* 29 (1873): 378–90.

———. "Gutachten über die Ertheilung des psychiatrischen Unterrichtes." *Psychiatrisches Zentralblatt* 6 (1876): 47–9, 57–9.

———. *Der klinische Unterricht in der Psychiatrie: Eine Studie.* Stuttgart: Enke, 1890.

Kretzschmar, F. *Die Unvollkommenheit der heutigen Psychiatrie und die Mangelhaftigkeit der deutschen Irrengesetzgebung mit Entwurf einer neuen Irrenprocessordnung. Ein Wort zur Irrenfrage an Laien, Aerzte und Juristen.* Leipzig: Uhlig, 1891.

Kreuser, [Heinrich]. "Ernst v. Zeller." *MCblWAL* 72 (1902): 776–9.

———. "Geschichtlicher Überblick über die Entwicklung des Irrenwesens in Württemberg." *MCblWAL* 72 (1902): 749–57.

Kurella, H[ans]. "Das preussische Irrenwesen im Lichte des Processes Mellage." *ZblNP* 18 (1895): 337–44.

——. "Pastor Bodelschwingh und die Nemesis." *ZblNP* 21 (1898): 54–7.

Lachner, E[ugen]. "Nekrolog: Solbrig." *CblDGPgP* 18 (1872): 186–94.

Laehr, Heinrich. *Über Irrsein und Irrenanstalten. Für Ärzte und Laien.* Halle: Pfeffer, 1852.

——. "Vorwort." *AZP* 15 (1858): 1–3.

——. "Bericht über die Versammlung der Irrenärzte in Dresden, am 15. und 16. September 1862." *AZP* 19 (1862): 587–93.

——. "Bericht über die Versammlungen deutscher Irrenärzte zu Frankfurt a.M. und Giessen im Jahre 1864." *AZP* 21, supplement (1864).

——. "Rundschau in Preussen." *AZP* 22 (1865): 312–28.

——. "Über die Aufnahmebedingungen in Irrenanstalten." *AZP* 22 (1865): 343–8.

——. "Die Irrenanstalten Deutschlands." *AZP* 22, nos. 5 and 6 (1865).

——. Review of *Das Projekt des Neubaues einer zweiten Heil- und Pflege-Anstalt im Großherzogtum Baden, vor den Landständen und den beiden medicinischen Facultäten,* by [Christian Friedrich Wilhelm] Roller and [Max] Fischer. *AZP* 24 (1867): 216–22.

——. "Bericht über die psychiatrische Versammlungen zu Dresden im September 1868." *AZP* 25, supplement (1868).

——. *Fortschritt?–Rückschritt! Reform-Ideen des herrn Geh. Rathes Prof. Dr. Griesinger in Berlin auf dem Gebiete der Irrenheilkunde.* 2 vols. Berlin: Oehmigke, 1868.

——. "Gegen einen Vorwurf Virchows." *AZP* 27 (1871): 751–3.

——. "Die Bildung von Vereinen Behufs Verbesserung der öffentlichen Fürsorge für Irre." *AZP* 30 (1874): 50–2.

——. "Privatanstalten im Dienst der öffentlichen." *AZP* 34 (1878): 102–6.

——. *Die Heil- und Pflegeanstalten für Psychisch-Kranke des deutschen Sprachgebietes.* 9th ed. Berlin: Reimer, 1882.

——. "Die Bedeutung der Psychiatrie für den ärztlichen Unterricht." *BKW* 34 (1897): 61–3, 86–7.

Laehr, Heinrich and Max Lewald. *Die Heil- und Pflege-Anstalten für Psychisch-Kranke des deutschen Sprachgebietes.* Berlin: Georg Reimer, 1899.

Leupoldt, J[ohann] M[ichael]. *Über Leben und Wirken und über psychiatrische Klinik in einer Irrenheilanstalt.* Nürnberg: Riegel & Wießner, 1825.

Lexis, W[ilhelm]. *Die Deutschen Universitäten.* Vol. 2. Berlin: Asher, 1893.

Leyden, E[rnst] v. "Die innere Klinik und die innere Medicin in den letzten 25 Jahren." *DMW* 26 (1900): 2–3.

Liepmann, H[ugo]. "Carl Wernicke." *ZblNP* 16 (1905): 564–72.

——. *Über Wernickes Einfluss auf die klinische Psychiatrie.* Berlin: S. Karger, 1911.

Lomer, Georg. "Ein psychiatrisches Nachrichtenbüro?" *PNW* 11 (1909/10): 177–9.

Löwenhardt, [Emil]. "Über den Zeitpunkt der Übersiedlung von Geistes- und Gemüthskranken in Irrenanstalten," *If* 1 (1859): 23–7.

Mann, Ludwig. "Bericht über die am 16. und 17. September 1898 zu Bonn abgehaltene Jahressitzung des Vereins der deutschen Irrenärzte." *MschrPN* 4 (1898): 331–42.

Mayer-Gross, W. "Die Entwicklung der klinischen Anschauungen Kraepelins." *AfPN* 87 (1929): 30–42.

Medizinische Fakultät an der Universität Heidelberg. "Bemerkungen über die Errichtung einer neuen Irrenanstalt im Grossherzogthume Baden." *Medicinische Annalen* 3 (1837): 161–80.

Medizinische Fakultät der Universität Freiburg. *Beleuchtung der Denkschrift des Herrn Geheimerath Dr. Roller über den Nothstand in den beiden Landes-Irrenanstalten und dessen Abhilfe durch Errichtung einer neuen Anstalt sowie das Bedürfniß der Universität Freiburg für den psychiatrischen Unterricht.* Freiburg: Wagner, 1876.

Mendel, Emanuel. *Die Progressive Paralyse der Irren: Eine Monographie.* Berlin: Hirschwald, 1880.

——. "Über Hirnbefunde bei der progressiven Paralyse der Irren." *BKW* 20 (1883): 249–52.

——. "Über paralytischen Blödsinn bei Hunden." *Sitzungsberichte der preussischen Akademie der Wissenschaften, math.-nat.wiss. Klasse* 20 (1884): 393–5.

——. "Syphilis und Dementia paralytica." *BKW* 22 (1885): 549–50, 679–81.

Meschede, Franz. "Über den Entwicklungsgang der Psychiatrie und über die Bedeutung des psychiatrischen Unterrichts für die wissenschaftliche und praktische Ausbildung der Ärzte." *DMW* 21 (1895): 37–9, 60–2.

Meyer, Ludwig. "Das Non-Restraint und die Deutsche Psychiatrie." *AZP* 20 (1863): 542–81.

——. "Lage der öffentlichen Irrenpflege in Hannover." *AfPN* 2 (1869): 1–28.

——. "Das ärztliche System der Marburger Irrenanstalt." *AfPN* 7 (1877): 224–30.

——. "Die psychiatrische Klinik der Königlichen Georg-August-Universität in Göttingen: Bericht für das Jahr 1887/88." *Klinisches Jahrbuch* 1 (1889): 212–17.

——. "Die Verbannung der Zwangsjacken aus der Irrenabteilung des alten allgemeinen Krankenhauses in Hamburg." *Die Irrenpflege* 1 (1897).

Meynert, Theodor. *Zur Mechanik des Gehirnbaues.* Vienna: Braumüller, 1874.

——. "Naturexperimente am Gehirn." *Jahrbücher für Psychiatrie* 10 (1892): 169–79.

Möbius, Paul Julius. *Über die Behandlung von Nervenkrankheiten und die Errichtung von Nervenheilstätten.* Berlin: Karger, 1896.

Moeli, C[arl]. *Zur Erinnerung an Carl Westphal.* Berlin: Hirschwald, 1890.

Mönkemöller, Otto. "Zur Geschichte der progressiven Paralyse." *ZgNP* 5 (1911): 500–90.

Müller, Anton. *Die Irrenanstalt in dem Königlichen Julius-Hospitale zu Würzburg.* Würzburg: Stahel, 1824.

Näcke, Paul. "Über den Wert der sog[enannten] Kurven-Psychiatrie." *AZP* 61 (1904): 280–95.

Nasse, [Friedrich]. "Über das Bedürfniß, daß mit der Vorbereitung zu dem ärztlichen Berufe auch jedesmal die zu dem ärztlichen Geschäft bei psychischen Kranken verbunden sei, und über die günstige Gelegenheit zu dieser Vorbereitung." *Zeitschrift für psychische Ärzte* 2 (1819): 325–62.

——. "Keine Irren in die klinischen Anstalten?" *Zeitschrift für psychische Ärzte* 5, no. 3 (1822): 172–201.

——. *Von der Stellung der Ärzte im Staate.* Leipzig: Cnobloch, 1823.

Naunyn, B[ernhard]. *Erinnerungen, Gedanken und Meinungen.* Munich: Bergmann, 1925.

Neisser, Clemens. "Die Bettbehandlung der Irren." *BKW* 27 (1890): 863–66.

——. "Noch einmal die Bettenbehandlung der Irren." *AZP* 50 (1894): 447–64.

Neumann, Heinrich. *Der Arzt und die Blödsinnigkeits-Erklärung.* Breslau: Goso-horsky, 1847.

——. *Gedanken über die Zukunft der schlesischen Irrenanstalten.* Wohlau: Leuckart, 1848.

——. *Lehrbuch der Psychiatrie.* Erlangen: Enke, 1859.

——. "Zum Non-Restraint." *AZP* 28 (1872): 677–90.

Nostiz und Jänkendorf, G. A. E. von. *Beschreibung der königl. Sächsischen Heil- und Pflegeanstalt Sonnenstein mit Bemerkungen über Anstalten für Herstellung oder Verwahrung der Geisteskranken.* 3 vols. Dresden: Walther, 1829.

Obersteiner, Heinrich. "Zur Kenntnis einiger Hereditätsgesetze." *Wiener Medizinische Jahrbücher* (1875): 179–88.

——. "Grundzüge einer Geschichte des Vereins für Psychiatrie und Neurologie in Wien in den ersten fünfzig Jahren seines Bestehens (1868–1918)." *Jahrbücher für Psychiatrie* 39 (1919): 1–46.

Offizieller Bericht über die Zweite Hauptversammlung des Deutschen Medizinalbeamten-Vereins zu Leipzig am 14. und 15. September 1903. Berlin: Fischer's Medizinische Buchhandlung, 1903.

Orth, Johannes. "Die Entwicklung des Unterrichts in der pathologischen Anatomie und allgemeinen Pathologie an der Berliner Universität." *BKW* 47 (1910): 1868–72.

Ortloff, Hermann. *Zur Irrengesetzgebung: ein sozial- und rechtspolitischer Bericht.* Weimar: Böhlaus, 1897.

Paetz, Albrecht. "Über die Einrichtung von Überwachungsstationen." *AZP* 44 (1888): 424–33.

Pándy, K[oloman]. *Irrenfürsorge in Europa: Eine vergleichende Studie.* Edited by E. Engelken. Berlin: Georg Reimer, 1908.

Parchappe de Vinay, Jean-Baptiste-Maximilian. *Des principes à suivre dans la fondation et la construction des asiles d'aliénés.* Paris: Masson, 1853.

Pelman, Carl. "Zur Geschichte des Deutschen Vereins für Psychiatrie." *MMW* 53 (1906): 760–1.

——. *Erinnerungen eines alten Irrenarztes.* Bonn: Friedrich Cohen, 1912.

Peretti, J[oseph]. "Über den Stand der Frage der Einrichtung von Nervenheilstätten und die Wege zu ihrer Lösung." *AZP* 56 (1899): 567–76.

Pieper. "Erwiederung gegen Pf[arrer] Hafner." *Evangelisches Gemeindeblatt für Rheinland und Westfalen* (No. 48, 1893). Reprinted in *AZP* 50 (1894): 854–5.

Purkyně, J[ohann]. "Mikroskop." In *Handwörterbuch der Physiologie,* edited by Rudolf Wagner, 411–41. Braunschweig: Vieweg, 1844.

Puschmann, Theodor. "Geschichte des klinischen Unterrichts." *Klinisches Jahrbuch* 1 (1889): 9–66.

——. *Geschichte des medizinischen Unterrichts.* Leipzig: Veit, 1889.

Quincke, [Heinrich]. "Zur Reform des medizinischen Unterrichts und der Prüfungsordnung." *DMW* 17 (1891).

Ramaer. "Übersicht der Theorien der Psychiatrie." *Tageblatt der 51. Versammlung der Gesellschaft deutscher Naturforscher und Ärzte in Cassel 1878.* 51 (1878): 280–81.

Redepennig. "Die psychiatrische Beobachtungstation für Fürsorgezöglinge in Göttingen." *AZP* 67 (1910): 520–39.

Reichardt, Martin. *Über die Untersuchung des gesunden und kranken Gehirns mittels der Waage.* Arbeiten aus der Königlichen psychiatrischen Klinik zu Würzburg, vol. 1. Jena: Fischer, 1906.

Reinhard, Herrmann. *Das Mikroskop und sein Gebrauch für den Arzt.* 2d ed. Leipzig: Winter, 1864.

Richarz, [Franz]. "Thesen, zu eventueller Vorlage nach der Diskussion über die Griesinger'schen Reformvorschläge in der Sitzung des psychiatrischen Vereins der Rheinprovinz vom 13. Juni 1868." *If* 10 (1868): 78–80.

Rieger, Konrad. "Psychiatrie als Examensfach." *ZblNP* 16 (1893): 493–500.

——. "Die neue psychiatrische Klinik der Universität Würzburg." *Klinisches Jahrbuch* 5 (1894): 145–56.

——. *Zusammenstellung einiger Begründungen, welche für die Notwendigkeit der Aufnahme der Psychiatrie in die medizinische Approbations-Prüfung des deutschen Reichs veröffentlicht worden sind.* Jena: Fischer, 1896.

——. "Die Psychiatrie in Würzburg seit dreihundert Jahren." In *Verhandlungen der physikalisch-medizinischen Gesellschaft zu Würzburg.* Vols. 29-31. Würzburg: Stahel'sche Verlags-Anstalt, 1898.

——. *Die Julius-Universität und das Julius-Spital.* Würzburg: Curt Kabitzsch, 1916.

——. "Konrad Rieger." In vol. 8 of *Die Medizin der Gegenwart in Selbstdarstellungen,* edited by L. R. Grote, 125–74. Leipzig: Felix Meiner, 1929.

Rigler, Johannes. *Das medicinische Berlin.* Berlin: Elwin Staude, 1873.

Risak, Erwin. *Der klinische Blick.* 2d ed. Vienna: Springer, 1938.

Ritterhaus, E. *Irrsinn und Presse.* Jena: Fischer, 1913.

Roller, C[hristian] F[riedrich] W[ilhelm]. *Die Irrenanstalt nach allen ihren Beziehungen.* Karlsruhe: Müller'sche Buchhandlung, 1831.

——. *Grundsätze für Errichtung neuer Irrenanstalten insbesondere der Heil- und Pflegeanstalt bei Achern im Großherzogthum Baden.* Karlsruhe: Müller'schen Buchhandlung, 1838.

——. "Das Studium der Psychiatrie." *AZP* 10 (1853): 73–88.

——. "Über Aufnahme-Bestimmungen in Irrenanstalten und Anstalts-Statuten überhaupt." *AZP* 24 (1867): 642–59.

——. *Psychiatrische Zeitfragen aus dem Gebiet der Irrenfürsorge in und ausser den Anstalten und ihren Beziehungen zum staatlichen und gesellschaftlichen Leben.* Berlin: Georg Reimer, 1874.

Samt, Paul. *Die naturwissenschaftliche Methode in der Psychiatrie.* Berlin: August Hirschwald, 1874.

Sander, Wilhelm. *Über Zählblättchen und ihre Benutzung bei statistischen Erhebungen der Irren.* Berlin: Sittenfeld, 1871.

Scheibe, [Oskar]. "Zweihundert Jahre des Charité-Krankenhauses zu Berlin." *CA* 34 (1910): 1–178.

Scholz, [Jean Paul Friedrich]. "Über Wachabteilungen in Irrenanstalten." *AZP* 45 (1889): 235–48.

Schüle, Heinrich. *Sektionsergebnisse bei Geisteskranken nebst Krankengeschichten und Epikrisen.* Leipzig: Duncker u. Humblot, 1874.

Schultze, B[ernhard] S[igmund]. *Über den Plan, den Besuch der psychiatrischen Klinik für die Studierenden der Medizin obligatorisch zu machen und ein Examen aus der Psychiatrie in die Approbationsprüfung der Aerzte einzureihen."* [Jena]: n.p., 1893.

——. *Die Psychiatrie: Prüfungsgegenstand für alle Aerzte? Eine Entgegnung an Herrn Professor Dr. Otto Binswanger.* Jena: Fischer, 1893.

——. *Mein Votum zur Revision der medizinischen Prüfungen.* Berlin: Mittler & Sohn, 1896.

——. *Die Psychiatrie: Prüfungsgegenstand für alle Aerzte? Vierter Aufsatz über das genannte Thema.* Jena: Fischer, 1896.

Schultze, Friedrich. "Neuropathologie und innere Medizin." *MMW* 51 (1904): 1301–3.

Schwalbe, J[ulius]. "Heilstätten für minderbemittelte Nervenkranke." *DMW* 24 (1898): 211–12.

Schwartz, [Oscar]. "Über die Stellung der Seelenheilkunde (Psychiatrie) zur Naturforschung und insbesondere zur praktischen Medicin." In *Amtlicher Bericht über die dreiunddreissigste Versammlung deutscher Naturforscher und Ärzte zu Bonn im September 1857,* edited by J. Noeggerath and H. F. Kilian, 66–70. Bonn: Carl Georgi, 1859.

Siemens, [Fritz] and [August] Zinn. "Psychiatrie und Seelsorge." In *Bericht über die von dem 'Verein der deutschen Irrenärzte in der Jahressitzung vom 25. Mai 1893 zu Frankfurt a/M. gepflogenen Verhandlungen und gefassten Beschlüsse,* edited by the Verein der deutschen Irrenärzte, 1–37. Munich: Lehmann, 1893.

——. "Zur Frage der Reform des Irrenwesens in Deutschland, insbesondere in Preussen." *AZP* 52 (1896): 818–39.

Siemens, Fritz. "Der ärztliche Nachwuchs für psychiatrische Anstalten." *PNW* 9 (1907): 77–81.

Siemerling, E[rnst]. *Bericht über die Wirksamkeit der psychiatrischen Universitätsklinik in Tübingen.* Tübingen: Franz Pietzcker, 1901.

——. *Zur Erinnerung an Friedrich Jolly.* Berlin: Hirschwald, 1904.

Smoler, [Moritz]. "Die Section für Psychiatrie und Staatsarzneikunde in Stettin." *CblDGPgP* 10 (1863): 294–309.

Snell, Ludwig [Daniel Christian]. "Über Monomanie als primäre Form der Seelenstörung." *AZP* 22 (1865): 368–81.

——. "Zur Erinnerung an Maximilian Jacobi." *AZP* 28 (1872): 414–24.

——. "Naturwissenschaftliche und ärztliche Standpunkte dem Unterrichtswesen unserer Zeit gegenüber." *AZP* 30 (1874): 689–96.

Solbrig, [August]. "Blicke auf die Entwickelung des Irrenanstaltswesens in Bayern im Laufe des letzten Decenniums." *AZP* 12 (1855): 401–24.

——. "Über psychiatrisch-klinischen Unterricht." *AZP* 18 (1861): 805–12.

——. *Verbrechen und Wahnsinn: Ein Beitrag zur Diagnostik zweifelhafter Seelenstörungen für Aerzte, Psychologen und Richter.* Munich: Cotta, 1867.

Sommer, Robert. "Die Wärterfrage." *ZblNP* 16 (1893): 603–8.

——. "Die Ausführung des Griesinger'schen Programms." *ZblNP* 16 (1893): 599–601; 17 (1894): 105–12.

——. *Diagnostik der Geisteskrankheiten für praktische Aerzte und Studierende.* Vienna: Urban-Schwarzenberg, 1894.

——. "Die klinische Untersuchung der Geisteskrankheiten." In *Die deutsche Klinik am Eingange des zwanzigsten Jahrhunderts,* edited by Ernst v. Leyden and Felix Klemperer, 1–58. Berlin: Urban, 1906.

——. "Die öffentliche Schlaf- und Ruhehallen bei der Internationalen Hygiene-Ausstellung in Dresden." *PNW* 13 (1911): 202–5.

——. "Die weitere Entwicklung der öffentlichen Ruhehallen." *Klinik für psychisch und nervöse Krankheiten* 6 (1911): 380.

Spamer, C[arl]. "Beobachtungen über Erblichkeit, besonders bei Psychosen und Neurosen." *BKW* 18 (1881): 202–3, 215–16.

Stier, Ewald. *Die Bedeutung der Psychiatrie für den Kulturfortschritt.* Jena: Fischer, 1911.

Tuczek, Franz. *Die wissenschaftliche Stellung der Psychiatrie.* Marburg: N. G. Elwert, 1906.

Tuke, Daniel Hack. *Chapters in the History of the Insane in the British Isles.* London: Kegan, Paul, Trench & Co., 1882.

Unger, Heinrich. *Die Irrengesetzgebung in Preussen nebst den Bestimmungen über das Entmündigungsverfahren sowie die Einrichtung und Beaufsichtigung der Irrenanstalten.* Berlin: Siemenroth & Troschel, 1898.

"Verhandlungen des XIX. deutschen Aerztetages zu Weimar am 22. und 23. Juni 1891." *Aerztliches Vereinsblatt* 18 (1891): 289–314, 332–60.

"Verhandlungen des XVIII. deutschen Aerztetages zu München am 23. und 24. Juni 1890." *Aerztliches Vereinsblatt* 17 (1890): 296–346.

Verhandlungen des Siebenundzwanzigsten Deutschen Juristentages (Innsbruck 1904). Berlin: Guttentag, 1905.

Vezin, Hermann. *Ueber Krankenhäuser, die Krankenpflege durch christliche Genossenschaften und über die Wirksamkeit französischer, englischer und russischer Frauen in den Hospitälern der Krim und der Turkei.* Münster: Theissing, 1858.

Virchow, Rudolf. "Über die Standpunkte in der wissenschaftlichen Medicin." *Archiv für Pathologische Anatomie und Physiologie und für klinische Medizin* 1 (1847): 3ff.

Viszánik, Michael. *Die Irrenheil- und Pflegeanstalten Deutschlands, Frankreichs, sammt der Cretinen-Anstalt auf dem Abendberge in der Schweiz.* Vienna: Gerold, 1845.

Vogt, H. "August Cramer." *AfPN* 50, no. 2 (1912): iii-xi.

Wagner von Jauregg, Julius. *Lebenserinnerungen.* Wien: Springer, 1950.

Waldeyer, W[ilhelm]. "Der Unterricht in den anatomischen Wissenschaften an der Universität Berlin im ersten Jahrhundert ihres Bestehens." *BKW* 47 (1910): 1864.

Walther, Ph[ilipp] Fr[anz] von. *Über klinische Lehranstalten in städtischen Krankenhäusern. Eine Principienfrage, zugleich in näherer Beziehung auf ihre gegenseitigen Verhältnisse in München.* Freiburg i.Br.: Herder, 1846.

Wassermann, A[ugust Paul]. "Die medizinische Fakultät." In *Die Universitäten im deutschen Reich,* edited by W. Lexis, 151–6. Berlin: Ascher, 1904.

Weber, Otto. *Das akademische Krankenhaus in Heidelberg, seine Mängel und die Bedürfnisse eines Neubaus.* Heidelberg: Mohr, 1865.

Wernicke, C[arl]. *Der aphasische Symptomencomplex: Eine psychologische Studie auf anatomischer Basis.* Breslau: Cohn & Weigert, 1874.

——. "Über den wissenschaftlichen Standpunkt in der Psychiatrie." In *Tageblatt der 53. Versammlung deutscher Naturforscher und Aerzte in Danzig 1880* 53 (1880): 128–35.

——. *Lehrbuch der Gehirnkrankheiten für Ärzte und Studierende.* Vol. 1. Kassel: Theodor Fischer, 1881.

——. "Über die Irrenversorgung der Stadt Breslau." *Breslauer Aerztliche Zeitschrift* 10 (1888): 169–72.

——. "Zweck und Ziel der Psychiatrischen Kliniken." *Klinisches Jahrbuch* 1 (1889): 218–23.

——. "Stadtasyle und psychiatrische Kliniken." *Klinisches Jahrbuch* 2 (1890): 186–93.

——. "Tagesfragen." *MschrPN* 1 (1897): 1–5.

Westphal, A[lexander], Robert Schulze, and A. H. Hübner. "Die neue Klinik für psychisch und Nervenkranke der Universität Bonn." *Klinisches Jahrbuch* 24 (1910): 227–50.

Westphal, Carl. "Über Erkrankungen des Rückenmarks bei der allgemeinen progressiven Paralyse der Irren." *Archiv für pathologische Anatomie und Physiologie und für klinische Medicin* 39 (1867): 90–115, 353–423, 592–606; and 40 (1867): 226–82.

———. "Nachrichten von der psychiatrischen Clinik zu Berlin." *AfPN* 1 (1868): 232–4.

———. "Einige Beobachtungen über die epileptiformen und apoplectischen Anfälle der paralytischen Geisteskrankheiten mit Rücksicht auf die Körperwärme." *AfPN* 1 (1868/69): 337–86.

———. "Über künstliche Erzeugung von Epilepsie bei Meerschweinchen." *BKW* 8 (1871): 460–3.

———. "Psychiatrische Klinik." *CA* 1 (1874): 453–64.

———. "Nerven-Klinik." *CA* 1 (1876): 421–452.

———. "Psychiatrische Kliniken." *AfPN* 7 (1877): 384–5.

———. *Psychiatrie und psychiatrischer Unterricht.* Berlin: Hirschwald, 1880.

———. "Vorschläge zur Abänderung der amtlichen Zählkarten für die Irrenanstalten." *AZP* 38 (1882): 717–9.

———. "Gutachten der Königlichen wissenschaftlichen Deputation für das Medizinalwesen betreffend die Überbürdung der Schüler in den höheren Lehranstalten." *Vierteljahresschrift für gerichtliche Medizin*, n.s., 40 (1884): 351–82.

———. *Gesammelte Abhandlungen.* Edited by A[lexander] Westphal. Berlin: Hirschwald, 1892.

Weygandt, W[ilhelm]. "Psychologie und Hirnanatomie mit besonderer Berücksichtigung der modernen Phrenologie." *DMW* 26 (1900): 657–61.

———. "Zur Frage der materialistischen Psychiatrie." *ZblNP* 24 (1901): 409–15.

Wille, Ludwig. "Vortrag zur Eröffnung der psychiatrischen Klinik in Basel im Sommersemester 1877." *AZP* 34 (1878): 395–403.

Wilmanns, Karl. "Die Entwicklung der badischen Irrenfürsorge mit besonderer Berücksichtigung der Universitäts-Kliniken." *AfPN* 87 (1929): 1–23.

Wollenberg, R[obert]. "Eduard Hitzig." *AfPN* 43 (1907): iii–xiv.

———. "Einweihungsfeier der Psychiatrischen- und Nervenklinik." *Strassburger Medizinische Zeitung* 8 (1911): 223–9.

———. *Erinnerungen eines alten Psychiaters.* Stuttgart: Enke, 1931.

Wunderlich, Carl August. *Geschichte der Medizin.* Stuttgart: Ebner & Seubert, 1859.

———. *Wilhelm Griesinger: Biographische Skizze.* Leipzig: Otto Wigand, 1869.

Zenker, W. "Irrenanstalten und die medizinische Fachpresse." *Ärztliches Vereinsblatt* 22 (1895): 638–41.

Ziehen, Th[eodor]. "Die Entwicklung des psychiatrischen und neuropathologischen Unterrichts an der Universität Berlin." *BKW* 47 (1910): 1882–3.

"Zur Charakteristik der psychiatrischen Section der Naturforscherversammlung zu Dresden." *BKW* 5 (1868): 447–8.

Secondary Sources

Abbott, Andrew. *The System of Professions: An Essay on the Division of Expert Labor.* Chicago: University of Chicago Press, 1988.

Ackerknecht, Erwin H. *Kurze Geschichte der Psychiatrie.* 2d ed. Stuttgart: Enke, 1967.
——. "Gudden, Huguenin, Hitzig: Hirnpsychiatrie im Burghölzli 1869–1879." *Gesnerus* 35 (1978): 66–78.
Alexander, Franz G. and Sheldon T. Selesnick. *The History of Psychiatry: An Evaluation of Psychiatric Thought and Practice from Prehistoric Times to the Present.* New York: Harper & Row, 1966.
Amberger, Renate Ulrike. "Haus Schönow: Von der Heilstätte für Nervenkranke zur Klinik für Akutgeriatrie." Med. diss., Free University Berlin, 2001.
Angst, Alfred E[rich]. "Die ersten psychiatrischen Zeitschriften in Deutschland." Med. diss., University of Würzburg, 1975.
Artelt, Walter. "Die Gründung und die ersten Jahrzehnte der Berliner Medizinische Fakultät." *Ciba-Zeitschrift* 7 (1956): 2571–81.
Auswahlbibliographie zur Geschichte des Bereichs Medizin (Charité) der Humboldt-Universität zu Berlin. Schriftenreihe der Universitätsbibliothek, vol. 50. Berlin: Universitätsbibliothek, 1985.
Baader, Gerhard. "Stadtentwicklung und psychiatrische Anstalten." In *'Gelêrter der arzenîê, ouch apotêker': Beiträge zur Wissenschaftsgeschichte,* edited by Gundolf Keil, 239–53. *Würzburger Medizinhistorische Forschungen,* vol. 24. Pattensen: Wellm, 1982.
Bakel, A. H. A. C. van. " 'Über die Dauer einfacher psychischer Vorgänge.' Emil Kraepelins Versuch einer Anwendung der Psychophysik im Bereich der Psychiatrie." In *Objekte, Differenzen und Konjunkturen: Experimentalsysteme im historischen Kontext,* edited by Michael Hagner, Hans-Jörg Rheinberger, and Bettina Wahrig-Schmidt, 83–105. Berlin: Akademie Verlag, 1994.
Beck, Clemens. "Die Geschichte der 'Heil- und Pflegeanstalt Illenau unter Chr. Fr. W. Roller (1802–1878)." Med. diss., University of Freiburg, 1984.
Beck, Hermann. "The Social Policies of Prussian Officials: The Bureaucracy in a New Light." *JMH* 64 (1992): 263–98.
Beddies, Thomas and Heinz-Peter Schmiedebach. "Die Diskussion um die ärztlich beaufsichtigte Familienpflege in Deutschland: Historische Entwicklung einer Maßnahme zur sozialen Integration psychisch Kranker." *Sudhoffs Archiv* 85 (2001): 82–107.
Benzenhöfer, Udo. *Bibliographie der zwischen 1975 und 1989 erschienenen Schriften zur Geschichte der Psychiatrie im deutschsprachigen Raum.* No. 4 of Hannoversche Abhandlungen zur Geschichte der Medizin und der Naturwissenschaften, edited by Wolfgang U. Eckart. Trecklenburg: Burgverlag, 1992.
——. *Psychiatrie und Anthropologie in der ersten Hälfte des 19. Jahrhunderts.* Hürtgenwald: Guido Pressler, 1993.
Berghof, Winfried. "Heinrich Damerow (1798–1866): Ein bedeutender Vertreter der deutschen Psychiatrie des 19. Jahrhunderts." Med. diss., University of Leipzig, 1990.
Berrios, G[erman] E. and R[enate] Hauser. "The Early Development of Kraepelin's Ideas on Classification—a Conceptual History." *Psychological Medicine* 18 (1988): 813–21.
Berrios, G[erman] E. and D[ominic] Beer. "The Notion of Unitary Psychosis: A Conceptual History." *HP* 5 (1994): 13–36.
Blackbourn, David and Geoff Eley. *The Peculiarities of German History: Bourgeois Society and Politics in 19th-Century Germany.* Oxford: Oxford University Press, 1984.

Blasius, Dirk. *Der verwaltete Wahnsinn: Eine Sozialgeschichte des Irrenhauses.* Frankfurt/M: Fischer, 1980.

——. *Umgang mit Unheilbarem: Studien zur Sozialgeschichte der Psychiatrie.* Bonn: Psychiatrie-Verlag, 1986.

——. *Friedrich Wilhelm IV, 1795–1861: Psychopathologie und Geschichte.* Göttingen: V&R, 1992.

——. *'Einfache Seelenstörungen': Geschichte der deutschen Psychiatrie, 1800–1945.* Frankfurt/M: Fischer, 1994.

Bleker, Johanna. "Die Stadt als Krankheitsfaktor: Eine Analyse ärztlicher Auffassungen im 19. Jahrhundert." *Medizinhistorisches Journal* 18 (1983): 118–36.

——. "Medical Students—to the Bed-side or to the Laboratory? The Emergence of Laboratory-training in German Medical Education 1870–1900." *Clio Medica* 21 (1987/8): 35–46.

Bleuler, M[anfred]. "Geschichte des Burghölzlis und der psychiatrischen Universitätsklinik." In *Züricher Spitalgeschichte,* edited by Canton Zurich, 2:377–425. Zurich: Berichthaus Zürich, 1951.

Bodamer, Joachim. "Zur Entstehung der Psychiatrie als Wissenschaft im 19. Jahrhundert." *Fortschritte der Neurologie, Psychiatrie und ihrer Grenzgebiete* 21 (1953): 511–35.

Bonner, Thomas Neville. *Becoming a Physician: Medical Education in Britain, France, Germany, and the United States, 1750–1945.* New York: Oxford University Press, 1995.

Brain, Robert M. "Bürgerliche Intelligenz." *Studies in History and Philosophy of Science* 26 (1995): 617–35.

Brakelmann, Günter, Martin Greschat, and Werner Jochmann. *Protestantismus und Politik: Werk und Wirkung Adolf Stöckers.* Hamburger Beiträge zur Social- und Zeitgeschichte, vol. XVII. Hamburg: Christians, 1982.

Braunsdorf, Annette. "Leben und Werk Otto Binswangers, Jena 1882–1919." Med. diss., University of Jena, 1988.

Breathnach, Caoimhghin S. "Eduard Hitzig, neurophysiologist and psychiatrist." *HP* 3 (1992): 329–338.

Burghardt, Harald. "Psychiatrische Universitätskliniken im deutschen Sprachraum (1828– 1914)." Med. diss., University of Cologne, 1985.

Burgmair, Wolfgang, Eric J. Engstrom, and Matthias M. Weber, eds. *Emil Kraepelin. Persönliches, Selbstzeugnisse.* Munich: Belleville, 2000.

——. *Emil Kraepelin. Kriminologische und forensische Schriften: Werke und Briefe.* Munich: Belleville, 2001.

——. *Emil Kraepelin. Briefe I, 1868–1886.* Munich: Belleville, 2002.

——. *Emil Kraepelin. Kraepelin in Dorpat, 1886–1891.* Munich: Belleville, 2003.

Burkhart, Elisabeth. "Ludwig Meyer (1827–1900): Leben und Werk. Ein Vertreter der deutschen Psychiatrie auf ihrem Weg zur medizinisch-naturwissenschaftlichen Fachdisziplin." Med. diss., Free University of Berlin, 1991.

Burnham, John C. *Jeliffe: American Psychoanalyst and Physician and his Correspondence with Sigmund Freud and C. G. Jung.* Chicago: University of Chicago Press, 1983.

Burrage, Michael, and Rolf Torstendahl, eds. *Professions in Theory and History: Rethinking the Study of the Professions.* Swedish Collegium for Advanced Study in the Social Sciences. London: Sage, 1990.

Busse, Gerd. "Schreber und Flechsig: der Hirnanatom als Psychiater." *Medizinhistorisches Journal* 24 (1989): 260–305.

Clarke, Edwin and L. Steven Jacyna. *Nineteenth-Century Origins of Neuroscientific Concepts.* Berkeley: University of California Press, 1987.

Cocks, Geoffrey. *Psychotherapy in the Third Reich: The Göring Institute.* Oxford: Oxford University Press, 1985.

Cocks, Geoffrey and Konrad Jarausch. *German Professions, 1800–1950.* New York: Oxford University Press, 1990.

Coleman, William. "Prussian Pedagogy: Purkyně at Breslau, 1823–1839." In *The Investigative Enterprise: Experimental Physiology in Nineteenth-Century Medicine,* edited by William Coleman and Frederic L. Holmes, 15–64. Berkeley: University of California Press, 1988.

Coleman, William and Frederic L. Holmes. *The Investigative Enterprise: Experimental Physiologie in Nineteenth-Century Medicine.* Berkeley: University of California Press, 1988.

Cunningham, Andrew and Perry Williams, eds. *The Laboratory Revolution in Medicine.* Cambridge: Cambridge University Press, 1992.

DeBrunner, Rudolf. "Alkoholabstinenz und Psychiatrie am Ende des 19. Jahrhunderts." Med. diss., University of Zurich, 1961.

Detlefs, Gerald. *Wilhelm Griesingers Ansätze zur Psychiatriereform.* Pfaffenweiler: Centaurus 1993.

Dickenson, Edward Ross. *The Politics of German Child Welfare from the Empire to the Federal Republic.* Harvard: Harvard University Press, 1996.

Dieckhöfer, Klemens. "Frühe Formen der Antipsychiatrie und die Reaktion der Psychiatrie." *Medizinhistorisches Journal* 19 (1984): 100–11.

Digby, Anne. *Madness, Morality, and Medicine: A Study of the York Retreat, 1796–1914.* Cambridge: Cambridge University Press, 1985.

Dörner, Klaus. "Psychiatrie und Gesellschaftstheorien." In *Psychiatrie der Gegenwart: Forschung und Praxis.* Grundlinien und Methoden der Psychiatrie, edited by K. P. Kisker et al., 1:771–809. 2d ed. Berlin: Springer 1979.

——. *Bürger und Irre: Zur Sozialgeschichte und Wissenschaftssoziologie der Psychiatrie,* 2d ed. Frankfurt/M: EVA, 1984.

——. "Wir verstehen die Geschichte der Moderne nur mit den Behinderten vollständig." *Leviathan* 22 (1994): 367–90.

——. "Wie gehören Behinderte zur Gesellschaft." *GuG* 20 (1994): 625–30.

Dowbiggin, Ian. *Inheriting Madness: Professionalization and Psychiatric Knowledge in Nineteenth-Century France.* Berkeley: University of California Press, 1991.

Drees, Annette. *Die Ärzte auf dem Weg zu Prestige und Wohlstand: Sozialgeschichte der württembergischen Ärzte im 19. Jahrhundert.* Vol. 9 of *Studien zur Geschichte des Alltags,* edited by Hans J. Teuteberg and Peter Borscheid. Münster: Coppenrath, 1988.

Dwyer, Ellen. *Homes for the Mad: Life inside Two Nineteenth-Century Asylums.* New Brunswick: Rutgers University Press, 1987.

Eberstadt, Elisabeth. "K[arl] A[ugust] von Solbrigs Liebe zu den Irren." In *Um die Menschenrechte der Geisteskranken,* edited by Werner Leibbrand, 31–49. Nürnberg: Die Egge, 1946.

Elm, Kaspar and Hans-Dietrich Loock, eds. *Seelsorge und Diakonie in Berlin: Beiträge zum Verhältnis von Kirche und Großstadt im 19. und beginnenden 20. Jahrhundert.* Berlin: de Gruyter, 1990.

Engstrom, Eric J. "Emil Kraepelin: Leben und Werk des Psychiaters im Spannungsfeld zwischen positivistischer Wissenschaft und Irrationalismus." Masters Thesis, University of Munich, 1990.

——. "Emil Kraepelin: psychiatry and public affairs in Wilhelmine Germany." *HP* 2 (1991): 111–32.

——. "Kraepelin." In *A History of Clinical Psychiatry: The Origin and History of Psychiatric Disorders,* edited by German E. Berrios and Roy Porter, 292–301. London: Athlone, 1995.

——. "Kulturelle Dimensionen von Psychiatrie und Sozialpsychologie: Emil Kraepelin und Willy Hellpach." In *Kultur und Kulturwissenschaften um 1900: Idealismus und Positivismus,* edited by Gangolf Hübinger, Friedrich Wilhelm Graf, and Rüdiger vom Bruch, 164–189. Stuttgart: Steiner, 1997.

——. "The Birth of Clinical Psychiatry: Power, Knowledge, and Professionalization in Germany, 1867–1914." Ph.D. Dissertation, University of North Carolina at Chapel Hill, 1997.

——. "Die Heidelberger psychiatrische Universitätsklinik am Ende des 19. Jahrhunderts: Institutionelle Grundlagen der klinischen Psychiatrie." *Jahrbuch für Universitätsgeschichte* 1 (1998): 49–68.

——. "Eduard Hitzigs 'Gutachten betreffend die Frage der Verbindung des akademischen Unterrichtes in der Psychiatrie und Neuropathologie an den preußischen Universitäten' (1889)." In *Neurologie in Berlin,* edited by Bernd Holdorff and Rolf Winau, 111–26. Berlin: De Gruyter, 2000.

——. "Disziplin, Polykratie und Chaos: Zur Wissens- und Verwaltungsökonomie der psychiatrischen und Nervenabteilung der Charité." *Jahrbuch für Universitätsgeschichte* 3 (2000): 162–80.

——. "Der Verbrecher als wissenschaftliche Aufgabe: Die kriminologischen und forensischen Schriften Kraepelins." In *Emil Kraepelin. Kriminologische und forensische Schriften: Werke und Briefe,* edited by Wolfgang Burgmair, Eric J. Engstrom, Matthias M. Weber, 353–90. Munich: Bellville, 2001.

Engstrom, Eric J. and Volker Hess, eds. *Zwischen Wissens- und Verwaltungsökonomie: Zur Geschichte des Berliner Charité Krankenhauses im 19. Jahrhundert.* In *Jahrbuch für Universitätsgeschichte* 3 (2000).

——. "Neurologie an der Charité zwischen medizinischer und psychiatrischer Klinik." In *Neurologie in Berlin,* edited by Bernd Holdorff and Rolf Winau, 99–110. Berlin: De Gruyter, 2000.

Engstrom, Eric J., Matthias Weber, and Wolfgang Burgmair. "Emil Kraepelin's Self-Assessment: Clinical Autography in Historical Context." *HP* 13 (2002): 89–119.

"Entwicklung der Universitäts-Nevenklinik Tübingen." TMs [photocopy]. University Psychiatric Clinic Tübingen.

Eulner, Hans-Heinz. "Eduard Hitzig (1838–1907)." *Wissenschaftliche Zeitschrift der Martin-Luther-Universität Halle Wittenberg, Mathematisch-Naturwissenschaftliche Reihe,* VI/5 (1957): 709–12.

——. *Die Entwicklung der medizinischen Spezialfächer an den Universitäten des deutschen Sprachgebietes.* Studien zur Medizingeschichte des neunzehnten Jahrhunderts, edited by W. Artelt and W. Rüegg, vol. 4. Stuttgart: Enke, 1970.

Eulner, Hans-Heinz and Walter Glatzel. "Die Psychiatrie an der Universität Halle." *Wissenschaftliche Zeitschrift der Martin-Luther-Universität Halle-Wittenberg, mathematisch-naturwissenschaftliche Reihe,* VII/2 (1958): 197–218.

Feger, Gabriele. "Die Geschichte des 'Psychiatrischen Vereins zu Berlin,' 1889–1920." Med. diss., Free University Berlin, 1983.

Feldmann, Renate. "Peter Willers Jessen (1793–1895): Eine Biographie, zugleich ein Beitrag zur Geschichte der Psychiatrie und der Irrenpflege in Schleswig-Holstein im 19. Jahrhundert." Med. diss., University of Kiel, 1983.

Foucault, Michel. *Madness and Civilization: A History of Insanity in the Age of Reason*. Translated by Richard Howard. New York: Random House, 1965.

——. *The Birth of the Clinic: An Archeology of Medical Perception*. Translated by A. M. Sheridan Smith. New York: Random House, 1973.

——. *Discipline and Punish: The Birth of the Prison*. Translated by Alan Sheridan. New York: Random House, 1977.

Frankenthal, Käte. *Jüdin, Intellektuelle, Sozialistin: Lebenserinnerungen einer Ärztin in Deutschland und im Exil*. Frankfurt/M: Campus, 1985.

Freeman, Hugh and German E. Berrios, eds. *150 Years of British Psychiatry, 1841–1991*. Vol. 2. London: Athlone Press, 1996.

Frevert, Ute. "Akademische Medizin und soziale Unterschichten im 19. Jahrhundert: Professionsinteressen—Zivilisationsmission—Sozialpolitik." *Jahrbuch des Instituts für Geschichte der Medizin der Robert Bosch Stiftung* 3 (1984): 41–59.

——. *Krankheit als politisches Problem 1770–1880: Soziale Unterschichten in Preußen zwischen medizinischer Polizei und staatlicher Sozialversicherung*. Göttingen: V&R, 1986.

Gadebusch Bondio, Mariacarla. *Die Rezeption der kriminalanthroplogischen Theorien von Cesare Lombroso in Deutschland von 1880–1914*. Abhandlungen zur Geschichte der Medizin und der Naturwissenschaften, edited by Rolf Winau and Heinz Müller-Dietz, vol. 70. Husum: Matthiesen Verlag, 1995.

Gast, Ursula. "Sozialpsychiatrische Traditionen zwischen Kaiserreich und Nationalsozialismus." *Psychiatrische Praxis* 16 (1989): 78–85.

Geduldig, Cordula. "Die Behandlung von Geisteskranken ohne physische Zwang: Die Rezeption des Non-Restraint im deutschen Sprachgebiet." Med. diss., University of Zurich, 1975.

Gerke, Wolfgang. "Die Reformanstalt Illenau und ihre Bedeutung für die badische Irrenfürsorge in der Ära Roller: eine psychiatriehistorische Studie anhand der Illenauer Krankengeschichten von 1826–1877." Med. diss., University of Freiburg, 1995.

Gispen, Kees. *New Profession, Old Order: Engineers and German Society, 1815–1914*. Cambridge: Cambridge University Press, 1989.

Goldberg, Ann. *Sex, Religion, and the Making of Modern Madness: The Ebersbach Asylum and German Society, 1815–1849*. New York: Oxford University Press, 1999.

——. "The Mellage Trial and the Politics of Insane Asylums in Wilhelmine Germany." JMH 74 (2002): 1–32.

Goldstein, Jan. "Foucault among the Sociologists: The 'Disciplines' and the History of the Professions." *History and Theory* 23 (1984): 170–92.

——. *Console and Classify: The French Psychiatric Profession in the Nineteenth Century*. Cambridge: Cambridge University Press, 1987.

——. "Framing Discipline with Law: Problems and Promises of the Liberal State," AHR 98 (1993): 364–75.

Goschler, Constantin. *Rudolf Virchow: Mediziner, Anthropologe, Politiker*. Cologne: Böhlau, 2002.

Graf, Oskar Maria. *Wir sind Gefangene: Ein Bekenntnis*. Munich: DTV, 1978.

Grefe, Jörg. "Die Vorstellungen zur Ätiologie der Progressiven Paralyse in der Allgemeinen Zeitschrift für Psychiatrie 1884–1913." Diss. med., University of Heidelberg, 1991.

Gruber, Georg B. "Zur Geschichte der Psychiatrie in Göttingen." *Sudhoffs Archiv* 40 (1956): 345–71.

Grünthal, Günther. "Das Ende der Ära Manteuffel." *Jahrbuch für die Geschichte Mittel- und Ostdeutschlands* 39 (1990): 179–219.

Gudden, Wolfgang. "Bernhard von Gudden: Leben und Werk." Med. diss., University of Munich, 1987.

Gülick, Bernhard van. "Die Geschichte des 'Psychiatrischen Vereins der Rheinprovinz' 1867–1930." Med. diss., Free University of Berlin, 1992.

Güse, Hans-Georg and Norbert Schmacke. *Psychiatrie zwischen bürgerlicher Revolution und Faschismus*, vol. 1. Kronberg: Athenäum, 1976.

Gutberlet, Susanne. "Die Vorgeschichte der Marburger Universitätspsychiatrie und die Berufung Heinrich Cramer's zum Direktor der Psychiatrie." Med. diss., University of Marburg, 1981.

Hagner, Michael. *Homo cerebralis: Der Wandel vom Seelenorgan zum Gehirn*. Berlin: Berlin Verlag, 1997.

Hagner, Michael and Bettina Wahrig-Schmidt. *Johannes Müller und die Philosophie*. Berlin: Akademie, 1992.

Haiduk, Anita. "Zur Geschichte der Psychiatrie in Mecklenburg und an der Universität Rostock." *Wissenschaftliche Zeitschrift der Universität Rostock*, Mat.-Nat. Series 21 (1972): 25–30.

Hamann, Peter. "Peter Willers Jessens ehemaliges Asyl Hornheim in Kiel: Ein Beitrag zur Psychiatriegeschichte Schleswig-Holsteins." *Historia Hospitalium* 12 (1977–8): 69–95.

Haraway, Donna. *Primate Visions: Gender, Race, and Nature in the World of Modern Science*. London: Verso, 1992.

Harndt, Ewald. "Die Stellung der medizinischen Fakultät an der preussischen Friedrich-Wilhelms-Universität zu Berlin als Beispiel für den Wandel des Geisteslebens im 19. Jahrhundert." *Jahrbuch für die Geschichte Mittel- und Ostdeutschlands* 20 (1971): 134– 160.

Haselbeck, H. "Zur Sozialgeschichte der 'Offenen Irren-Fürsorge': Vom Stadtasyl zum Sozialpsychiatrischen Dienst." *Psychiatrische Praxis* 12 (1985): 171–9.

Hausen, Karin. "Frauenräume." In *Frauengeschichte—Geschlechtergeschichte*, edited by Karin Hausen and Heide Wunder. Frankfurt/M: Campus, 1992.

Heine, Eva. *Die Anfänge einer organisierten ärztlichen Fortbildung im Deutschen Reich*. Schriftenreihe der Münchener Vereinigung für Geschichte der Medizin, vol. 17. Gräfelfing: Demeter-Verl., 1985.

Heischkel, Edith. "Die Entwicklung der klinischen Anstalten 1810–1933." In *Das Universitätsklinikum in Berlin: Seine Ärzte und seine wissenschaftliche Leistungen 1810–1933*, edited by Paul Diepgen and Paul Rostock, 16–52. Leipzig: Barth, 1939.

Henseler, Heinz. "Die 'Analytische Methode' des Psychiaters Heinrich Wilhelm Neumann." Med. diss., University of Munich, 1959.

Herold, Carola. "Untersuchungen zur Organisations-Geschichte der Psychiatrie in Deutschland." Med. diss., University of Marburg, 1972.

Herzog, Gunter. *Krankheitsurtheile: Logik und Geschichte in der Psychiatrie*. Rehburg-Loccum: Psychiatrie-Verlag, 1984.

Hess, Volker. *Der wohltemperierte Mensch: Wissenschaft und Alltag des Fiebermessens (1850–1900)*. Frankfurt/M: Campus, 2000.

Hildebrandt, Helmut. "Der psychologische Versuch in der Psychiatrie: Was wurde aus Kraepelins (1895) Program?" *Psychologie und Geschichte* 5 (1993): 5–30.

Hilf, Eric. "Zur Geschichte der Charitédirektion im 19. Jahrhundert: Aufbau, Struktur und Personen der Charitéverwaltung zwischen 1820 und 1870." *Zeitschrift für Universitätsgeschichte* 3 (2000): 49–68.

Hoff, Paul. "Emil Kraepelin und die Psychiatrie als klinische Wissenschaft: Ein Beitrag zum Selbstverständnis psychiatrischer Forschung." Habilitation, Munich, 1992.

Höll, Thomas and Paul-Otto Schmidt-Michel. *Irrenpflege im 19. Jahrhundert: Die Wärterfrage in der Diskussion der deutschen Psychiater*. Bonn: Psychiatrie Verlag, 1989.

Huerkamp, Claudia. *Der Aufstieg der Ärzte im 19. Jahrhundert. Vom gelehrten Stand zum professionellem Experten: Das Beispiel Preußens*. Kritische Studien zur Geschichtswissenschaft, edited by Helmut Berding, Jürgen Kocka and Hans-Ulrich Wehler, vol. 68. Göttingen: V&R, 1985.

Hummel, Stephan. "Zur medikamentösen Therapie in der Psychiatrie in den Jahren 1844 bis 1914: Eine Analyse anhand deutschsprachiger psychiatrischer Fachzeitschriften." Med. diss., University of Leipzig, 1987.

Jacobsen, Ulf. "Wissenschaftsbegriff und Menschenbild bei Wilhelm Griesinger: Ein Beitrag zur Geschichte des ärztlichen Selbstverständnisses im 19. Jahrhundert." Med. diss., University of Heidelberg, 1986.

Janzarik, Werner. "Hundert Jahre Heidelberger Psychiatrie." In *Psychologie als Grundlagenwissenschaft*, edited by Werner Janzarik, 1–18. Klinische Psychologie und Psychopathologie, edited by Helmut Remschmidt, vol. 8. Stuttgart: Enke, 1979.

——. "Die klinische Psychopathologie zwischen Greisinger und Kraepelin im Querschnitt des Jahres 1878." In *Psychologie als Grundlagenwissenschaft*, edited by Werner Janzarik, 51–61. Klinische Psychologie und Psychopathologie, edited by Helmut Remschmidt, vol. 8. Stuttgart: Enke, 1979.

Jarausch, Konrad. *The Unfree Professions: German Lawyers, Teachers, and Engineers, 1900–1950*. New York: Oxford University Press, 1990.

Jarausch, Konrad and Larry E. Jones, eds. *In Search of a Liberal Germany: Studies in the History of German Liberalism from 1789 to the Present*. New York: Berg, 1990.

Jerns, Gerd Udo. "Die neurologisch-psychiatrischen Vorträge in der Abteilung für Neurologie und Psychiatrie der Gesellschaft Deutscher Naturforscher und Ärzte von 1886 bis 1913." Med. diss., Free University Berlin, 1991.

Jetter, Dieter. *Zur Typologie des Irrenhauses in Frankreich und Deutschland (1780–1840)*. Wiesbaden: Steiner, 1971.

——. *Grundzüge der Geschichte des Irrenhauses*. Darmstadt: WBG, 1981.

Johnson, Jeffrey Allan. *The Kaiser's Chemists: Science and Modernization in Imperial Germany*. Chapel Hill: University of North Carolina Press, 1990.

Jones, Colin and Roy Porter, eds. *Reassessing Foucault: Power, Medicine and the Body*. London: Routledge, 1994.

Kastner, Ingrid. "Die Geschichte der Versorgung psychisch Kranker im Rheinland unter besonderer Berücksichtigung des Köln-Bonner Raumes im 19. Jahrhundert." Med. diss., University of Cologne, 1977.

Katzenstein, Rafael. *Karl Ludwig Kahlbaum und sein Beitrag zur Entwicklung der Psychiatrie*. Zurich: Juris, 1963.

Kaufmann, Doris. *Aufklärung, Bürgerliche Selbsterfahrung und die 'Erfindung' der Psychiatrie in Deutschland, 1770–1850.* Veröffentlichungen des Max-Planck-Institutes für Geschichte, vol. 122. Göttingen: V&R, 1995.

Keil, Gundolf. "Deutsche psychiatrische Zeitschriften des 19. Jahrhunderts." In *Psychiatrie auf dem Wege zur Wissenschaft,* edited by Gerhardt Nissen and Gundolf Keil, 28–35. Stuttgart: Thieme, 1985.

Kersting, Franz-Werner. "Medical Profession and Lunatic Asylums: The case of Westphalia, 1890–1945. In *Proceedings of the 1st European Congress on the History of Psychiatry and Mental Health Care,* edited by Leonie de Goei and Joost Vijselaar, 204–12. Rotterdam: Erasmus, 1993.

——. *Anstaltsärzte zwischen Kaiserreich und Bundesrepublik: Das Beispiel Westfalen.* Forschungen zur Regionalgeschichte, edited by Karl Teppe, vol. 17. Paderborn: Schöningh, 1996.

Kersting, Franz-Werner, Karl Teppe, and Bernd Walter. "Gesellschaft—Psychiatrie—Nationalsozialismus: Historisches Interesse und gesellschaftliches Bewußtsein." In *Nach Hadamar: Zum Verhältnis von Psychiatrie und Gesellschaft im 20. Jahrhundert,* edited by Karl Teppe, 9–61. Paderborn: Schöningh, 1993.

Keyserlingk, Hugo v. "Die Jenaer Nervenklinik im Wandel der Zeit." *Wissenschaftliche Zeitschrift der Friedrich-Schiller-Universität Jena, Mathematisch-Naturwissenschaftliche Reihe,* 2 (1952–3): 17–23.

Kindt, Hildberg. *Vorstufen der Entwicklung zur Kinderpsychiatrie im 19. Jahrhundert: Zur Wertung von Hermann Emminghaus und seiner 'Psychische Störungen des Kindesalters' (1887).* Freiburger Forschungen zur Medizingeschichte, edited by Eduard Seidler et al., vol. 1. Freiburg i.Br.: Hans Ferdinand Schulz, 1971.

Klinkenberg, Norbert. "Die sozialpolitische Isolierung des Krankenhauses im 19. Jahrhundert auf dem Hintergrund der katholisch-bürgerlichen Sozialbestrebungen." *Historia Hospitalium* 15 (1983–4): 213–25.

Köhler, Ernst. *Arme und Irre: Die liberale Fürsorgepolitik des Bürgertums.* Berlin: Wagenbach, 1977.

Koselleck, Reinhart. *Preußen zwischen Reform und Revolution: Allgemeines Landrecht, Verwaltung und soziale Bewegung von 1791–1848.* 3d ed. Munich: DTV, 1981.

Koshar, Rudy. "Foucault and Social History: Comments on Combined Underdevelopment." *AHR* 98 (1993): 354–63.

Kramer, Cheryce. "A Fool's Paradise: The Psychiatry of Gemüth in a Biedermeier Asylum." Ph.D. Dissertation, University of Chicago, 1998.

Kremer, Richard L. "Building Institutes of Physiology in Prussia, 1836–1846: Contexts, Interests and Rhetoric." In *The Laboratory Revolution in Medicine,* edited by Andrew Cunningham and Perry Williams, 72–109. Cambridge: Cambridge University Press, 1992.

Kretschmann, Karl-Ernst. "Friedrich Althoffs Nachlaß als Quelle für die Geschichte der medizinischen Fakultät in Halle von 1882–1907." Med. diss., University of Halle, 1959.

Kreuter, Alma. *Deutschsprachige Neurologen und Psychiater: Ein biographisch-bibliographisches Lexikon von den Vorläufern bis zur Mitte des 20. Jahrhunderts.* 3 vols. Munich: K. G. Saur, 1996.

Kuhn, Roland. "Griesingers Auffassung der psychischen Krankheiten und seine Bedeutung für die weitere Entwicklung der Psychiatrie." *Bibliotheca psychiatrica et neurologica* 100 (1957): 41–67.

Kuratorium Gedenkstätte Sonnenstein, e.V., ed. *Geschichte der Heil- und Pflegeanstalt Pirna-Sonnenstein (1811–1939)*. Vol. 1. Sonnenstein: Beiträge zur Geschichte des Sonnensteins und der Sächsischen Schweiz. Lampertswalde: Stoba, 1998.

Küster, Thomas, ed. *Quellen zur Geschichte der Anstaltspsychiatrie in Westfalen.* Forschungen zur Regionalgeschichte, edited by Karl Teppe, vol. 26. Paderborn: Schöningh, 1998.

Kutzer, Michael. "Der pathologisch-anatomische Befund und seine Auswertung in der deutschen Psychiatrie der ersten Hälfte des 19. Jahrhunderts." *Medizinhistorisches Journal* 26 (1991): 214–35.

——. "Die Irrenheilanstalt in der ersten Hälfte des 19. Jahrhunderts: Anmerkungen zu den therapeutischen Zielsetzungen." In *Vom Umgang mit Irren: Beiträge zur Geschichte psychiatrischer Therapeutik,* edited by Johann Glatzel, Steffan Haas and Heinz Schott, 63–82. Regensburg: S. Roderer, 1990.

Labisch, Alfons. "Stadt und Krankenhaus: Das Allgemeine Krankenhaus in der kommunalen Sozial- und Gesundheitspolitik des 19. Jahrhunderts." In *'Einem jeden Kranken in einem Hospitale sein eigenes Bett': Zur Sozialgeschichte des Allgemeinen Krankenhauses in Deutschland im 19. Jahrhundert,* edited by Alfons Labisch and Reinhard Spree, 253–96. Frankfurt/M: Campus, 1996.

Labisch, Alfons and Reinhard Spree, eds. *Medizinische Deutungsmacht im sozialen Wandel des 19. und frühen 20. Jahrhunderts.* Bonn: Psychiatrieverlag, 1989.

——. *'Einem jeden Kranken in einem Hospitale sein eigenes Bett': Zur Sozialgeschichte des Allgemeinen Krankenhauses in Deutschland im 19. Jahrhundert.* Frankfurt/M: Campus, 1996.

Labisch, Alfons and Florian Tennstedt. *Der Weg zum 'Gesetz über die Vereinheitlichung des Gesundheitswesens vom 3. Juli 1934: Entwicklungslinien und -momente des staatlichen und kommunalen Gesundheitswesens in Deutschland.* Düsseldorf: Akademie für Öffentliches Gesundswesen, 1985.

——. "Die Allgemeinen Krankenhäuser der Städte und der Religionsgemeinschaften Ende des 19. Jahrhunderts: Statistische und juristische Anmerkungen am Beispiel Preußens (1877–1903)." In *'Einem jeden Kranken in einem Hospitale sein eigenes Bett': Zur Sozialgeschichte des Allgemeinen Krankenhauses in Deutschland im 19. Jahrhundert,* edited by Alfons Labisch and Reinhard Spree, 297–319. Frankfurt/M: Campus, 1996.

Lachmund, Jens and Gunnar Stollberg. "The Doctor, his Audience, and the Meaning of Illness: The Drama of Medical Practice in the Late 18th and Early 19th Centuries." *MGG* supplement 1 (1992): 53–65.

Lampe, Hermann. *Die Entwicklung und Differenzierung von Fachabteilungen auf den Versammlungen von 1828 bis 1913: Bibliographie zur Erfassung der Sektionsvorträge mit einer Darstellung der Entstehung der Sektionen und ihrer Problematik.* Schriftenreihe zur Geschichte der Versammlungen deutscher Naturforscher und Ärzte, edited by Hans Querner, vol. 2. Hildesheim: Gerstenberg, 1975.

Lanczik, Mario. "Heinrich Neumann und seine Lehre von der Einheitspsychose." *Fundamenta Psychiatrica* (1989): 49–54.

——. *Der Breslauer Psychiater Carl Wernicke: Werkanalyse und Wirkungsgeschichte als Beitrag zur Medizingeschichte Schlesiens.* Schlesische Forschungen, vol. 2. Sigmaringen: Thorbecke, 1988.

Langer, Karin. "Heinrich Laehr und das Asyl Schweizerhof in Zehlendorf bei Berlin." Med. diss., Free University of Berlin, 1966.

Langewiesche, Dieter. *Liberalismus in Deutschland.* Frankfurt/M: Suhrkamp, 1988.

Latour, Bruno. *Science in Action: How to Follow Scientists or Engineers through Society.* Cambridge: Harvard University Press, 1987.

Ledford, Kenneth E. *From General Estate to Special Interest: German Lawyers 1878–1933.* Cambridge: Cambridge University Press, 1995.

Leibbrand, Werner, and Annemarie Wettley. *Der Wahnsinn: Geschichte der abendländischen Psychopathologie.* Munich: Karl Albers, 1961.

Leibbrand-Wettley, Annemarie. "Die Stellung des Geisteskranken in der Gesellschaft des 19. Jahrhunderts." In *Der Arzt und der Kranke in der Gesellschaft des neunzehnten Jahrhunderts,* edited by Walter Artelt and Walter Rüegg, 50–69. Stuttgart: Enke, 1967.

Lemke, Rudolf. "150jähriges Jubiläum der Nervenklinik an der Friedrich-Schiller-Universität Jena." *Wissenschaftliche Zeitschrift der Friedrich-Schiller-Universität Jena, Mathematisch-Naturwissenschaftliche Reihe* 4 (1954–5): 363–72.

Lengwiler, Martin. *Zwischen Klinik und Kaserne. Die Geschichte der Militärpsychiatrie in Deutschland und der Schweiz, 1870–1914.* Zurich: Chronos, 2000.

Lenoir, Timothy. "Science for the Clinic: Science Policy and the Formation of Carl Ludwig's Institute in Leipzig." In *The Investigative Enterprise: Experimental Physiology in Nineteenth-Century Medicine,* edited by William Colemann and Frederic L. Holmes, 139–78. Berkeley: University of California Press, 1988.

———. "Laboratories, Medicine and Public Life in Germany, 1830–1849: Ideological Roots of the Institutional Revolution." In *The laboratory revolution in medicine,* edited by Andrew Cunningham and Perry Williams, 14–71. Cambridge: Cambridge University Press, 1992.

———. *Instituting Science: The Cultural Production of Scientific Disciplines.* Stanford: Stanford University Press, 1997.

Leopoldt, Margarete. "Carl Friedrich Flemming (1799–1880): ein Vertreter der deutschen Psychiatrie des neunzehnten Jahrhunderts." Med. diss., Free University Berlin, 1983.

Light, Donald. *Becoming Psychiatrists: The Professional Transformation of Self.* New York: W. W. Norton, 1980.

Linke, Robert. "Psychiatrische und Neurologische Zeitschriften im 19. Jahrhundert." Med. diss., University of Düsseldorf, 1979.

Lohff, Brigitte. "Johannes Müller (1801–1858) als akademischer Lehrer." Med. Diss., University of Hamburg, 1977.

Lunbeck, Elizabeth. *The Psychiatric Persuasion: Knowledge, Gender, and Power in Modern America.* Princeton: Princeton University Press, 1994.

Luther, B., I. Wirth, and C[hristian] Donalies. "Zur Entwicklung der Neurologie/Psychiatrie in Berlin, insbesondere am Charité-Krankenhaus." *CA,* n.s., 2 (1982): 275–90.

Macmillan, Malcolm. "Experimental and clinical studies of localisation before Flourens." *Journal of the History of the Neurosciences* 4 (1995): 139–54.

Mann, Gunther. "Dekadenz, Degeneration, Untergangsangst im Lichte der Biologie des 19. Jahrhunderts." *Medizinhistorisches Journal* 20 (1985): 6–35.

Marx, Otto M. "Nineteenth-Century Medical Psychology: Theoretical Problems in the Work of Griesinger, Meynert, and Wernicke." *ISIS* 61 (1970): 355–70.

———. "Wilhelm Griesinger and the History of Psychiatry: A Reassessment," *Bulletin of the History of Medicine* 46 (1972): 519–44.

———. "German Romantic Psychiatry," *HP* 1 (1990): 351–81 and 2 (1991): 1–25.

McClelland, Charles. *The German Experience of Professionalization: Modern Learned Professions and Their Organizations from the early Nineteenth Century to the Hitler Era.* Cambridge: Cambridge University Press, 1991.

Mette, Alexander. *Wilhelm Griesinger: Der Begründer der wissenschaftlichen Psychiatrie in Deutschland.* Vol. 26. Biographien hervorragender Naturwissenschaftlicher, Techniker und Mediziner. Leipzig: BSB B. G. Teubner Verlagsanstalt, 1976.

Micale, Mark and Roy Porter, eds. *Discovering the History of Psychiatry.* New York: Oxford University Press, 1994.

Middelhof, Hans Dieter. "C. F. W. Roller und die Vorgeschichte der Heidelberger Psychiatrischen Klinik." In *Psychologie als Grundlagenwissenschaft,* edited by Werner Janzarik, 33–50. Klinische Psychologie und Psychopathologie, edited by Helmut Remschmidt, vol. 8. Stuttgart: Enke, 1979.

Müller, Christian. *Vom Tollhaus zum Psychozentrum: Vignetten und Bausteine zur Psychiatriegeschichte in zeitlicher Abfolge.* Schriften zur Wissenschaftsgeschichte, edited by Armin Geus and Guido Pressler, vol. 12. Hürtgenwald: Guido Pressler, 1993.

Müller, Christoph. "Die Jenaer Nervenklinik zwischen 1859 und 1882 und ihre Direktoren Franz Xaver Schöman und Friedrich Siebert." Med. diss., University of Jena, 1990.

Müller, Christoph and Valentin Wieczorek. "Die Jenaer 'Irrenanstalt' zwischen 1859 und 1882 unter Franz Xaver Schöman und Friedrich Siebert." In *Medizinprofessoren und ärztliche Ausbildung: Beiträge zur Geschichte der Medizin,* edited by G. Wagner and G. Wessel, 132–44. Jena: Universitätsverlag, 1992.

Münch, Ragnhild. *Gesundheitswesen im 18. und 19. Jahrhundert: Das Berliner Beispiel.* Berlin: Akademie Verlag, 1995.

Nauck, E[rnst] Th[eodor]. *Zur Geschichte des medizinischen Lehrplans und Unterrichts der Universität Freiburg i.Br.* Beiträge zur Freiburger Wissenschafts- und Universitätsgeschichte, edited by Johannes Vincke, vol. 2. Freiburg i. Br.: Eberhard Albert, 1952.

——. "Die ersten Jahrzehnten des psychiatrischen und neurologischen Unterrichts in Freiburg i.Br." *Berichte der Naturforschenden Gesellschaft zu Freiburg i.Br.* 46 (1956): 63–84.

Neues, Horst. *Die Geschichte der privaten Heil- und Pflegeanstalt der neusser Alexianer-Bruder in den Jahren 1869–1932.* Herzogenrath: Murken-Altrogge, 1991.

Neumärker, Klaus-Jürgen. *Karl Bonhoeffer: Leben und Werk eines deutschen Psychiaters und Neurologen in seiner Zeit.* Berlin: Springer, 1990.

Nipperdey, Thomas. *Deutsche Geschichte 1866–1918.* Vol. 1. Munich: Beck, 1990.

Olesko, Kathryn M. "Commentary: On Institutes, Investigations, and Scientific Training." In *The Investigative Enterprise: Experimental Physiology in Nineteenth-Century Medicine,* edited by William Coleman and Frederic L. Holmes, 295–332. Berkeley: University of California Press, 1988.

——. *Physics as a Calling: Discipline and Practice in the Königsberg Seminar for Physics.* Cornell History of Science Series, edited by L. Pearce Williams. Ithaca: Cornell University Press, 1991.

Oosterhuis, Harry. *Stepchildren of Nature: Krafft-Ebing, Psychiatry, and the Making of Sexual Identity.* Chicago: University of Chicago Press, 2000.

Orth, Linda, et al. *Pass op, sonst küss de bei de Pelman: Das Irrenwesen im Rheinland des 19. Jahrhundert.* Bonn: Grenzenlos, [1994].

Ortmann, Frank. "Die Entstehung der Psychiatrie in Jena." Med. diss., University of Jena, 1983.

Osborne, Thomas. "On Anti-Medicine and Clinical Reason." In *Reassessing Foucault: Power, Medicine and the Body,* edited by Colin Jones and Roy Porter, 28–47. London: Routledge, 1994.

Panse, Fr[iedrich] et al. *Das psychiatrische Krankenhauswesen: Entwicklung, Stand, Reichweite und Zukunft.* Schriftenreihe aus dem Gebiete des öffentlichen Gesundheitswesens, edited by Josef Stralau and Bernhard Zoller, vol. 19. Stuttgart: Thieme, 1964.

Pantel, J. "Von der Nervenabteilung zur Neurologischen Klinik—die Etablierung des Heidelberger Lehrstuhls für Neurologie 1883–1969." *Fortschritte der Neurologie und Psychiatrie* 59 (1991): 468–76.

Pauleikhoff, Bernhard. *Das Menschenbild im Wandel der Zeit: Ideengeschichte der Psychiatrie und der klinischen Psychologie.* 2 Vols. Hürtgenwald: Guido Pressler, 1987.

Pernice, Andreas. "Family Care and Asylum Psychiatry in the Nineteenth Century: The Controversy in the *Allgemeine Zeitschrift für Psychiatrie* between 1844 and 1902." *HP* 6 (1995): 55–68.

Pfeffer, Rolf. "Professor Franz von Rinecker." Med. diss., University of Würzburg, 1981.

Pfetsch, Frank R. *Zur Entwicklung der Wissenschaftspolitik in Deutschland, 1750–1914.* Berlin: Duncker & Humblot, 1974.

Plessner, Helmut. *Die verspätete Nation: Über die politische Verführbarkeit bürgerlichen Geistes.* Stuttgart: Kohlhammer, 1959.

Porep, Rüdiger and Christel Porep-Böhme. "Die Vorgeschichte und die Anfänge der Psychiatrischen und Nervenklinik der Christian-Albrechts-Universität zu Kiel." *Christiana Albertina* 13 (1973): 11–23.

Prüll, Cay-Rüdiger. "Zum Selbstbild der deutschen Psychiater im 20. Jahrhundert: Theodor Kirchhoffs 'Deutsche Irrenärzte' von 1921." In *Selbstbilder des Arztes im 20. Jahrhundert: Medizinhistorische und medizinethische Aspekte,* edited by Karl-Heinz Leven and Cay-Rüdiger Prüll, 97–128. Freiburger Forschungen zur Medizingeschichte, vol. 16. Freiburg: Hans Ferdinand Schulz, 1994.

———. "Zwischen Krankenversorgung und Forschungsprimat: Die Pathologie an der Berliner Charité im 19. Jahrhundert." *Zeitschrift für Universitätsgeschichte* 3 (2000): 87–109.

Rabinbach, Anson. *The Human Motor: Energy, Fatigue, and the Origins of Modernity.* New York: Basic Books, 1990.

Radkau, Joachim. *Das Zeitalter der Nervosität: Deutschland zwischen Bismarck und Hitler.* Munich: Hanser, 1998.

Rautenberg, E. C. *Verminderte Schuldfähigkeit: Ein besonderer, fakultativer Strafmilderungsgrund?* Kriminologische Schriftenreihe, vol. 85. Heidelberg: Kriminalistik Verlag, 1984.

Reichert, Brigitte. "Hermann Emminghaus. Ein Pionier der Kinder und Jugendpsychiatrie: Leben, Werk und Wirkungsgeschichte." Med. diss., University of Würzburg, 1989.

Reisby, Niels. "An Anti-Psychiatry Debate of the 1890's." In *The Department of Psychiatry: Kommunehospitalet Copenhagen, 1875–1975,* edited by Fini Schulsinger et al., 15–20. Acta Psychiatrica Scandinavica, Supplementum 261. Copenhagen: Munksgaard, 1975.

Reiser, Stanley Joel. *Medicine and the Reign of Technology*. Cambridge: Cambridge University Press, 1977.

Riese, Reinhard. *Die Hochschulen auf dem Wege zum wissenschaftlichen Großbetrieb: Die Universität Heidelberg und das badische Hochschulwesen, 1860–1914*. Industrielle Welt, edited by Werner Conze, vol. 19. Stuttgart: Ernst Klett, 1977.

Risse, Guenter B. *Mending Bodies, Saving Souls: A History of Hospitals*. New York: Oxford University Press, 1999.

Ritter, Gerhard A. *Sozialversicherung in Deutschland und England: Entstehung und Grundzüge im Vergleich*. Munich: Beck, 1983.

Roberts, James S. *Drink, Temperance, and the Working Class in Nineteenth-Century Germany*. Boston: Allen & Unwin, 1984.

Roelcke, Volker. "Die wissenschaftliche Vermessung der Geisteskranken. Emil Kraepelins Lehre von den endogenen Psychosen." In *Meilensteine der Medizin*, edited by Heinz Schott, 389–95. Dortmund: Harenberg, 1996.

——. "Biologizing Social Facts. An Early 20th Century Debate on Kraepelin's Concepts of Culture, Neurasthenia, and Degeneration." *Culture, Medicine and Psychiatry* 21 (1997): 383–403.

——. *Krankheit und Kulturkritik: Psychiatrische Gesellschaftsdeutungen im bürgerlichen Zeitalter (1790–1914)*. Frankfurt/M: Campus, 1999.

Rössler, A[lice]. "Zur Geschichte der Universitäts-Nervenklinik Erlangen." In *Psychiatrie in Erlangen: Festschrift zur Eröffnung des Neubaus der Psychiatrischen Universitätsklinik Erlangen*, edited by E. Lungershausen and R. Baer. Erlangen: perimed, 1985.

Rose, Nikolas. *Inventing Our Selves: Psychology, Power, and Personhood*. Cambridge Studies in the History of Psychology, edited by Mitchell G. Ash and William R. Woodward. Cambridge: Cambridge University Press, 1998.

Rothman, David. *The Discovery of the Asylum: Social Order and Disorder in the New Republic*. Boston: Little and Brown, 1971.

Rouse, Joseph. *Knowledge and Power: Toward a Political Philosophy of Science*. Ithaca: Cornell University Press, 1987.

Sachße, Christoph and Florian Tennstedt. *Geschichte der Armenfürsorge in Deutschland*. Vol. 2. Stuttgart: Kohlhammer, 1988.

Sammet, Kai. *Ueber Irrenanstalten und deren Weiterentwicklung in Deutschland: Wilhelm Griesinger im Streit mit der konservativen Anstaltspsychiatrie 1865–1868*. Hamburger Studien zur Geschichte der Medizin, vol. 1. Hamburg: Lit, 2000.

Scherg-Zeisner, Christiane. "Die ärztliche Ausbildung an der königlich-bayerischen Julius-Maximilians-Universität Würzburg, 1814–1872." Diss. med., University of Würzburg, 1973.

Schimmelpennig, Gustav W. "Alfred Erich Hoche. Das wissenschaftliche Werk: 'Mittelmäßigkeit'? (Hinweise zu methodologischen Problemen der Medizingeschichte)." In *Berichte aus den Sitzungen der Joachim Jungius-Gesellschaft der Wissenschaften e.V., Hamburg*, vol. 8, no. 3. Göttingen: V&R, 1990.

Schindler, Thomas-Peter. "Psychiatrie im Wilhelminischen Deutschland im Spiegel der Verhandlungen des 'Vereins der deutschen Irrenärzte' (ab 1903: 'Deutscher Verein für Psychiatrie') von 1891–1914." Med. diss., Free University Berlin, 1990.

Schmidt, Paul-Otto. *Asylierung oder familiale Versorgung: Die Vorträge auf der Sektion Psychiatrie der Gesellschaft Deutscher Naturforscher und Ärzte bis 1885*. Abhandlungen zur Geschichte der Medizin und der Naturwissenschaften, vol. 44. Husum: Matthiesen, 1982.

Schmidt-Degenhard, Michael. "Ludwig Snell (1817–1892): Ein bedeutender Hildesheimer Arzt und Wissenschaftler des 19. Jahrhunderts." *Jahrbuch für Stadt und Stift Hildesheim* 60 (1989): 83–98.

——. "Melancholie-Behandlung im Lichte der Psychiatriegeschichte." In *Klinische Diagnostik und Therapie der Depression,* edited by M. Wolfersdorf et al., 35–63. Roderer: Regensburg, 1989.

——. "Einheitspsychose—Begriff und Idee." In *Für und Wider der Einheitspsychose,* edited by C[hristoph] Mundt and H[ans-Martin] Saß, 1–11. Stuttgart: Thieme, 1992.

Schmiedebach, H[einz]-P[eter]. "Zum Verständniswandel der 'psychopathischen' Störungen am Anfang der naturwissenschaftlichen Psychiatrie in Deutschland." *Nervenarzt* 56 (1985): 140–45.

——. *Psychiatrie und Psychologie im Widerstreit: Die Auseinandersetzung in der Berliner medicinisch-psychologischen Gesellschaft (1867–1899).* Abhandlungen zur Geschichte der Medizin und der Naturwissenschaften, edited by Rolf Winau and Heinz Müller-Dietz, vol. 51. Husum: Matthiesen, 1986.

——. "Wilhelm Griesinger." In *Berlinische Lebensbilder: Mediziner,* edited by Wolfgang Treue and Rolf Winau, 109–31. Vol. 60 of Einzelveröffentlichungen der historischen Kommission zu Berlin. Berlin: Colloquium, 1987.

——. "Mensch, Gehirn und wissenschaftliche Psychiatrie: Zur therapeutischen Vielfalt bei Wilhelm Griesinger." In *Vom Umgang mit Irren: Beiträge zur Geschichte psychiatrischer Therapeutik,* edited by Johann Glatzel, Steffan Haas and Heinz Schott, 83–105. Regensburg: S. Roderer, 1990.

——. "Eine 'antipsychiatrische Bewegung' um die Jahrhundertwende." In *Medizinkritische Bewegungen im deutschen Reich (ca. 1870 bis ca. 1933),* Medizin, Geschichte und Gesellschaft, edited by Martin Dinges, supplement no. 9, 127–59. Stuttgart: Steiner, 1996.

Schmitt, Wolfram. "Das Modell der Naturwissenschaft in der Psychiatrie im Übergang vom 19. zum 20. Jahrhundert." *BWG* 6 (1983): 89–101.

——. "Biologismus und Psychopathologie: Die Heidelberger Schule." In *Vom Umgang mit Irren: Beiträge zur Geschichte psychiatrischer Therapeutik,* edited by Johann Glatzel, Steffan Haas and Heinz Schott, 121–31. Regensburg: S. Roderer, 1990.

Schneck, Peter and Hans-Uwe Lammel, eds. *Die Medizin an der Berliner Universität und an der Charité zwischen 1810 und 1850.* Abhandlungen zur Geschichte der Medizin und der Naturwissenschaften, vol. 67. Berlin: Matthiesen, 1995.

Schrenk, Martin. *Über den Umgang mit Geisteskranken: Die Entwicklung der psychiatrischen Therapie vom 'moralischen Regime' in England und Frankreich zu den 'psychischen Curmethoden' in Deutschland.* Berlin: Springer, 1973.

Schröer, Heinz. *Carl Ludwig: Begründer der messenden Experimentalphysiologie 1816–1895.* Grosse Naturforscher, edited by Heinz Degen, vol. 33. Stuttgart: Wissenschaftliche Verlagsgesellschaft, 1967.

Schulze, Heinz and Christian Donalies. "100 Jahre Psychiatrie und Neurologie im Rahmen der Berliner Gesellschaft für Psychiatrie und Neurologie und der Nervenklinik der Charité." *Wissenschaftliche Zeitschrift der Humboldt Universität zu Berlin,* Math.-Nat. Series 17 (1968): 5–10.

Schwarz, Thomas. "Anton Bumm (1849–1903)." Med. diss., University of Munich, 1982.

Scull, Andrew. *Museums of Madness: The Social Organization of Insanity in Nineteenth-Century England.* New York: St. Martin's Press, 1979.

———. "The Domestication of Madness." *Medical History* 27 (1983): 233–48.

———. "Psychiatry and Social Control in the Nineteenth and Twentieth Centuries." *HP* 2 (1991): 149–69.

Scull, Andrew, Charlotte MacKenzie, and Nicholas Hervey. *Masters of Bedlam: The Transformation of the Mad-Doctoring Trade.* Princeton: Princeton University Press, 1996.

Seige, Max. "Erinnerungen an Otto Binswanger." *Wissenschaftliche Zeitschrift der Friedrich-Schiller-Universität Jena, Mathematisch-Naturwissenschaftliche Reihe* 4 (1954–5): 373–78.

Sheehan, James J. *German Liberalism in the 19th Century.* Chicago: University of Chicago Press, 1978.

Siadek, Silvia. "Psychiatrische Gesamtversorgung einer Region in Deutschland um die Jahrhundertwende am Beispiel der Stadt Göttingen." Med. diss., University of Göttingen, 1987.

Siemann, Wolfram. *Gesellschaft im Aufbruch: Deutschland, 1849–1871.* Frankfurt/M: Suhrkamp, 1990.

Simmer, Hans H. "Principles and Problems of Medical Undergraduate Education in Germany during the Nineteenth and early Twentieth Centuries." In *The History of Medical Education,* edited by C. D. O'Malley, 173–200. UCLA Forum in Medical Sciences, vol. 12. Berkeley: University of California Press, 1970.

Spiske, Hilmar. *Bibliographie zur Geschichte der Anstaltspsychiatrie.* Kieler Beiträge zur Geschichte der Medizin und Pharmazie, edited by Gerhard Rudolph and Fridolf Kudlien, vol. 14. Neumünster: Karl Wachholtz, 1975.

Spree, Reinhard. "Krankenhausentwicklung und Sozialpolitik in Deutschland während des 19. Jahrhunderts." *HZ* 260 (1995): 75–105.

———. "Sozialer Wandel im Krankenhaus während des 19. Jahrhunderts: Das Beispiel des Münchener Allgemeinen Krankenhauses." *Medizinhistorisches Journal* 33 (1998): 245–291.

Starr, Paul. *The Social Transformation of American Medicine.* New York: Basic Books, 1982.

Steiner, Andreas. *'Das nervöse Zeitalter': Der Begriff der Nervosität bei Laien und Ärzten in Deutschland und Österreich um 1900.* Zurich: Juris, 1964.

Steinberg, Holger. *Kraepelin in Leipzig: Eine Begegnung von Psychiatrie und Psychologie.* Bonn: Ed. das Narrenschiff, 2001.

Stollberg, Gunnar. "Zur Geschichte der Pflegeklassen in deutschen Krankenhäusern." In *'Einem jeden Kranken in einem Hospitale sein eigenes Bett': Zur Sozialgeschichte des Allgemeinen Krankenhauses in Deutschland im 19. Jahrhundert,* edited by Alfons Labisch and Reinhard Spree, 374–98. Frankfurt/M: Campus, 1996.

Störmer, Norbert. *Innere Mission und geistige Behinderung. Von den Anfängen der Betreuung geistig behinderter Menschen bis zur Weimarer Republik.* Münster: Lit, 1991.

Stürzbecher, Manfred. "Aus der Geschichte des städtischen Krankenhauses Moabit." In *1872–1972: Städtisches Krankenhaus Moabit, Festschrift zum 100-jährigen Bestehen,* edited by Bezirksamt Tiergarten, 13–17. Berlin: n.p., 1972.

——. "Zur Berufung Johannes Müllers an die Berliner Universität." *Jahrbuch für die Geschichte Mittel- und Ostdeutschlands* 21 (1972): 184–226.

——. "Allgemeine und Spezialkrankenhäuser, insbesondere Privatkrankenanstalten im 19. Jahrhundert in Berlin." In *Studien zur Krankenhausgeschichte im 19. Jahrhundert im Hinblick auf die Entwicklung in Deutschland,* edited by Hans Schadewaldt, 105–120. Studien zur Medizingeschichte im 19. Jahrhundert, vol. 7. Göttingen: V&R, 1976.

Tennstedt, Florian. *Sozialgeschichte der Sozialpolitik in Deutschland: Vom 18. Jahrhundert bis zum Ersten Weltkrieg.* Göttingen: V&R, 1981.

Teuscher, Ursula. "Die Irrenpflege in der Rheinprovinz im 19. Jahrhundert am Beispiel Aachens." Med. diss., Rheinisch-Westphälische Technische Hochschule Aachen, 1979.

Thiele, R[udolf]. "Über Griesingers Satz: 'Geisteskrankheiten sind Gehirnkrankheiten'," *MschrPN* 63 (1927): 294–313.

Thom, Achim. "Erscheinungsformen und Widersprüche des Weges der Psychiatrie zu einer medizinischen Disziplin im 19. Jahrhundert." In *Zur Geschichte der Psychiatrie im 19. Jahrhundert,* edited by Achim Thom, 11–32. Berlin: VEB Verlag Volk und Gesundheit, 1984.

Trenckmann, Ulrich. "Zur halleschen Hirnpsychiatrie im ausgehenden 19. Jahrhundert: pro memoria Carl Wernicke (1848–1905)." *Wissenschaftliche Beiträge der Martin-Luther-Universität Halle-Wittenberg* 29(1980): 46–52.

Trollenburg, Heinz. "Die Entwicklung des Bezirkskrankenhauses für Neurologie und Psychiatrie Uchtspringe." Med. diss., University of Leipzig, 1970.

Tuchman, Arleen M. "From the Lecture to the Laboratory: The Institutionalization of Scientific Medicine at the University of Heidelberg." In *The Investigative Enterprise: Experimental Physiology in Nineteenth-Century Medicine,* edited by William Coleman and Frederic L. Holmes, 65–99. Berkeley: University of California Press, 1988.

——. *Science, Medicine, and the State in Germany: The Case of Baden, 1815–1871.* Oxford: Oxford University Press, 1993.

——. "Institutions and Disciplines: Recent Work in the History of German Science." *JMH* 69 (1997): 298–319.

Tümmler, Fred. "Veröffentlichungen aus dem Gebiet der Psychiatrie in der Münchener Medizinischen Wochenschrift von 1854–1914." Med. diss., University of Munich, 1979.

Turner, Trevor. " 'Not Worth Powder and Shot': The Public Profile of the Medico-Psychological Association, c. 1851–1914." In *150 Years of British Psychiatry, 1841–1991,* edited by Hugh Freeman and German Berrios, 3–16. London: Athlone Press, 1991.

Van Helden, Albert and Thomas L. Hankins. *Instruments.* Osiris, vol. 9. Chicago: University of Chicago Press, 1994.

Van Hetern, Godelieve. "Clinical Education in Nineteenth-Century Germany: A Theatre of Knowledge." *Bulletin of the Society for the Social History of Medicine* 41 (1987): 41–5.

Vanja, Christina. "Madhouses, Children's Wards, and Clinics: The Development of Insane Asylums in Germany." In *Institutions of Confinement: Hospitals, Asylums, and Prisons in Western Europe and North America, 1500–1950,* edited by Norbert Finzsch and Robert Jütte. Cambridge: Cambridge University Press, 1996.

Verwey, Gerlof. *Psychiatry in an Anthropological and Biomedical Context: Philosophical Presuppositions and Implications of German Psychiatry, 1820–1870.* Studies in the History of Modern Science, edited by Robert Cohen, Erwin Hiebertand Everett Mendelsohn, vol. 15. Dordrecht: Reidel, 1985.

vom Bruch, Rüdiger. "Bürgerliche Sozialreform im deutschen Kaiserreich." In *Weder Kommunismus noch Kapitalismus: Bürgerliche Sozialreform in Deutschland vom Vormärz bis zur Ära Adenauer,* edited by Rüdiger vom Bruch, 61–179. Munich: Beck, 1985.

Wahrig-Schmitt, Bettina. *Der junge Wilhelm Griesinger im Spannungsfeld zwischen Philosophie und Physiologie: Anmerkungen zu den philosophischen Würzeln seiner frühen Psychiatrie.* Tübingen: Günther Narr, 1985.

Weber, Matthias. *Ernst Rüdin: Eine kritische Biographie.* Berlin: Springer, 1993.

———. *Die Entwicklung der Psychopharmakologie im Zeitalter der naturwissenschaftlichen Medizin: Ideengeschichte eines psychiatrischen Therapiesystems.* Angewandte Neurowissenschaft, vol. 4. Munich: Urban & Vogel, 1999.

Weber, Matthias and Eric J. Engstrom. "Kraepelin's Diagnostic Cards: The Confluence of Empirical Research and Preconceived Categories." *HP* 8 (1997): 375–385.

Wehler, Hans-Ulrich. *Deutsche Gesellschaftsgeschichte.* 3 vols. Munich: Beck, 1987–1995.

Weindling, Paul. *Health, Race, and German Politics between National Unification and Nazism.* Cambridge: Cambridge University Press, 1989.

Weingart, Peter, Jürgen Kroll, and Kurt Bayertz. *Rasse, Blut, und Gene: Geschichte der Eugenik und Rassenhygiene in Deutschland.* Frankfurt/M: Suhrkamp, 1992.

Wenig, Hans-Günter. "Medizinische Ausbildung im 19. Jahrhundert." Med. diss., University of Bonn, 1969.

Wetzell, Richard. *Inventing the Criminal: A History of German Criminology, 1880–1945.* Studies in Legal History, edited by Thomas A. Green and Hendrik Hartog. Chapel Hill: University of North Carolina Press, 2000.

Wieczorek, Valentin. "Zur Entwicklung der Universitäts-Nervenklinik seit der Gründung im Jahre 1804." *Wissenschaftliche Zeitschrift der Friedrich-Schiller-Universität Jena, Mathematisch-Naturwissenschaftliche Reihe* 30/1 (1981): 7–22.

———. "Die Nervenklinik Jena im 19. und zu Beginn des 20. Jahrhunderts: Gestaltung der Ausbildung im Fach Psychiatrie/Neurologie unter D. G. Kieser, O. Binswanger und H. Berger." In *Jenaer Hochschullehrer der Medizin: Beiträge zur Geschichte des Medizinstudiums,* edited by Günther Wagner, 62–90. Jena: Friedrich-Schiller-Universität, 1988.

Wiese, Klaus. "Vom hirnpsychiatrischen Paradigma zu einer humanwissenschaftlichen Psychiatrie." *Wissenschaftliche Zeitschrift der Karl-Marx-Universität Leipzig, Mathematisch-Naturwissenschaftliche Reihe* 31 (1982): 139–49.

Winau, Rolf. *Medizin in Berlin.* Berlin: Walter de Gruyter, 1987.

Windholz, George. "Psychiatric Treatment and the Condition of the Mentally Disturbed at Berlin's Charité in the Early Decades of the Nineteenth Century." *HP* 6 (1995): 157–76.

Witzler, Beate. *Großstadt und Hygiene: Kommunale Gesundheitspolitik in der Epoche der Urbanisierung.* Medizin, Gesellschaft und Geschichte, edited by Robert Jütte, vol. 5. Stuttgart: Steiner, 1995.

Young, Robert M. "Fritsch and Hitzig and the Localized Electrical Excitability of the Cerebral Hemispheres." In *Mind, Brain and Adaptation in the Nineteenth Century:*

Cerebral Localization and its Biological Context from Gall to Ferrier, 224–33. Oxford: Clarendon Press, 1970.

Zeller, Gerhart. "Von der Heilanstalt zur Heil- und Pflegeanstalt: Ein Beitrag zur Geschichte des psychiatrischen Krankenhauswesens." *Fortschritte der Neurologie und Psychiatrie* 49 (1981): 121–7.

Zloczower, Awraham. *Career Opportunities and the Growth of Scientific Discovery in 19th-Century Germany.* New York: Arno Press, 1981.

Index

Milton Keynes UK
Ingram Content Group UK Ltd.
UKHW010424250424
441649UK00004B/89/J